FIRST AID™
CASES
FOR THE
USMLE STEP 1
Second Edition

TAO LE, MD, MHS

Assistant Clinical Professor of Medicine and Pediatrics
Chief, Section of Allergy and Immunology
Department of Medicine
University of Louisville

VINITA TAKIAR, MS, MPhil

Medical Scientist Training Program
Yale University School of Medicine
Class of 2010

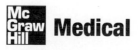 **Medical**

New York / Chicago / San Francisco / Lisbon / London / Madrid / Mexico City
Milan / New Delhi / San Juan / Seoul / Singapore / Sydney / Toronto

First Aid™ Cases for the USMLE Step 1, Second Edition

Copyright © 2009 by Tao Le. All rights reserved. Printed in the United States of America. Except as permitted under the United States Copyright Act of 1976, no part of this publication may be reproduced or distributed in any form or by any means, or stored in a data base or retrieval system, without the prior written permission of the publisher.

Previous edition copyright © 2006 by Tao Le.

First Aid™ is a trademark of The McGraw-Hill Companies, Inc.

1 2 3 4 5 6 7 8 9 0   QPD/QPD   12 11 10 9

ISBN 978-0-07-160135-1
MHID 0-07-160135-X
ISSN 1559-5757

NOTICE

Medicine is an ever-changing science. As new research and clinical experience broaden our knowledge, changes in treatment and drug therapy are required. The authors and the publisher of this work have checked with sources believed to be reliable in their efforts to provide information that is complete and generally in accord with the standards accepted at the time of publication. However, in view of the possibility of human error or changes in medical sciences, neither the authors nor the publisher nor any other party who has been involved in the preparation or publication of this work warrants that the information contained herein is in every respect accurate or complete, and they disclaim all responsibility for any errors or omissions or for the results obtained from use of the information contained in this work. Readers are encouraged to confirm the information contained herein with other sources. For example and in particular, readers are advised to check the product information sheet included in the package of each drug they plan to administer to be certain that the information contained in this work is accurate and that changes have not been made in the recommended dose or in the contraindications for administration. This recommendation is of particular importance in connection with new or infrequently used drugs.

This book was set in Electra LH by Rainbow Graphics.
The editors were Catherine A. Johnson and Regina Brown.
The production supervisor was Phil Galea.
Project management was provided by Rainbow Graphics.
Quebecor World Dubuque was printer and binder.

This book is printed on acid-free paper.

To the contributors to this and future editions, who took time to share their knowledge, insight, and humor for the benefit of all those who yearn to pass their boards.

and

To our families, friends, and loved ones, who encouraged and assisted us in the task of assembling this guide.

CONTENTS

Contributing Authors   xv

Senior Reviewers   xvii

Preface   xix

Acknowledgments   xxi

How to Contribute   xxiii

| SECTION I | GENERAL PRINCIPLES | 1 |

Behavioral Science   **3**

Case 1: Alcohol Withdrawal   4

Case 2: Benzodiazepine Overdose   5

Case 3: Anorexia Nervosa   6

Case 4: Bias   8

Case 5: Confidentiality and Its Exceptions   9

Case 6: Core Ethical Principles   10

Case 7: Delirium   11

Case 8: Drug Intoxication   12

Case 9: Evaluation of Diagnostic Tests   13

Case 10: Infant Development   14

Case 11: Malpractice   15

Case 12: Operant Conditioning   16

Case 13: Opioid Withdrawal   17

Case 14: Sleep Physiology   18

Case 15: Sleep Stages   19

Biochemistry   **21**

Case 1: Alkaptonuria   22

Case 2: Cyanide Poisoning   23

Case 3: DiGeorge Syndrome   24

Case 4: Familial Hypercholesterolemia   25

Case 5: Down Syndrome   26

Case 6: Ehlers-Danlos Syndrome   28

Case 7: Fragile X Syndrome   30

Case 8: Fructose Intolerance   31

Case 9: Homocystinuria   32

Case 10: Hurler's Syndrome   33

Case 11: I-cell Disease   34

Case 12: Kartagener's Syndrome 35

Case 13: Lesch-Nyhan Syndrome 36

Case 14: McArdle's Disease 37

Case 15: Phenylketonuria 38

Case 16: Pyruvate Dehydrogenase Deficiency 39

Case 17: Tay-Sachs Disease 40

Case 18: Vitamin B_1 (Thiamine) Deficiency 41

Case 19: von Gierke's Disease 42

Microbiology and Immunology **43**

Case 1: *Acanthamoeba* Infection 45

Case 2: *Actinomyces* vs *Nocardia* 46

Case 3: Anthrax 47

Case 4: Ascariasis 48

Case 5: Aspergillosis 49

Case 6: Botulism 50

Case 7: Candidiasis 51

Case 8: Chagas' Disease 52

Case 9: Cholera 53

Case 10: Chronic Granulomatous Disease 54

Case 11: *Clostridium difficile* Infection 55

Case 12: Congenital Syphilis 56

Case 13: Creutzfeldt-Jakob Disease 57

Case 14: Cryptococcal Meningitis 58

Case 15: Cysticercosis 59

Case 16: Cytomegalovirus Infection 60

Case 17: Dengue Fever 62

Case 18: Diphtheria 63

Case 19: Elephantiasis 64

Case 20: Giardiasis 65

Case 21: Gonorrhea with Septic Arthritis 66

Case 22: Group B *Streptococcus* in Infant 68

Case 23: Hand, Foot, and Mouth Disease 69

Case 24: Herpes Simplex Virus Type 2 70

Case 25: Hookworm 72

Case 26: Influenza 73

Case 27: Isolated IgA deficiency 74

Case 28: Kaposi's Sarcoma 76

Case 29: Leishmaniasis 77

Case 30: *Legionella* Infection 78

Case 31: Leprosy 80

Case 32: *Listeria* Meningitis 82

Case 33: Liver Cysts/*Echinococcus* 83

Case 34: Malaria 84

Case 35: Lyme Disease 86

Case 36: Measles 87

Case 37: Mononucleosis 88

Case 38: Mucormycosis 89

Case 39: Mumps 90

Case 40: *Neisseria meningitidis* Meningitis 91

Case 41: Onchocerciasis 92

Case 42: Osteomyelitis 93

Case 43: Pinworm 94

Case 44: *Pneumocystis jiroveci* Pneumonia 95

Case 45: Poison Ivy 96

Case 46: Polio 97

Case 47: *Pseudomonas aeruginosa* Infection 98

Case 48: Rabies 99

Case 49: Ringworm 100

Case 50: Rocky Mountain Spotted Fever 101

Case 51: Rotavirus Infection 102

Case 52: Schistosomiasis 103

Case 53: *Shigella* and Hemolytic-Uremic Syndrome 104

Case 54: Shingles 105

Case 55: Strongyloidiasis 107

Case 56: Systemic Mycoses 108

Case 57: Toxic Shock Syndrome 109

Case 58: Toxoplasmosis 111

Case 59: Transplant Reaction 112

Case 60: Yellow Fever 113

Case 61: Tuberculosis 114

Pharmacology **117**

Case 1: Acetaminophen Overdose 118

Case 2: Agranulocytosis Secondary to Drug Toxicity 119

Case 3: Barbiturate vs. Benzodiazepine 120

Case 4: Benzodiazepine Overdose 121

Case 5: β-Adrenergic Second Messenger Systems 122

Case 6: Cholinergic Drugs 123

Case 7: Drug Development 124

Case 8: Drug-Induced Lupus 126

Case 9: Ethylene Glycol Poisoning 128

Case 10: Lead Poisoning 129

Case 11: Pharmacodynamics 130

Case 12: Neuromuscular Blocking Agents 132

Case 13: Pharmacokinetics 133

Cardiovascular   **137**

Case 1: Abdominal Aortic Aneurysm   138

Case 2: Aortic Stenosis   139

Case 3: Atherosclerosis   140

Case 4: Atrial Fibrillation   141

Case 5: Atrial Myxoma   142

Case 6: Atrioventricular Block   144

Case 7: Coarctation of the Aorta   145

Case 8: Congenital Rubella   146

Case 9: Coronary Artery Disease   148

Case 10: Congestive Heart Failure   150

Case 11: Deep Venous Thrombosis   151

Case 12: Dilated Cardiomyopathy   152

Case 13: Endocarditis   154

Case 14: Hypertrophic Cardiomyopathy   156

Case 15: Hypertension   158

Case 16: Kawasaki's Disease   159

Case 17: Mitral Valve Prolapse   160

Case 18: "Monday Disease"   161

Case 19: Myocardial Infarction   162

Case 20: Pericarditis   163

Case 21: Obstruction of Superior Mesenteric Artery/Inferior Mesenteric Artery   164

Case 22: Patent Ductus Arteriosus   166

Case 23: Polyarteritis Nodosa   168

Case 24: Rheumatic Heart Disease   169

Case 25: Temporal Arteritis   170

Case 26: Tetralogy of Fallot   171

Case 27: Truncus Arteriosus   172

Case 28: Wolff-Parkinson-White Syndrome   174

Case 29: Wegener's Granulomatosis   176

Endocrine   **177**

Case 1: 11β-Hydroxylase Deficiency   178

Case 2: 21β-Hydroxylase Deficiency   180

Case 3: Addison's Disease   181

Case 4: Conn's Syndrome   183

Case 5: Cushing's Syndrome   184

Case 6: Diabetes Mellitus   185

Case 7: Gigantism   186

Case 8: Gout   188

Case 9: Graves' Disease   189

Case 10: Hyperparathyroidism   190

Case 11: Hypothyroidism   191

Case 12: Metabolic Syndrome 192

Case 13: Multiple Endocrine Neoplasia Type IIA 194

Case 14: Non-Insulin-Dependent (Type 2) Diabetes 196

Case 15: Pheochromocytoma 198

Case 16: Pseudohypoparathyroidism 199

Case 17: Sheehan's Syndrome 200

Case 18: Thyroglosssal Duct Cyst 201

Case 19: Thyroid Cancer 202

Case 20: Thyroidectomy 203

Case 21: Toxic Multinodular Goiter 204

Gastrointestinal 207

Case 1: Achalasia 208

Case 2: Acute Pancreatitis 209

Case 3: Alcoholic Cirrhosis 210

Case 4: Appendicitis 212

Case 5: Barrett's Esophagus 213

Case 6: Choledocholithiasis 214

Case 7: Crigler-Najjar Syndrome 216

Case 8: Diverticulitis 218

Case 9: Cholangitis 220

Case 10. Esophageal Atresia/Fistula 221

Case 11: Gastrinoma 222

Case 12: Hemochromatosis 223

Case 13: Hepatitis B Virus Infection 224

Case 14: Hepatitis C Virus Infection 225

Case 15: Hepatocellular Carcinoma 226

Case 16: Hyperbilirubinemia 227

Case 17: Inflammatory Bowel Disease 228

Case 18: Lower Gastrointestinal Bleeding 229

Case 19: Meckel's Diverticulum 230

Case 20: Painless Jaundice 232

Case 21: Pellagra 233

Case 22: Primary Biliary Cirrhosis 234

Case 23: Pseudomembranous Colitis/*Clostridium difficile* Infection 236

Case 24: Pyloric Stenosis 237

Case 25: Reye's Syndrome 238

Case 26: Short Bowel Syndrome/Malabsorption 239

Case 27: Stomach Cancer 240

Case 28: Upper Gastrointestinal Tract Bleeding 241

Case 29: Vitamin B_{12} Deficiency 242

Case 30: Zollinger-Ellison Syndrome 244

Hematology and Oncology 245

Case 1: Acute Intermittent Porphyria 247

Case 2: Acute Lymphoblastic Leukemia   248

Case 3: Acute Myelogenous Leukemia   250

Case 4: Aplastic Anemia   251

Case 5: β-Thalassemia   252

Case 6: Autoimmune Hemolytic Anemia   254

Case 7: Breast Cancer   255

Case 8: Carcinoid Syndrome   256

Case 9: Burkitt's Lymphoma   258

Case 10: Chronic Myelogenous Leukemia   259

Case 11: Colorectal Cancer   260

Case 12: Disseminated Intravascular Coagulation   261

Case 13: Gastric Cancer   262

Case 14: Glioblastoma Multiforme   263

Case 15: Glucose-6-Phospate Dehydrogenase Deficiency   264

Case 16: Head and Neck Cancer   265

Case 17: Hemochromatosis   266

Case 18: Hodgkin's Lymphoma   268

Case 19: Hemophilia   270

Case 20: Teratoma   271

Case 21: Idiopathic Thrombocytopenic Purpura   272

Case 22: Lead Poisoning   274

Case 23: Lung Cancer (Pancoast's Syndrome)   275

Case 24: Macrocytic Anemia   276

Case 25: Microcytic Anemia   277

Case 26: Neuroblastoma   278

Case 27: Multiple Myeloma   280

Case 28: Oligodendroglioma   281

Case 29: Ovarian Cancer (Sertoli-Leydig Tumor)   282

Case 30: Pancreatic Cancer   283

Case 31: Polycythemia   284

Case 32: Retinoblastoma   285

Case 33: Sickle Cell Anemia   286

Case 34: Small Cell Lung Carcinoma   288

Case 35: Spherocytosis   289

Case 36: Splenic Injury   290

Case 37: Testicular Cancer   291

Case 38: Thrombotic Thrombocytopenic Purpura/Hemolytic-Uremic Syndrome   292

Case 39: von Willebrand's Disease   293

Musculoskeletal   **295**

Case 1: Costochondritis   296

Case 2: Cutaneous Squamous Cell Carcinoma   297

Case 3: Gunshot Wound to Left Flank   298

Case 4: Ewing's Sarcoma   300

Case 5: Hip Fracture   301

Case 6: Inguinal Hernia   302

Case 7: Knee Pain   303

Case 8: Melanoma   304

Case 9: Muscular Dystrophy   305

Case 10: Osteoarthritis   306

Case 11: Neurofibromatosis   308

Case 12: Osteogenesis Imperfecta   309

Case 13: Rheumatoid Arthritis   310

Case 14: Osteoporosis   312

Case 15: Subclavian Stab Wound   313

Case 16: Rotator Cuff Tear   314

Case 17: Systemic Lupus Erythematosus   316

Case 18: Systemic Sclerosis (Scleroderma)   317

Neurology   **319**

Case 1: Alzheimer's Disease   321

Case 2: Brown-Séquard Syndrome   322

Case 3: Amyotrophic Lateral Sclerosis   324

Case 4: Corneal Abrasion/Eye Injury   325

Case 5: Central Cord Syndrome   326

Case 6: Craniopharyngioma   328

Case 7: Damage to Recurrent Laryngeal Nerve   329

Case 8: Femoral Neuropathy   330

Case 9: Glaucoma   331

Case 10: Glioblastoma Multiforme   332

Case 11: Guillain-Barré Syndrome   334

Case 12: Horner's Syndrome   336

Case 13: Hydrocephalus   338

Case 14: Huntington's Disease   340

Case 15: Macular Degeneration   341

Case 16: Homonymous Hemianopia   342

Case 17: Medulloblastoma   344

Case 18: Meningioma   345

Case 19: Middle Ear Infection/Ear Anatomy   346

Case 20: Metastatic Brain Tumor   348

Case 21: Migraine   349

Case 22: Multiple Sclerosis   350

Case 23: Neurofibromatosis Type 1   352

Case 24: Myasthenia Gravis   354

Case 25: Parkinson's Disease   355

Case 26: Neurofibromatosis Type 2   356

Case 27: Pituitary Adenoma   358

Case 28: Seizures/Status Epilepticus   359

Case 29: Stroke   360

Case 30: Spinal Cord Compression   362

Case 31: Sturge-Weber Syndrome   363

Case 32: Subarachnoid Hemorrhage   364

Case 33: Subdural Hematoma   366

Case 34: Syncope   367

Case 35: Transient Ischemic Attack   368

Case 36: Tuberous Sclerosis   370

Case 37: Ulnar Nerve Damage   372

Case 38: Vascular Dementia   373

Case 39: Vestibulo-ocular Reflexes   374

Case 40: Viral Meningitis   376

Case 41: von Hippel–Lindau Disease   378

Case 42: Wernicke-Korsakoff Syndrome   379

Psychiatry   **381**

Case 1: Attention Deficit Hyperactivity Disorder   382

Case 2: Autism   383

Case 3: Bipolar Disorder   384

Case 4: Depression   385

Case 5: Generalized Anxiety Disorder   386

Case 6: Obsessive-Compulsive Disorder   387

Case 7: Obsessive-Compulsive Personality Disorder   388

Case 8: Panic Disorder   389

Case 9: Posttraumatic Stress Disorder   390

Case 10: Rett's Disorder   391

Case 11: Schizophrenia   392

Case 12: Somatoform Disorder   393

Case 13: Steroid-Induced Mania   394

Case 14: Tardive Dyskinesia   395

Case 15: Tourette's Disorder   396

Renal   **397**

Case 1: Acute Tubular Necrosis   398

Case 2: Autosomal Dominant Polycystic Kidney Disease   399

Case 3: Alport's Syndrome   400

Case 4: Drug-Induced Acute Interstitial Nephritis   401

Case 5: Fanconi's Syndrome   403

Case 6: Goodpasture's Syndrome   405

Case 7: Henoch-Schönlein Purpura   407

Case 8: Hypercalcemia   408

Case 9: Hypokalemia   410

Case 10: Hyponatremia   411

Case 11: Hypophosphatemic (Vitamin D–Resistant) Rickets   412

Case 12: Metabolic Acidosis with Respiratory Alkalosis   414

Case 13: Metabolic Alkalosis   416

Case 14: Minimal Change Disease   417

Case 15: Nephrotic Syndrome 418
Case 16: Pyelonephritis 419
Case 17: Rapidly Progressive Glomerulonephritis 420
Case 18: Renal Artery Stenosis/Hypertension/Renin-Angiotensin-Aldosterone Axis 422
Case 19: Renal Calculi 423
Case 20: Syndrome of Inappropriate Secretion of ADH 425
Case 21: Transplant Immunology 426
Case 22: Urinary Reflux 427

Reproductive **429**
Case 1: Abruptio Placentae 430
Case 2: Androgen Insensitivity Syndrome 432
Case 3: Bacterial Vaginosis 433
Case 4: Benign Prostatic Hyperplasia 434
Case 5: Breast Mass 435
Case 6: Ectopic Pregnancy 436
Case 7: Endometriosis 438
Case 8: Erectile Dysfunction 440
Case 9: Fitz-Hugh and Curtis Syndrome 441
Case 10: Gestational Diabetes 442
Case 11: Klinefelter's Syndrome 443
Case 12: Leiomyoma 444
Case 13: Menopause 445
Case 14: Molar Pregnancy and Choriocarcinoma 446
Case 15: Ovarian Cancer 447
Case 16: Paget's Disease of the Breast 448
Case 17: Preeclampsia 449
Case 18: Testicular Torsion 451
Case 19: Turner's Syndrome 452

Respiratory **453**
Case 1: Acute Respiratory Distress Syndrome/Diffuse Alveolar Damage 454
Case 2: Asbestosis 455
Case 3: Asthma 456
Case 4: Atelectasis 457
Case 5: Bronchiectasis 458
Case 6: Chronic Obstructive Pulmonary Disease 459
Case 7: Community-Acquired Pneumonia 460
Case 8: Congenital Cystic Adenomatoid Malformation of the Lung 462
Case 9: Cystic Fibrosis 463
Case 10: Emphysema 464
Case 11: Epiglottitis Due to *Haemophilus influenzae* Infection 465
Case 12: Malignant Mesothelioma 467
Case 13: Malignant Pleural Effusion 468
Case 14: *Mycoplasma Pneumoniae* Pneumonia 469

Case 15: Pulmonary Embolism   470

Case 16: Respiratory Acidosis   472

Case 17: Sarcoidosis   474

Case 18: Small Cell Carcinoma   475

Case 19: Spontaneous Pneumothorax   476

Case 20: Thoracic Outlet Obstruction (Klumpke's Palsy)   477

Appendix   **479**

Index   **487**

About the Authors   **503**

CONTRIBUTING AUTHORS

Rakesh Razdan Ahuja
Yale University School of Medicine
Class of 2010

Mamie Air
Yale University School of Medicine
Class of 2009

Justin Brent Cohen
Yale University School of Medicine
Class of 2009

Jennifer Giltnane, MD, PhD
Resident
Department of Pathology
Vanderbilt Hospital

Kelvin Lau, MD
Resident
Department of Pediatrics
Children's Hospital of Philadelphia

Leah McNally
Yale University School of Medicine
Class of 2009

Jennifer Pluznick, PhD
Postdoctoral Fellow
Department of Cellular and Molecular Physiology
Yale University School of Medicine

Christina L. Shenvi, PhD
Yale University School of Medicine
Class of 2009

Paul Charles Walker, MD
Resident
Department of Otolaryngology
University of Iowa

SENIOR REVIEWERS

Sumit Bhargava, MD
Assistant Professor of Pediatrics
Section of Respiratory Medicine
Department of Pediatrics
Yale University School of Medicine

Sheldon Campbell, MD, PhD
Associate Professor
Department of Laboratory Medicine
Yale University School of Medicine

Joseph Craft, MD
Professor of Internal Medicine and Rheumatology
Chief of Rheumatology and Immunobiology
Yale University School of Medicine

John P. Geibel, MD, DSc
Vice Chairman
Department of Surgery
Yale University School of Medicine

Stephanie Halene, MD
Associate Research Scientist
Department of Internal Medicine
Yale University School of Medicine

Sandra Iragorri, MD
Assistant Clinical Professor of Pediatrics Nephrology
Department of Pediatrics
Yale University School of Medicine

Nisha Manickam, DO
Clinical Fellow Internal Medicine Infectious Disease
Yale University School of Medicine

Geoffey Miller, MD
Professor of Pediatrics and Neurology
Department of Pediatrics
Yale University School of Medicine

Jennifer Myer, MD
Assistant Clinical Professor
Department of Psychiatry
Yale University School of Medicine

Errol Norwitz, MD, PhD
Associate Professor
Department of Obstetrics and Gynecology
Yale University School of Medicine

Edward Perry, MD
Assistant Professor
Department of Psychiatry
Yale University School of Medicine

George A. Porter, MD, PhD
Assistant Professor
Department of Pediatrics
Yale University School of Medicine

Sanziana Roman, MD
Surgeon, Assistant Professor
Department of Surgery
Yale University School of Medicine

Mark Solomon, MD
Professor
Molecular Biophysics and Biochemistry
Yale University School of Medicine

Louis Trevisan, MD
Assistant Clinical Professor
Department of Psychiatry
Yale University School of Medicine

PREFACE

With *First Aid Cases for the USMLE Step 1*, 2nd edition, we continue our commitment to providing students with the most useful and up-to-date preparation guides for the USMLE Step 1. This edition represents an outstanding effort by a talented group of authors and includes the following:

- Commonly asked question stems on the USMLE Step 1 integrated into a single USMLE-style case.
- Concise yet complete explanations.
- Two-column format for easy self-quizzing.
- High-yield images, diagrams, and tables to complement the questions and answers.
- Organized as a perfect supplement to *First Aid for the USMLE Step 1*.

We invite you to share your thoughts and ideas to help us improve *First Aid Cases for the USMLE Step 1*. See "How to Contribute," on p. xxiii.

Louisville	Tao Le
New Haven	Vinita Takiar

ACKNOWLEDGMENTS

This has been a collaborative project from the start. We gratefully acknowledge the thoughtful comments and advice of the residents, international medical graduates, and faculty who have supported the authors in the development of *First Aid Cases for the USMLE Step 1*, 2nd edition.

For support and encouragement throughout the process, we are grateful to Thao Pham and Selina Bush. Thanks to our publisher, McGraw-Hill, for the valuable assistance of their staff. For enthusiasm, support, and commitment to this challenging project, thanks to our editor, Catherine A. Johnson. For outstanding editorial work, we thank Emma D. Underdown, Isabel Nogueira, and Michael Shelton. A special thanks to Rainbow Graphics for remarkable production work.

Louisville	Tao Le
New Haven	Vinita Takiar

HOW TO CONTRIBUTE

To continue to produce a high-yield review source for the USMLE Step 1 exam, we invite you to submit any suggestions or corrections. We also offer **paid internships** in medical education and publishing ranging from three months to one year (see below for details). Please send us your suggestions for the following:

- High-yield USMLE Step 1 cases.
- New facts, mnemonics, diagrams, and illustrations.
- Low-yield cases to remove.

For each entry incorporated into the next edition, you will receive a $10 gift certificate, as well as personal acknowledgment in the next edition. Diagrams, tables, partial entries, updates, corrections, and study hints are also appreciated, and significant contributions will be compensated at the discretion of the authors. Also let us know about material in this edition that you feel is low yield and should be deleted.

The preferred way to submit entries, suggestions, or corrections is via our blog:

www.firstaidteam.com

Otherwise, please send entries, neatly written or typed or on disk (Microsoft Word), to:

First Aid Team
914 North Dixie Avenue, Suite 100
Elizabethtown, KY 42701
Attention: Step 1 Casebook

All entries become property of the authors and are subject to editing and reviewing. Please verify all data and spellings carefully. In the event that similar or duplicate entries are received, only the first entry received will be used. Include a reference to a standard textbook to facilitate verification of the fact. Please follow the style, punctuation, and format of this edition if possible.

INTERNSHIP OPPORTUNITIES

The author team is pleased to offer part-time and full-time paid internships in medical education and publishing to motivated medical students and physicians. Internships may range from three months (e.g., a summer) up to a full year. Participants will have an opportunity to author, edit, and earn publication credit on a wide variety of projects, including the popular *First Aid* series. Writing/editing experience, familiarity with Microsoft Word, Internet access, and a passion for education are desired. Go to our blog www.firstaidteam.com to apply for an internship. A sample of your work or a proposal of a specific project is helpful.

General Principles

- ► Behavioral Science
- ► Biochemistry
- ► Microbiology and Immunology
- ► Pharmacology

Behavioral Science

Case 1	4
Case 2	5
Case 3	6
Case 4	8
Case 5	9
Case 6	10
Case 7	11
Case 8	12
Case 9	13
Case 10	14
Case 11	15
Case 12	16
Case 13	17
Case 14	18
Case 15	19

▶ **Case 1**

A 58-year-old man is brought to the emergency department by his supervisor after he was found stumbling and confused at work. On physical examination, the patient appears slightly sedated and admits to recent heavy drinking, but says his last drink was 1–2 days earlier. He also says he vomited three times earlier that morning. He denies chest and abdominal pain. He is afebrile but tremulous. CT scan of the head is negative for mass lesions or bleeding. Relevant laboratory findings are as follows:

Aspartate aminotransferase: 57 U/L
Alanine aminotransferase: 18 U/L
Lactate dehydrogenase: 398 U/L

■ What is the most likely diagnosis?	Alcohol withdrawal.
■ What is the pathophysiology of this condition?	Alcohol is a central nervous system depressant that causes neuronal changes, including the downregulation of α-aminobutyric acid receptors when chronically abused. Alcohol withdrawal can lead to neuronal hyperactivity via a decrease in cortical inhibition. Additionally, increased serum norepinephrine and altered serotonin levels have been implicated in both alcohol craving and tolerance.
■ What are the symptoms of this condition?	Minor symptoms (occurring 6–36 hours after the last drink) include: ■ Diaphoresis ■ Gastrointestinal upset ■ Headache ■ Nausea and vomiting ■ Palpitations ■ Tremulousness Seizures can occur within 6–48 hours of the last drink. Visual (or less commonly, tactile or auditory) hallucinations can occur within 12–48 hours of the last drink, and delirium tremens may occur within 48–96 hours.
■ What is delirium tremens?	About 5% of patients with alcohol withdrawal symptoms develop **delirium tremens**, which is a collection of symptoms that includes delirium, tachycardia, hypertension, agitation, low-grade fever, and diaphoresis. If untreated, the mortality rate of patients who develop delirium tremens is around 20%; major causes of death include arrhythmia and infection.
■ What is the most appropriate treatment for this condition?	**Benzodiazepines**, particularly lorazepam or diazepam, are the treatment of choice for all types of alcohol withdrawal symptoms, including withdrawal seizures and delirium tremens. Barbiturates and propofol are used if the patient is refractory to benzodiazepines.

A 24-year-old woman is brought to the emergency department with confusion, blurred vision, dizziness, and somnolence. Her friend states the woman is generally healthy, but is taking medication for occasional episodes of intense fear, sweating, nausea, and abdominal and chest pain. Physical examination reveals a respiratory rate of 8 breaths per minute.

■ What is the most likely diagnosis?	Benzodiazepine toxicity, as characterized by respiratory depression, confusion, and other symptoms of central nervous system depression.
■ What class of drugs might be responsible for this patient's symptoms?	Her friend's description is consistent with a diagnosis of panic disorder. Benzodiazepines (such as clonazepam, lorazepam, and alprazolam) are commonly used in the short-term treatment of panic disorder.
■ What treatment was likely administered to this patient in the emergency department?	Flumazenil, a competitive antagonist at the α-aminobutyric acid (GABA) receptor, is effective in reversing symptoms of benzodiazepine overdose.
■ How does the mechanism of action of benzodiazepines differ from that of barbiturates?	Normally, $GABA_A$ receptors respond to GABA binding by opening chloride channels, which leads to hyperpolarization. Binding of benzodiazepines to α subunits or to an area of the α unit influenced by the α unit facilitates channel opening, but does not directly initiate chloride current. Both benzodiazepines and barbiturates enhance the affinity of GABA for $GABA_A$ receptors. Benzodiazepines act by increasing the **frequency** of opening of chloride channels. In contrast, barbiturates act by increasing the **duration** of opening of chloride channels.
■ What are the advantages of using benzodiazepines vs. using barbiturates?	Benzodiazepines have a lower risk of dependence, P450 system involvement, respiratory depression, coma, and loss of rapid eye movement sleep. They are considered to be much safer than barbiturates in cases of overdose.
■ What drugs, when taken with benzodiazepines, increase the likelihood of developing toxicity?	■ Acetaminophen ■ Alcohol ■ Cimetidine ■ Disulfiram ■ Isoniazid ■ Valproic acid

► **Case 3**

A 17-year-old girl presents to her physician with right foot pain. She states she has been exercising quite frequently recently. She has not had menses for several months now. Upon further questioning, she reluctantly states that she is afraid of gaining weight and eats only cereal and vegetables. Her weight is currently 44.1 kg (97 lb) and her body mass index is 17 kg/m². An x-ray of her foot is taken (see Figure 1-1). Relevant laboratory findings are as follows:

Hemoglobin: 10.8 g/dL
Hematocrit: 33.5%
Mean corpuscular volume (MCV): 78.5 fl

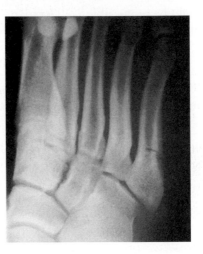

FIGURE 1-1. (Courtesy of Alan B. Storrow, MD, as published in Knoop KJ. Stack LB, Storrow AB. *Atlas of Emergency Medicine*, 2nd ed. New York: McGraw-Hill, 2002: 343.)

▪ What is the most likely diagnosis?	Anorexia nervosa.
▪ What other symptoms of this condition are common at presentation?	Patients typically present with severe weight loss and clinical manifestations of multiple nutritional deficiencies. Dental caries and erosions (see Figure 1-2) may be present if patients are also vomiting. Additional purging via laxative abuse may cause palpitations, lightheadedness, or chest pain due to electrolyte abnormalities.
▪ What diagnosis would be of concern if this patient were of normal weight?	**Bulimia nervosa** can present with similar findings. Its hallmark is uncontrollable binge eating followed by purging. These patients are usually of normal weight and have irregular menses. Nutritional deficiencies, however, are uncommon.
▪ What kind of anemia does this patient likely have?	Low hematocrit and low MCV suggest a **microcytic anemia**, most likely due to iron deficiency, a common feature in these patients. Inadequate vitamin B_{12} and folate intake cause a **macrocytic anemia**. Some patients may have an overall **normocytic anemia** due to the combined microcytic and macrocytic anemias.
▪ What nutritional deficiency may contribute to the radiographic findings in Figure 1-1?	Fractures of the fifth metatarsal bone in these patients are often related in part to osteopenia or osteoporosis secondary to vitamin D and calcium deficiency.

■ What region of the brain regulates appetite and is thought to play a role in eating disorders?

The "feeding center" is located in the lateral nucleus of the hypothalamus. When stimulated, it promotes eating/appetite. The "satiety center" is located in the ventromedial nucleus. When stimulated, it signals the body to stop eating. Lesions to this area cause hyperphagia and obesity.

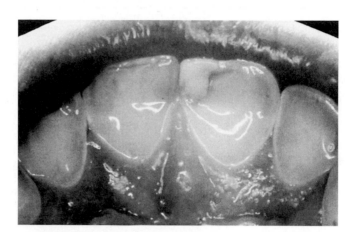

FIGURE 1-2. Dental erosions in patients with vomiting. (Courtesy of David P. Kretzschmar, DDS, MS, as published in Knoop KJ. Stack LB, Storrow AB. *Atlas of Emergency Medicine,* 2nd ed. New York: McGraw-Hill, 2002: 175.)

GENERAL PRINCIPLES

BEHAVIORAL SCIENCE

▶ **Case 4**	An overseer of clinical trials is given an application for the study of a new drug that is intended to independently lower weight. The company seeking to test this drug wants to distribute it to volunteer members of local fitness clubs for 3 weeks and then contact each participant in 3 months to follow up on their results.
▪ **What is bias?**	Bias refers to any source of error in the determination of association between the exposure (drug use in this case) and outcome (weight loss in this case).
▪ **What types of bias can be found in this study?**	There are three types of bias in this drug company's proposal: ▪ **Sampling bias:** All the subjects tested are members of a fitness club and are therefore more likely to lose weight than are members of the general population. For this reason, the results of the trial cannot be generalized to the targeted population as a whole. ▪ **Selection bias:** All the subjects tested were able to choose whether or not they wanted to try the new drug. Because of this nonrandomly assigned study group, there is no way to eliminate the placebo effects of the drug. ▪ **Recall bias:** The company that distributes the drug plans to contact all the participants 3 months after the study is completed. As a result of knowing what is expected of them, the subjects may be more likely to claim that they have lost weight.
▪ **What is another important type of bias found in the research design of some studies?**	Late-look bias, which pertains to information being gathered at an inappropriate time, is another type of bias; one example would be following up on results after another intervention outside of the study has taken place.
▪ **What are some ways in which bias can be reduced?**	Bias can be reduced by using placebos; randomizing the subjects who are using the drug; using a double-blind study; and using a crossover study in which the subject acts as his or her own control.

▶ **Case 5**

A 27-year-old woman comes to the emergency department with bruises on her wrists and forearms. x-ray of the chest shows the woman to have three broken ribs. While taking the history, the woman tells the physician that her boyfriend got upset with her because she overcooked his steak. She claims that she provoked the incident by not preparing his food correctly and asks the doctor not to tell the police or anyone else.

▪ **What should the physician do in this scenario?**	Because the patient is not considered to be a minor or an elderly patient, defined as being aged 65 years or more, the patient's right to confidentiality must ultimately be respected. Although the physician should make all resources available to her such as a battered women's home, the ethical principles of patient autonomy and privacy must be followed.
▪ **Should the physician contact members of the woman's family or close friends mentioned when taking the social history?**	No, the physician should not. Disclosing this information when clearly told not to by the patient would break the principle of autonomy. Also, the physician is bound by the privacy rule of the Health Insurance Portability and Accountability Act (HIPAA).
▪ **What are the exceptions to confidentiality?**	There are a number of exceptions to confidentiality other than the age measures put in place to protect minors and the elderly population. These exceptions rely on the physician's judgment of the situation. If the potential harm to self or others is great or serious, then confidentiality may be violated in order to preserve the principle of beneficence. It is the responsibility of physicians to take steps to prevent harm if there are no alternative means to protect those at risk.
▪ **What is the *Tarasoff* decision?**	This is a law requiring a physician to **directly** inform and protect potential victims from harm. For example, if the woman told the physician that she had a gun and was going to go back home and kill her boyfriend for abusing her, the physician would have a duty to inform the boyfriend and detain the patient.
▪ **What is the physician's duty if a patient has a serious infectious disease and is putting others at risk of infection?**	Physicians have a duty to warn public officials and other identifiable persons at risk if a patient has certain infectious diseases. These diseases include hepatitis A and B, salmonella, shigella, syphilis, measles, mumps, AIDS, rubella, tuberculosis, chickenpox, and gonorrhea.

A 67-year-old man presents with a crushing, substernal chest pain that he claims used to occur only on exertion, but now occurs at random times throughout the day. His wife is very concerned about her husband's welfare and asks the attending physician what he thinks can be done. The attending physician meets with the patient and his wife and discusses the diagnosis of unstable angina and its association with myocardial infarction. The physician then describes the option of bypass surgery and asks the patient if he would like to have this surgery.

■ If the patient, with full mental capacity, decides that he would not like to have this surgery, what should the physician do?	Under the core ethical principle of **autonomy**, physicians have an obligation to respect and honor the medical care preferences of their patients.
■ If the physician believed that not going ahead with this surgery was not in his patient's best interest, what should the physician do?	Although physicians have a fiduciary duty to act in the patient's best interest under the ethical principle of **beneficence**, if the patient can make an informed decision, the patient ultimately has the right to decide what type of treatment he is willing to undergo.
■ What ethical principle is violated in all surgeries?	Because the benefits of a surgical intervention often outweigh the risks, the principle of **nonmaleficence** or "do no harm" is often broken as a means to a better end.
■ What final ethical principle must physicians follow that has not been discussed?	The last of the four core ethical principles is **justice**, which is to treat all persons fairly without exception.

A 65-year-old diabetic man is admitted to the hospital for repair of a hip fracture. On postoperative day 4, his wife reports that he seems very confused and he could not remember her name. Evaluation reveals the patient is inattentive and generally confused. However, his nurse notes that he was fine both the day before and 3 hours earlier. The patient has been taking morphine, and is continuing to take his previously prescribed β-blocker and angiotensin-converting enzyme inhibitor for hypertension. He is afebrile, and his blood pressure is 105/51 mm Hg. Relevant laboratory findings are as follows:

Sodium: 133 mEq/L   Phosphate: 3.0 mg/dL
Calcium: 8.9 mg/dL   Blood urea nitrogen: 18 mg/dL
Potassium: 3.9 mEq/L   Creatinine: 1.5 mg/dL
Chloride: 99 mEq/L   Glucose: 58 mg/dL
Magnesium: 1.9 mg/dL   Urinalysis: unremarkable
Bicarbonate: 25.1 mEq/L

■ What is the most likely diagnosis?

Delirium. The *Diagnostic and Statistical Manual of Mental Disorders*, 4th edition, lists the key features of delirium as:
- Altered consciousness with reduced attention.
- Altered cognition of perceptual disturbance not accountable for by dementia.
- Development over a short time with waxing and waning.
- Evidence that the change is caused by a medical condition, drug, or other substance.

■ What is the differential diagnosis of this condition?

Delirium should be distinguished from depression, psychotic illness, and dementia. This is difficult because delirium is often superimposed on dementia, and is often mistaken for dementia in elderly persons. The acuity of presentation and the waxing and waning course are the most helpful ways to differentiate delirium from dementia. Furthermore, delirium is caused by a medical or pharmacological entity. This cause must be excluded before a change in mental status can be labeled as something other than delirium.

■ What risk factors are associated with this condition?

- Advanced age
- Dehydration
- Hypoglycemia
- Institutionalization
- Metabolic and electrolyte disturbances
- Particular medications
- Postoperative state

■ What are the most common drugs that cause this condition?

Major classes of drugs that commonly cause delirium are opioids (especially morphine and meperidine), anticholinergic agents (including benztropine used to treat parkinsonian side effects of antipsychotic medications), anticonvulsants (phenytoin), antidepressants (tricyclic antidepressants, selective serotonin reuptake inhibitors), β-blockers, digoxin, corticosteroids, dopamine agonists, H_2-receptor blockers, and sedative hypnotics. This list is not complete, as many more drugs can cause delirium.

■ What are the most appropriate treatments for this condition?

The key to treating delirium is to treat the underlying etiology. The most common disturbances include fluid and electrolyte imbalances, infections (especially urinary tract infections), drug or alcohol toxicity, alcohol withdrawal, psychoactive drug withdrawal, metabolic disorders, and low perfusion states. The first step in treatment should be thorough medication review and a reversal of any metabolic abnormalities.

▶ **Case 8**

A 19-year-old male college student is brought to the emergency department by his roommate, who found him sitting outside their room breathing very shallowly. The patient is difficult to understand because he is intoxicated, has slurred speech, and is drowsy. Physical examination reveals pinpoint pupils. The roommate admits they were both at a party earlier in the evening, but he lost track of the patient and is not sure what he could have taken.

■ What drugs of abuse could be involved in this case?	■ Alcohol ■ Amphetamines ■ Benzodiazepines or barbiturates ■ Cocaine ■ Heroin (opioids) ■ Lysergic acid diethylamide (LSD) ■ Phencyclidine (PCP)
■ What signs and symptoms are associated with alcohol intoxication and withdrawal?	■ Intoxication: disinhibition, decreased cognition, unsteady gait. ■ Withdrawal: tremor, seizures, delirium tremens (benzodiazepines).
■ What signs and symptoms are associated with opioid intoxication and withdrawal?	■ Intoxication: intense euphoria, drowsiness, slurred speech, decreased memory, pupil constriction, decreased respirations. ■ Withdrawal: nausea, vomiting, pupil dilation, insomnia.
■ What signs and symptoms are associated with benzodiazepine or barbiturate intoxication and withdrawal?	■ Intoxication: respiratory and cardiac depression, disinhibition, unsteady gait. ■ Withdrawal: agitation, anxiety, depression, tremor, seizures, delirium.
■ What signs and symptoms are associated with PCP and LSD intoxication and withdrawal?	■ PCP intoxication: intense psychosis, violence, rhabdomyolysis, hyperthermia. ■ LSD intoxication: increased sensation, colors richer, tastes heightened, visual hallucinations. ■ Withdrawl from PCP occurs due to reabsorption of the drug in the small intestines. ■ There are no withdrawal symptoms from LSD.

A breakout of a virulent bacterial infection has occurred in a small city outside Tehran, Iran. In an effort to isolate those people who are infected from those who are not, scientists have devised a new test to determine whether a host has been infected and have applied it to 400 persons. Although 57 people are actually infected, the test was positive in only 30 cases. Of those who are not infected, the test was negative in 300 cases.

■ What is the sensitivity of this diagnostic test?	**Sensitivity** is defined as the percentage of those with an infection who test positive for it. Therefore, the sensitivity of this test is 30/57, or 52.6% (see Table 1-1).
■ What is the specificity of this diagnostic test?	**Specificity** is defined as the percentage of those who do not have an infection and test negative for it. Therefore, the specificity of this test is 300/343, or 87.5%.
■ What is the positive predictive value (PPV) of this test?	**PPV** is defined as the proportion of those who actually have an infection in relation to those who tested positive for it. Therefore, the PPV of this test is 30/73, or 41.1%.
■ What is the negative predictive value (NPV) of this test?	**NPV** is defined as the proportion of those who do not have an infection in relation to those who tested negative for it. Therefore, the NPV of this test is 300/327, or 91.7%.
■ What is the prevalence of this new outbreak in the population tested?	**Prevalence** is defined as the proportion of people who actually have the infection in relation to the total population at a point in time. Therefore, the prevalence of this disease is 57/400, or 14.3%.

TABLE 1-1. Determining Diagnostic Test Data

	THOSE WITH INFECTION	THOSE WITHOUT INFECTION	NUMBER OF PERSONS TESTED
Test positive	30	43	73
Test negative	27	300	327
Total	57	343	400

▶ **Case 10**

A mother of 15-month-old fraternal male twins consults her pediatrician because she is concerned about the development of one twin. Her concern lies in the fact that the older twin began to walk at approximately 12 months of age, but the younger twin still is unable to walk by himself. Physical examination reveals no significant issues.

▪ Is it appropriate that the younger twin has not yet walked?	Yes. The approximate age children achieve the motor milestone of walking is 15 months. However, the child should be able to sit alone, a milestone that should occur between 6 and 9 months of age.
▪ By what age should the infant reflexes have disappeared?	These reflexes normally disappear within the first year. They include the Moro reflex (extension of limbs when startled), the rooting reflex (nipple seeking when cheek brushed), the palmar reflex (grasps objects in palm), and the Babinski reflex (large toe dorsiflexes with plantar stimulation).
▪ What cognitive/social milestones should these infants have reached?	Social smile (3 mo), recognizes people (4–5 mo), stranger anxiety (7–9 mo), orients to voice (7–9 mo), separation anxiety (15 mo), and the ability to speak a few words (15 mo).
▪ When evaluating the development of the twins, the physician was interested in the brothers' Apgar scores at birth. What are the components of the Apgar score?	Apgar is a useful acronym for the scoring system—Appearance, Pulse, Grimace, Activity, and Respiration (see Table 1-2). Each category is scored from 0–2, with 10 being a perfect score. The scoring is done at 1 and 5 minutes after birth.
▪ What upcoming motor and social milestones should the mother expect to see?	Upcoming motor milestones include climbing stairs (12–24 mo), the ability to stack 6 blocks (18–24 mo), riding a tricycle (3 yrs), simple drawings (4 yrs), and hopping on one foot (4 yrs). Upcoming cognitive/social milestones include object permanence (12–24 mo), parallel play (24–48 mo), core gender identity (24–36 mo), toilet training (30–36 mo), group play (3 yrs), and cooperative play (4 yrs).

TABLE 1-2. Apgar Scoring System

CATEGORY	SCORE 0	SCORE 1	SCORE 2
Appearance (color)	Blue/pale	Trunk pink	All pink
Pulse	None	<100	>100
Grimace (reflex irritability)	None	Grimace	Grimace + cough
Activity (muscle tone)	Limp	Some	Active
Respiration (effort)	None	Irregular	Regular

A 40-year-old woman in Miami visits a plastic surgeon, who was referred to her by a friend, for abdominal liposuction. After the surgeon fully explains the procedure and its possible complications, the woman agrees to continue with the operation and is scheduled for surgery the following week. Approximately 3 weeks after the liposuction, the woman's abdominal skin becomes dimpled in the area where the procedure took place. Extremely upset with the outcome, she goes to her plastic surgeon and threatens to file a malpractice suit against him if he does not repair her abdomen.

■ **What is a malpractice suit and what does it require in order to be justifiable?**

A malpractice suit is a civil suit under negligence that requires four fundamental things, also referred to as the "four D's." First, it must be understood that the physician had a **duty** or responsibility to the patient. Second, the physician must have breached that duty, which is called **dereliction**. Third, the patient must suffer some sort of harm or **damage**. Finally, the harm caused must be **directly** a cause of the dereliction. Therefore, the four D's are duty, dereliction, damage, and direct.

■ **In this particular case, if the physician decides not to perform a reparative procedure, are the grounds for malpractice justified?**

It depends. Although the duty and damage are clearly present in this situation, one must question whether the physician committed dereliction, a neglect of his duty, and if the patient's abdomen dimple is the result of neglect. Specifically for liposuction, patients should be advised to maintain regular exercise and dieting after the surgery to prevent tissue scarring and to allow for proper healing. If, for example, the patient did not do these things even though she was told to do so to prevent complications, the physician's actions would not be the cause of the harm incurred. If, however, he had in some way not followed the standard of care in her treatment and this had resulted in her complication, the woman would have better justification for her lawsuit.

■ **What is the difference between a criminal suit and a malpractice suit with respect to the burden of proof?**

In a criminal suit, the burden of proof must be "beyond a reasonable doubt," whereas in a malpractice suit, the burden of proof is more along the lines of "more likely than not."

■ **What is the most common reason for a litigation process to ensue between the patient and a physician?**

The number one factor leading to litigation is poor communication between the physician and the patient.

■ **What action should the physician take?**

The physician should try to find the reason for the dimpling of the abdomen. If the reason found is that he had made a mistake in the surgery, then he should immediately apologize to the patient for it. Studies have shown that if a physician is honest and up front about an error, he or she is less likely to be sued by the patient. Furthermore, if miscommunication were found to be the reason for this outcome, then the physician should make every effort to avoid such miscommunication with his future patients.

GENERAL PRINCIPLES

BEHAVIORAL SCIENCE

► **Case 12**   A couple is eating dinner at home with their quiet 6-year-old son. The couple gets into an argument and the father starts to yell at his son, who begins to cry. His mother gives the child candy, which temporarily relieves the crying. His mother continues to give him candy every time the child cries. The father then yells at the child and takes away the candy because children who cry should not be given candy.

▪ **What defense mechanism is the father using?**	**Displacement**, characterized by transferral of feelings from one object to another. In this case, the father's anger at the mother is displaced onto the child.
▪ **What type of reinforcement is the child using on the mother?**	This is an example of **positive reinforcement**, in which the consequences of a response increase the likelihood that the response will recur. Specifically, the child cries because crying makes it more likely the mother will continue to give him candy.
▪ **How does negative reinforcement differ from punishment?**	In **negative reinforcement**, behavior is encouraged or reinforced so as to remove an aversive stimulus. In **punishment**, behavior is discouraged and reduced by administration of an aversive stimulus.
▪ **Which method of conditioning is the father using by removing the reward?**	The father is employing **extinction**, characterized by elimination of a behavior by nonreinforcement. The child may stop crying after discovering that there is no reward for the behavior.

A male newborn was delivered at home is brought to the emergency department by his grandmother 30 minutes after his birth. The grandmother says the baby "isn't acting right." The baby weighs 2700 g (about 6 pounds) and was born at 38 weeks' gestational age. However, the baby is limp, unresponsive, and breathing infrequently, with bluish skin and pupils 2 mm in diameter. The infant is immediately resuscitated and stabilized for transfer to the neonatal intensive care unit (NICU) for monitoring. By day 3 of life, his nurse reports the infant is vomiting, has diarrhea, and cries excessively. Physical examination reveals tachycardia, tachypnea, dilated pupils, diaphoresis, tremors, increased muscle tone, and piloerection.

■ **What is the most likely diagnosis for the newborn's presentation in the ED?**	Opioid intoxication, heralded by the triad of (1) respiratory depression, (2) central nervous system depression, and (3) pinpoint pupils. Importantly, **pinpoint pupils** due to opioid intoxication will be present despite opioid tolerance.
■ **What pharmacologic treatment should this patient receive in the ED to specifically target the cause of his symptoms?**	Naloxone, an opioid antagonist, will reverse the effects of opioid agonists in this patient by selectively binding to opioid receptors.
■ **What is the most likely diagnosis on day 3 of life?**	The newborn is demonstrating symptoms of opiate withdrawal, also known as **neonatal abstinence syndrome**. Tachycardia, dilated pupils, diaphoresis, and other opiate withdrawal symptoms are related to sympathetic hyperactivity.
■ **What is the most appropriate long-term treatment for this patient?**	An opioid agonist, such as methadone, will relieve symptoms of acute opiate withdrawal. Methadone administration can then be tapered as the baby is weaned.
■ **What opioid drugs are most commonly used to treat this condition?**	■ Codeine ■ Fentanyl ■ Hydromorphone ■ Meperidine ■ Methadone ■ Morphine ■ Oxycodone ■ Buprenorphine

GENERAL PRINCIPLES

BEHAVIORAL SCIENCE

17

► **Case 14**

A 21-year-old man and his mother visit the clinic because his daytime sleepiness is starting to interfere with his studies. The man is slightly obese and has a history of pulmonary hypertension. His mother mentions he was prescribed a medication "for sleep," but he does not use it. On questioning, the man says he has a prescription for amphetamines and is taking sertraline. His mother also mentions that while they were sitting in the waiting room for their appointment, the young man said he heard "bells ringing," which no one else heard. Shortly thereafter, the young man fell asleep during their conversation.

▪ **Why does the patient have a prescription for amphetamines?**	The hallucinations, sudden onset of sleep, and amphetamine treatment is consistent with a diagnosis of **narcolepsy**. This condition has a strong genetic component.
▪ **What kind of hallucinations is the patient having?**	Hallucinations prior to falling asleep are termed **hypnagogic hallucinations** ("gogic"—"go" to sleep). **Hypnopompic hallucinations**, which occur during waking, are also associated with narcolepsy.
▪ **What stage of sleep is this patient likely to experience immediately upon falling asleep?**	Narcolepsy is associated with rapid eye movement (REM) sleep within 10 minutes of falling asleep.
▪ **What other electroencephalographic (EEG) abnormalities might be expected in this patient?**	Sertraline, a selective serotonin reuptake inhibitor, suggests the possibility of depression. **Depression** is associated with decreased REM latency and decreased stage 4, slow-wave sleep. Effective treatment with antidepressants, however, usually reverses any EEG abnormalities caused by major depression.
▪ **What other common sleep abnormality might account for poor quality of sleep?**	Obesity and pulmonary hypertension are associated with **sleep apnea**, which can be very disruptive and can lead to significant daytime fatigue. Arrhythmias and loud snoring are also associated with sleep apnea.

GENERAL PRINCIPLES

BEHAVIORAL SCIENCE

► **Case 15**

An 8-year-old boy who has been consistently incontinent at night has been diagnosed with primary nocturnal enuresis. After several months of unsuccessful nonpharmacologic therapy, the child is brought back to the pediatrician. The boy will be going to a 3-week-long summer camp in 1 month, and his parents are concerned about the social and psychological implications of his enuresis. They are interested in pharmacologic therapy to prevent his bed-wetting while he is at summer camp.

■ In what stage of sleep is this patient's enuresis occurring?	Enuresis occurs during stage 4 sleep, which is the deepest non–rapid eye movement (non-REM) sleep (see Table 1-3).
■ What pharmacologic treatment is most appropriate for this patient?	Imipramine is a tricyclic antidepressant that has been successfully used to treat primary nocturnal enuresis in children. It works by decreasing the duration of stage 4 sleep.
■ Which neurotransmitters influence sleep?	Serotonin (from the raphe nucleus) initiates sleep. Acetylcholine is the principal neurotransmitter promoting REM sleep. Conversely, norepinephrine reduces REM sleep.
■ What physiologic changes occur in REM sleep?	Pulse increases in rate and variability, REMs occur, blood pressure rises and has increased variability, and penile or clitoral tumescence occurs. The percentage of sleep spent in REM sleep decreases with increasing age.
■ What class of drugs is useful for treating night terrors and sleepwalking?	Benzodiazepines are useful for this purpose. Night terrors and sleepwalking occur during stage 4 sleep, and benzodiazepines shorten stage 4 sleep.

TABLE 1-3. Stages of Sleep

STAGE (% OF SLEEP)	DESCRIPTION	EEG WAVEFORM
Awake	Active mentally, alert	Beta (highest frequency, lowest amplitude)
Awake/eyes closed		Alpha
Stage 1 (5%)	Light sleep	Theta
Stage 2 (45%)	Deeper sleep	Sleep spindles and K complexes
Stage 3–4 (25%)	Deepest non-REM sleep	Delta (lowest frequency, highest amplitude; slow-wave sleep)
REM (25%)	Dreaming, loss of motor tone, increased brain oxygen use; may represent a memory processing function	Beta

Biochemistry

Case 1	22
Case 2	23
Case 3	24
Case 4	25
Case 5	26
Case 6	28
Case 7	30
Case 8	31
Case 9	32
Case 10	33
Case 11	34
Case 12	35
Case 13	36
Case 14	37
Case 15	38
Case 16	39
Case 17	40
Case 18	41
Case 19	42

▶ **Case 1**

A 45-year-old man comes to a community health clinic for his annual physical examination. He has no major complaints other than his chronic arthritis, which is worsening and is affecting his lower back, hips, and knees. On physical examination, the patient's sclerae are noted to be brownish-blue, and his ear cartilage is similarly discolored. An x-ray of the spine reveals disk degeneration and dense calcification that is most prominent in the lumbar region. Upon voiding for urinalysis, the man's urine is a normal color; however, after standing, the urine turns dark.

▪ What is the most likely diagnosis?	Alkaptonuria (ochronosis).
▪ What is the biochemical defect in this condition?	This disease is characterized by the absence of **homogentisate oxidase**, an enzyme of tyrosine metabolism that catalyzes the conversion of homogentisate to maleylacetoacetate (see Figure 2-1). The accumulation of homogentisate in cartilage leads to arthritis as well as to the discoloration of sclerae and other areas of the body.
▪ The metabolite that accumulates in this condition is derived from an essential amino acid. Which amino acid is this?	Homogentisate is derived from phenylalanine. Homogentisate oxidase is necessary for the metabolism of this amino acid, which is both glucogenic and ketogenic. Homogentisate is normally metabolized to acetoacetate (a ketone) and fumarate (part of the tricarboxylic acid cycle).
▪ Given this patient's extent of joint disease, how might his mental functioning be affected?	Alkaptonuria has no effect on cognitive functioning. Aside from its effects on joints and discoloration of sclerae and skin, the disease is benign.
▪ What is the most appropriate treatment for this condition?	There are no known ways to prevent the build-up of homogentisate. Dietary restriction of tyrosine and phenylalanine will reduce the production of homogentisate, but there has been no demonstrated benefit to this approach. Treating the symptoms of the patient's arthritis is the only recommended therapy in this case.

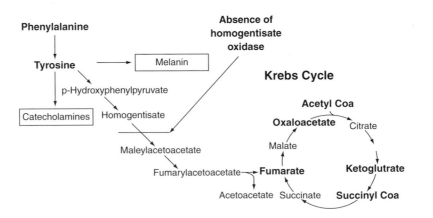

FIGURE 2-1. Flow chart showing conversion of homogentisate to maleylacetoacetate in phenylalanine metabolism.

▶ **Case 2**

A 37-year-old chemist with a 20-year history of bipolar disorder is rushed to the emergency department by his wife, who found him lying unconscious in the living room of their home. The man's skin is bright red, and he is breathing rapidly. Upon presentation, his breath smells like bitter almonds.

▪ What is the most likely diagnosis?	This man has ingested cyanide (the "bitter almond" breath is pathognomonic).
▪ What biochemical process is disrupted in this condition?	Cyanide is a direct inhibitor of one step in the electron transport chain (see Figure 2-2). Cyanide inhibits cytochrome oxidase.
▪ Does this patient have a greater-than-normal or lower-than-normal proton concentration in the intermembrane space of his mitochondria?	The man will have a lower proton concentration. The electron transport chain fuels the transport of protons from the mitochondrial matrix to the intermembrane space. Because this patient has ingested cyanide and has thus inhibited this process, his proton gradient is weakened, and therefore he will have a lower concentration of protons in the intermembrane spaces of his mitochondria.
▪ What is the most appropriate treatment for this condition?	Amyl nitrite is used to treat cyanide poisoning. Amyl nitrate oxidizes hemoglobin to methemoglobin. This is normally undesirable because this form of hemoglobin binds oxygen less avidly. However, methemoglobin strongly binds cyanide, preventing it from further disrupting electron transport.
▪ What other substances inhibit the electron transport chain?	Amytal, rotenone, antimycin A, azide, and **carbon monoxide** also inhibit the electron transport chain.
▪ What other substances act within the mitochondria and reduce synthesis of adenosine triphosphate (ATP)?	▪ Oligomycin is an example of a chemical that can directly inhibit mitochondrial ATP synthase. Although the proton gradient forms, ATP is not produced. As a result, electron transport ceases. ▪ Uncoupling agents such as 2,4-dinitrophenol (2,4-DNP) allow protons to cross the inner mitochondrial membrane. Electron transport is not disrupted, but protons are able to flow into the matrix from the intermembrane space. This reduces the proton gradient that drives ATP formation.

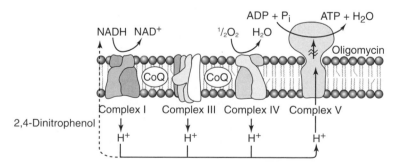

FIGURE 2-2. Cyanide inhibition of oxidative phosphorylation in the electron transport chain. (Reproduced, with permission, from Le T, Bhushan V, Rao DA. *First Aid for the USMLE Step 1: 2008.* New York: McGraw-Hill, 2008: 97.)

▶ **Case 3**

A 6-month old boy with a history of frequent infections is brought to the emergency department because of stiff muscles and difficulty feeding. On examination he is found to have a carpopedal spasm, and tapping on his facial nerve leads to spasm of the facial muscle.

▪ **What is the most likely diagnosis?**	This child has DiGeorge syndrome (22q11 syndrome), which is characterized by hypoparathyroidism and T-cell deficiency.
▪ **What is the etiology of this condition?**	DiGeorge syndrome is caused by a developmental defect involving the third and fourth pharyngeal arches. It results in a hypoplastic thymus and parathyroid glands. Laboratory tests of this patient would show hypocalcemia and low T-cell count. The hypocalcemia causes tetany and carpopedal spasm. Chvostek's sign involves tapping on the facial nerve and observing spasm of the facial muscle. It is another indication of hypocalcemia.
▪ **This patient is at risk for developing what type of infections?**	Because of the aplastic thymus, patients with this disorder have ineffective T cells and are particularly susceptible to viral and fungal infections.
▪ **What abnormality may be observed on an x-ray of the chest in this patient?**	An x-ray of the chest in a child with DiGeorge syndrome may show a reduced thymic shadow.
▪ **What other abnormalities are associated with this condition?**	**CATCH 22** is a mnemonic for the 22q11 syndrome, which involves a deletion in this region of chromosome **22**. Clinical manifestations include **C**ardiac abnormalities, **A**bnormal facies, **T**hymic hypoplasia, **C**left palate, and **H**ypocalcemia.

A 27-year-old man with little prior medical care was brought to the emergency department because of chest pain followed by sudden collapse. Resuscitation attempts were unsuccessful. On autopsy, he was found to have thick atherosclerotic plaques in his arteries, including the coronary arteries, aorta (see Figure 2-3), and renal arteries. He also had small, raised yellow/brown lesions on the extensor surfaces of his arms.

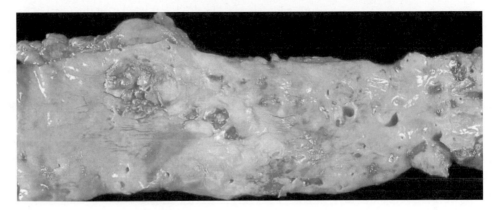

FIGURE 2-3. Severe atherosclerosis of the aorta. (Reproduced from the Center for Disease Control Public Health Image Library, [http://phil.cdc.gov].)

■ What is the most likely diagnosis?	This patient had familial hypercholesterolemia (FH), an inherited disorder characterized by extremely high serum cholesterol levels.
■ What is the genetic pattern of this condition?	FH is inherited in an autosomal manner. Heterozygotes typically have high cholesterol, around 370 mg/dL, and are at increased risk of myocardial infarctions. Homozygotes frequently have extremely high cholesterol levels, up to 1000 mg/dL. They frequently die before 30 years of age due to cardiovascular disease. For reference, normal total cholesterol is less than 200 mg/dL, and levels over 240 mg/dL are considered elevated.
■ What is the molecular basis of this condition?	In FH there is a mutation in the low-density lipoprotein (LDL) receptor gene. This results in a smaller number of functional LDL receptors. Normally, LDL circulates in the blood and binds to its receptor on hepatocyte membranes and is then taken up into the liver and metabolized. In patients with FH, LDL is taken up by the hepatocytes less efficiently, leading to elevated LDL levels in the blood.
■ What would be found on microscopic examination of the lesions on his arms?	Cholesterol deposits in the skin are termed xanthomas. They form when there is a persistently elevated LDL level. They are composed largely of lipid-laden macrophages.
■ Statin drugs are frequently used to treat this condition. What is the mechanism of action of these drugs?	Statins inhibit 3-hydroxy-3-methylglutaryl coenzyme A (HMG CoA) reductase, a hepatic enzyme that catalyzes the rate-determining step in cholesterol synthesis. They reduce the amount of endogenous cholesterol synthesized by the liver.

GENERAL PRINCIPLES

BIOCHEMISTRY

► **Case 5**

A 2-day-old boy is brought to the emergency department by his mother because of frequent vomiting. He was delivered at home by a midwife. His mother is 40 years old, and received no prenatal care. The mother reports that since birth the boy has been unable to keep food down, vomiting greenish material soon after eating. He has also become lethargic and progressively less responsive. On examination the boy is found to have several abnormalities, including prominent epicanthal folds, upslanting palpebral fissures, and macroglossia. He also has thick skin at the nape of his neck.

■ **What is the likely diagnosis and cause of the vomiting?**

This child most likely has Down syndrome, which can be associated with gastrointestinal disorders such as duodenal atresia or stenosis, annular pancreas, tracheoesophageal defects, and anal atresia. Duodenal atresia below the sphincter of Oddi would give rise to bilious vomiting as seen in this patient.

■ **What is the most common cytogenetic abnormality in patients with this condition?**

Individuals with Down syndrome most commonly have trisomy 21, which results from nondisjunction of chromosome 21 during meiotic anaphase 1 or anaphase 2. The risk of nondisjunction increases with maternal age.

■ **What other medical abnormalities are seen in children with this condition?**

A number of abnormalities are seen in children with Down syndrome, including a single palmar crease; small, folded ears; a short neck; Brushfield spots (pale yellow spots on the iris); and a gap between the first and second toes. These children also suffer from heart disease, most often cardiac cushion malformations (see Figure 2-4), and may have ophthalmologic problems, gastrointestinal tract malformations, poor hearing, and mental retardation. Males with Down syndrome are almost always infertile. Individuals with Down syndrome have a shorter life expectancy than the general population.

■ **What screening is available in utero for this condition?**

Reduced levels of α-fetoprotein and elevated levels of β-human chorionic gonadotropin (β-hCG) in the maternal blood are both markers of Down syndrome. Ultrasound measurements of nuchal lucency are also used. A definitive diagnosis can be made via karyotype analysis of fetal cells obtained via amniocentesis. The only cases that may not be detectable by karyotyping are the 1% caused by fetal mosaicism.

■ **What is the risk that this couple will have a second child with this condition?**

Because 95% of cases of Down syndrome are due to spontaneous nondisjunction during meiosis, the child's parents would have a very low probability of having another child with Down syndrome. However, 5% of cases are inherited and caused by a Robertsonian translocation between chromosomes 14 and 21. The parent carrying the translocation may display mild symptoms. Karyotype analysis of the parents can establish whether there is a translocation. In such cases the theoretical risk of conceiving an embryo with the affected chromosome is 1 in 3, but the incidence of live birth of affected babies is actually lower (15%).

- **Later on in life, what disorders is this baby at risk of developing?**

Older individuals with trisomy 21 have a very high risk of developing early Alzheimer's disease. This may be related to the fact that the amyloid-β (Aβ) protein implicated in Alzheimer's disease is encoded on chromosome 21. They are also at increased risk of hematologic disorders, particularly acute leukemias, most commonly acute lymphoblastic leukemia.

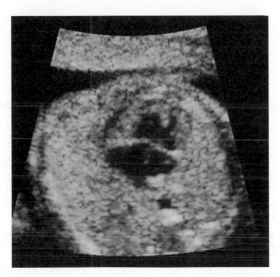

FIGURE 2-4. Ultrasound image of a fetal heart with large atrial septal defect and ventricular septal defect as indicated by the missing "cross" or crux of the heart, also known as an endocardial cushion defect. This anomaly is commonly associated with Down syndrome. (Courtesy of Wesley Lee, MD.)

► **Case 6**

A 5-year-old boy is brought to his pediatrician because of frequent bruising. His mother explains that he develops bruises after even minor trauma (see Figure 2-5). Other than one episode of shoulder dislocation, his medical history is unremarkable. On examination the child has many bruises at different stages of healing. He also has hyperextensible joints.

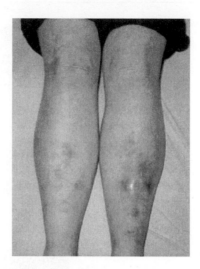

FIGURE 2-5. Bruising on the lower extremities. Poor wound healing gives rise to "cigarette paper" scars. (Reproduced, with permission, from Lichtman MA, Shafer MS, Felgar RE, Wang N. *Lichtman's Atlas of Hematology.* New York: McGraw-Hill, 2007: Figure XI.A.38.)

■ In a child who presents with many bruises, what study should be done to determine whether the bruising may be the result of child abuse?	A whole-body bone x-ray study should be performed to assess for multiple fractures or fractures in unusual locations. Children who are victims of child abuse may show multiple fractures at different stages of healing. This can also be observed in osteogenesis imperfecta.
■ What hereditary disorders can give rise to joint hypermobility?	Marfan's syndrome and Ehlers-Danlos syndrome are two hereditary connective tissue disorders that can cause joint hypermobility.
■ What is the most likely diagnosis?	Ehlers-Danlos syndrome is most likely. While Marfan's syndrome can cause joint hypermobility, it is unlikely to cause easy bruising.
■ What is the etiology of the easy bruising in this child?	Ehlers-Danlos syndrome is caused by different mutations that affect the formation of type III collagen. Most forms of the disorder are inherited as autosomal dominant mutations. The defect may prevent proper synthesis or posttranslational modification of collagen.
■ What other abnormalities may be present in individuals with this condition?	Other clinical manifestations include thin, fragile skin; abnormal scar formation; aortic aneurysms; rupture of large arteries; and rupture of the bowel and uterus (pregnancy increases the risk of uterine rupture).

- **Describe the stages of collagen synthesis.**

- Protein translation on ribosomes in the rough endoplasmic reticulum (RER).
- Hydroxylation of proline and lysine residues in the ER. This step requires vitamin C.
- Glycosylation of lysine residues to form α chains. Three α chains form a triple helix of procollagen in the Golgi apparatus.
- The procollagen is secreted by exocytosis.
- Extracellular enzymes cleave the terminal regions of the procollagen to form tropocollagen.
- Many tropocollagen units line up in a staggered arrangement and cross-link to form the final collagen fibrils.

- **Where are the four major types of collagen found in the body?**

- Type I is found in bone, skin, tendons, fascia, dentin, and the cornea.
- Type II is in cartilage, nucleus pulposus, and the vitreous body.
- Type III is reticular collagen, found in skin, blood vessels, the uterus, granulation tissue, and fetal tissue.
- Type IV collagen is found in basement membranes.

GENERAL PRINCIPLES

BIOCHEMISTRY

► **Case 7**

A 6-year-old boy is followed by his pediatrician for delayed language acquisition and behavioral problems at school. His mother reports a normal pregnancy with adequate prenatal care and adds that she did not use drugs or alcohol during the pregnancy. Genetic analysis reveals a normal 46,XY karyotype but an abnormal-appearing X chromosome. Polymerase chain reaction (PCR) analysis reveals an abnormal region on the X chromosome with 200 CGG trinucleotide repeats.

■ **What is the most likely diagnosis?**

This boy has fragile X syndrome. This disease occurs in individuals who have an expansion of a CGG trinucleotide repeat sequence on the X chromosome. This expansion results in hypermethylation of DNA in the 5′ region of the *FMR1* gene, which silences the gene by inhibiting its transcription. The FMR1 protein is an RNA-binding protein.

■ **What is PCR?**

Polymerase chain reaction is a laboratory method used to amplify DNA in order to facilitate detection. First, the patient's DNA is denatured by heat, causing strand separation. During cooling, primers specific for the target gene (in this case the *FMR1* gene) anneal to the patient's DNA. These primers are subsequently elongated using a heat-stable DNA polymerase. The number of copies of the gene is thus doubled. Repeated cycles of heating, annealing, and elongation in a thermocycler produce an exponential increase in copies of the target gene, thereby generating enough DNA so that the region of interest can be reliably sequenced.

■ **What is the inheritance pattern of this condition?**

Fragile X syndrome is an X-linked genetic disorder. It is the most common inherited cause of mental retardation. The hallmark of X-linked disorders is the absence of father-to-son disease transmission. These disorders are much more common in males than in females. However, mild symptoms of fragile X syndrome are apparent in a significant minority of female carriers. Fragile X syndrome is not fully penetrant, and many families show a maternal transmission pattern.

■ **What physical abnormalities are associated with this condition?**

Individuals with fragile X syndrome frequently have long, narrow faces, with a large jaw and ears, and a prominent forehead. Most postpubertal males also have macroorchidism.

■ **What are other trinucleotide repeat disorders, and why are they associated with "permutations"?**

Other disorders attributable to trinucleotide repeat expansion include: Huntington's disease (CAG expansion on chromosome 4), myotonic dystrophy, and Friedreich's ataxia. Typically, higher numbers of trinucleotide repeats result in more severe and earlier onset of the phenotypic expression of disease. Patients with an intermediate number of repeats are said to have a **permutation** because, while they themselves are clinically normal, their children are at risk of having an increased number of repeats, and therefore an increased risk of expressing clinical disease. This feature of worsening disease through generations is termed **anticipation**.

■ **What are the major preventable causes of mental retardation?**

In utero infections, maternal drug or alcohol use, and nutritional deficiencies are preventable causes of mental retardation in the fetus.

A 5-month-old girl is brought to the pediatrician by her parents because she has been very sleepy lately and has been vomiting and sweating profusely at night. The infant's mother remarks that their daughter was doing fine during the first months of life, but began showing these changes shortly after she began weaning from breast milk. Laboratory testing reveals a serum glucose level of 30 mg/dL, and urinalysis is positive for reducing sugar but negative for glucose.

▪ What is the most likely diagnosis?	Fructose intolerance.
▪ What intermediate is elevated within the liver cells in this condition?	Fructose-1-phosphate is elevated in fructose intolerance.
▪ What enzyme is deficient in this condition?	Aldolase B is deficient in this disorder.
▪ How does this condition cause hypoglycemia?	Aldolase B catalyzes the conversion of fructose-1-phosphate into glyceraldehyde and dihydroxyacetone phosphate (DHAP) (see Figure 2-6). Its absence results in accumulation of fructose-1-phosphate in liver cells and a consequent depletion of adenosine triphosphate (ATP). A low cellular supply of ATP inhibits glycogenolysis and gluconeogenesis, and therefore leads to very low serum glucose. Excess fructose is lost in the urine.
▪ What is the most appropriate treatment for this condition?	The condition is treated through the removal of fructose, sucrose (a disaccharide of glucose and fructose), and sorbitol from the diet.
▪ Why did the infant exhibit no symptoms while exclusively fed breast milk?	Carbohydrates in breast milk are largely from lactose rather than fructose.

FRUCTOSE METABOLISM (LIVER)

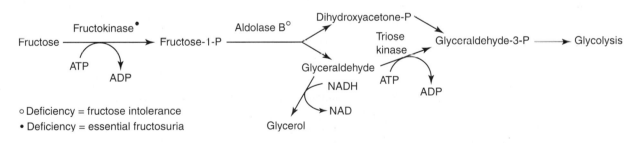

FIGURE 2-6. **Aldolase B splitting fructose-1-phosphate into glyceraldehyde and DAP.** (Reproduced, with permission, from Le T, Bhushan V, Rao DA. *First Aid for the USMLE Step 1: 2008.* New York: McGraw-Hill, 2008: 99.)

▶ **Case 9**

A 12-year-old mentally retarded boy is brought into a health clinic in Peru. His parents have noted that he seems to have difficulty with his vision. Physical examination reveals bilateral dislocated lenses and a marfanoid body habitus. Laboratory studies show increased levels of serum methionine and serum homocysteine.

▪ What is the most likely diagnosis?	Homocystinuria.
▪ What is the biochemical defect in this condition?	The most common form of inherited homocystinuria results from reduced activity of **cystathionine synthase**, an enzyme that converts homocysteine to cystathionine (see Figure 2-7).
▪ What vitamin supplementation would be appropriate in this condition?	**Vitamin B$_6$** (pyridoxine) is a necessary cofactor with cystathionine synthase. Vitamin B$_6$ supplementation has been successful in many patients with this enzyme deficiency.
▪ In addition to vitamin supplementation, what other dietary changes should be made?	The absence of cystathionine synthase means that cysteine cannot be formed from methionine. Therefore, cysteine becomes an essential amino acid. This child should be given a diet low in methionine and high in cysteine.
▪ This boy has a marfanoid body habitus, and lens subluxation, two characteristics of this condition. For which other conditions is this patient at greatly increased risk?	This child is at increased risk for **cardiovascular disease** Elevated plasma homocysteine leads to an increased risk of coronary artery disease, stroke, and peripheral artery disease. He is also at risk for **osteoporosis.** Homocysteine inhibits collagen cross-linking and over time can cause osteoporosis.
▪ What enzyme deficiency is most likely to be found in a patient with increased serum homocysteine but decreased serum methionine?	This could be caused by a deficiency of methionine synthase. This enzyme catalyzes the conversion of homocysteine to methionine. Like patients with cystathionine synthase deficiency, these patients often have central nervous system dysfunction and vascular disease.

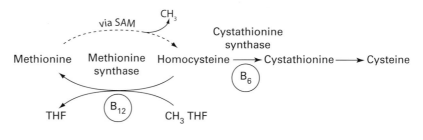
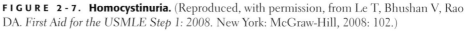

FIGURE 2-7. Homocystinuria. (Reproduced, with permission, from Le T, Bhushan V, Rao DA. *First Aid for the USMLE Step 1: 2008.* New York: McGraw-Hill, 2008: 102.)

► Case 10

A 1-year-old boy is brought to the pediatrician because his parents have recently noted a number of abnormalities. Although the child was normal at birth, he does not interact with others as his older sister did at the same age. His parents also note that he has coarse facial features. Physical examination reveals skeletal abnormalities and an umbilical hernia. Funduscopic examination shows corneal clouding. Additionally, the baby's liver and spleen are enlarged, and his joints are stiff.

■ What is the most likely diagnosis?	Hurler's syndrome.
■ What is the pathophysiology of this condition?	This syndrome results from a defect in α-L-iduronidase, an enzyme essential to the degradation of dermatan sulfate and heparan sulfate. This disease is one of the **mucopolysaccharidoses**, a group of hereditary disorders characterized by defects in glycosaminoglycan (GAG) metabolism. In Hurler's syndrome, the GAGs are not appropriately degraded in the lysosomes and are therefore deposited in various tissues. The disease is inherited in an autosomal recessive manner.
■ What disease has a similar presentation, but is typically milder?	**Hunter's syndrome** is another mucopolysaccharidosis. It is due to a deficiency of iduronate sulfatase and has X-linked inheritance. Unlike Hurler's syndrome, Hunter's syndrome does not present with corneal clouding, but affected patients may exhibit aggressive behavior.
■ What are the typical findings on electron microscopy?	The lysosomal vesicles appear swollen. This is due to accumulation of partially degraded polysaccharides.
■ What key modification must be made in the Golgi apparatus in order for lysosomal enzymes such as α-L-iduronidase to be properly targeted to lysosomes?	Lysosomal enzymes must be covalently modified with mannose-6-phosphate (M6P) as they pass through the *cis* Golgi network in order to be targeted to the lysosomes. These M6P groups are then recognized by M6P receptor proteins in the *trans* Golgi network.

▶ **Case 11**

A 2-year-old boy with a history of mental retardation and restricted joint movement is brought to his primary care physician for a routine checkup. He is the full-term product of an uncomplicated pregnancy. A careful family history reveals that his parents are first cousins. On examination he has coarse facial features and clouded corneas. Blood tests revealed elevated lysosomal enzymes in the serum.

■ What is the significance of the consanguinity between the child's parents?	In consanguineous relationships there is an increased risk of a child's inheriting the same genetic mutation from both of his parents. There is therefore a higher incidence of autosomal recessive disorders in this population.
■ What is the most likely diagnosis?	This patient is suffering from I-cell disease, which is characterized by coarse facial features, poor tone, kyphosis, and mental retardation. Death usually occurs in infancy or early childhood.
■ What is the fundamental molecular defect in this condition?	In I-cell disease there is a mutation in the enzyme found in the Golgi apparatus that is responsible for adding a mannose-6-phosphate group to proteins destined for lysosomes. Instead of trafficking to lysosomes, these lysosomal enzymes are secreted from the cell, and high levels are found in the blood. Because the lysosomes lack the normal hydrolytic enzymes, material accumulates in the lysosomes and is not effectively broken down.
■ What abnormalities would be evident by electron microscopy of cells in an affected patient?	This patient's cells would contain many vacuoles. These consist of lysosomes filled with material that could not be degraded.
■ What proteins direct movement of vesicles between the endoplasmic reticulum (ER) and Golgi apparatus?	The Golgi apparatus is responsible for modifying many different proteins and directing their trafficking. COP I proteins mediate retrograde movement of vesicles from the Golgi apparatus to the ER, while COP II proteins mediate anterograde transport from the ER to the Golgi apparatus.

► **Case 12**

A 35-year-old man visits a fertility specialist along with his 27-year-old wife. They have been trying to conceive for over 13 months but have been unsuccessful. The husband has no previous children but the wife has two children from a prior marriage. Their past medical history is largely unremarkable except for repeated sinus infections and a chronic cough in the husband.

■ **What is the most likely diagnosis?**	The fact that the wife has had prior children suggests that the cause of infertility may lie in the male. Given the history, Kartagener's syndrome is most likely. This is a genetic disorder with an autosomal recessive inheritance pattern.
■ **What is the cause of their infertility?**	In men with Kartagener's syndrome there is an abnormality in dynein function. Dynein is an ATPase that acts as a molecular motor. Dynein is responsible for retrograde transport of material along microtubules. In addition, it is required for movement of cilia and flagella. If this enzyme is not functional, it results in immotile sperm.
■ **What is the cause of the husband's recurrent sinus infections?**	The cilia of the respiratory epithelium require functional dynein for motility. Therefore, they are unable to transport bacteria and particles out of the respiratory tract. The retained particles and bacteria can lead to infections as well as a chronic cough with sputum production.
■ **What abnormality might be observed on x-ray of the chest?**	Situs inversus can also be seen in individuals with Kartagener's syndrome. On an x-ray of the chest, the heart would be found predominantly on the right side of the thorax. In addition, he may have evidence of bronchiectasis on the x-ray, with signs of dilated bronchioles.
■ **What condition is caused by a mutation in microtubule polymerization?**	Chédiak-Higashi syndrome is an autosomal recessive disorder caused by a defect in microtubule polymerization. It results in impaired migration of immune cells such as neutrophils, and impaired lysosome fusion, which results in large granules visible within the cytoplasm (see Figure 2-8). These both contribute to immune deficiency. Patients present with recurrent bacterial infections with staphylococci and streptococci. They also frequently have partial albinism and neuropathies.
■ **There are a number of antimicrobial drugs that inhibit microtubule function. What are some examples?**	Mebendazole and related drugs inhibit microtubule activity in helminths. Griseofulvin is an antifungal that acts on microtubules. A number of chemotherapeutic agents also interfere with microtubule function, such as vincristine, vinblastine, and taxols such as paclitaxel.

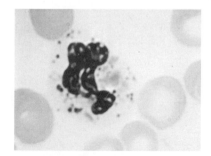

FIGURE 2-8. A neutrophil with large granules. (Reproduced, with permission, from Lichtman MA, Beutler E, Kipps TJ, Seligsohn U, Kaushansky K, Prchal JT. *Williams Hematology*, 7th ed. New York: McGraw-Hill, 2006: Fig. 66-5.)

A 2-year-old boy is brought to the pediatrician by his mother, who is visibly upset. The mother reports that her son has recently been biting his fingers and scratching his face incessantly. She says he was normal for the first few months of his life, but has become increasingly irritable since about 3 months of age. The mother also mentions that her son often has "orange-colored sand" in his diapers. Laboratory studies reveal a serum uric acid level of 55 mg/dL. Urinalysis reveals crystalluria and microscopic hematuria.

▪ What is the most likely diagnosis?	Lesch-Nyhan syndrome.
▪ What is the biochemical defect in this condition?	Lesch-Nyhan syndrome is characterized by a deficiency in hypoxanthine-guanine phosphoribosyltransferase (HGPRT).
▪ What is the function of the deficient enzyme?	HGPRT plays a key role in the purine salvage pathway (see Figure 2-9), recycling hypoxanthine and guanine to the purine nucleotide pool. In the absence of this enzyme, these purine bases are degraded into uric acid, thus causing hyperuricemia. Uric acid crystals in the urine give rise to the crystalluria.
▪ What is the most appropriate treatment for this condition?	Allopurinol is a drug that inhibits xanthine oxidase, thus preventing the formation of uric acid from the more soluble hypoxanthine and xanthine. Hypoxanthine and xanthine can more easily be excreted in the urine. Doses should be titrated to normalize serum uric acid levels.
▪ What other conditions can be expected if this disease is not treated?	Kidney stones, renal failure, gouty arthritis, and subcutaneous tophus deposits will result if the disorder is left untreated.

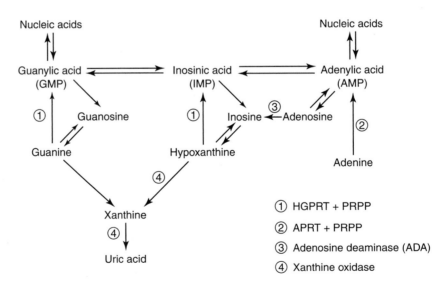

① HGPRT + PRPP
② APRT + PRPP
③ Adenosine deaminase (ADA)
④ Xanthine oxidase

FIGURE 2-9. Purine salvage pathway. (Reproduced, with permission, from Le T, Bhushan V, Rao DA. *First Aid for the USMLE Step 1: 2008.* New York: McGraw-Hill, 2008: 103.)

A 19-year-old college student comes to the university health clinic complaining of muscle aches. She recently began an exercise program in an attempt to lose the 6–8 kg (13–17 lb) that she had gained over the past year. After her first day of weightlifting, however, she became extremely sore. Several hours later, her urine was the color of "cherry soda pop." Physical examination is unremarkable. Laboratory tests reveal a serum creatine kinase level of 93970 IU/L. Urinalysis is negative for blood and positive for myoglobin.

■ What is the most likely diagnosis?	McArdle's disease (type V glycogen storage disease).
■ What is the biochemical defect in this condition?	McArdle's disease is caused by a deficiency of muscle glycogen phosphorylase. Although glycogen formation is not affected, glycogen cannot be broken back down to glucose (glycogenolysis) because the α-1,4-glycosidic bonds cannot be broken in the muscle to release glucose-1-phosphate.
■ What are the most likely findings on biopsy of the liver and muscle?	A liver biopsy will be normal, as the defective enzyme is present only in muscle. Muscle biopsy will show accumulation of glycogen.
■ After the patient completes an exercise tolerance test, her lactic acid levels do not increase normally. Why?	Lactic acid is a product of anaerobic glucose metabolism. Failure of lactic acid levels to elevate after exercise is an indication of a defect in the metabolism of glycogen or glucose to lactate. This response can be seen in other disorders of glycogenolysis or glycolysis as well.
■ What accounts for the color of her urine?	Her muscles begin to break down during exercise because of the lack of glucose. This causes myoglobinuria as well as elevated creatine kinase.
■ What is the most appropriate treatment for this condition?	Oral ingestion of sucrose before exercise has been demonstrated to improve exercise tolerance and reduce the risk of myoglobinuria.

GENERAL PRINCIPLES

BIOCHEMISTRY

▶ **Case 15**

A 2-year-old boy is brought to a health clinic in Mexico because of poor development, as well as vomiting, irritability, and a skin rash. The boy's mother also notes that his urine has a strange "mousy" odor. Physical examination reveals the child has an eczema-like rash, is hyperreflexive, and has increased muscle tone. He is surprisingly fair-skinned in comparison to the rest of his family. Laboratory studies reveal a serum phenylalanine level of 28 mg/dL.

■ What is the most likely diagnosis?	Phenylketonuria (PKU).
■ What is the pathophysiology of this condition?	PKU is caused by a defect in the metabolism of **phenylalanine** (see Figure 2-10). Normally, this essential amino acid is converted to tyrosine by phenylalanine hydroxylase. However, when phenylalanine hydroxylase activity is reduced or absent, phenlalanine builds up. This leads to excess phenylketones in the blood, and results in the symptoms seen in this patient. PKU is inherited in an autosomal recessive fashion.
■ What additional physical characteristics are common at presentation?	Other physical findings include failure to thrive, mental retardation, microcephaly, large cheek and upper jaw bones, and widely spaced teeth with poorly developed enamel.
■ What is the cofactor for the defective enzyme in this disease that, when deficient, can also lead to increased levels of phenylalanine in the blood?	A deficiency in tetrahydrobiopterin can also lead to increased blood levels of phenylalanine.
■ What is the most appropriate treatment for this condition?	PKU should be treated with decreased dietary phenylalanine (which is contained in many foods, including artificial sweeteners). In patients with PKU, tyrosine cannot be derived from phenylalanine, so it becomes an essential amino acid. Therefore, the patient should also receive dietary tyrosine supplementation.

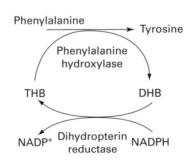

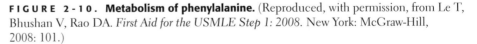

FIGURE 2-10. Metabolism of phenylalanine. (Reproduced, with permission, from Le T, Bhushan V, Rao DA. *First Aid for the USMLE Step 1: 2008.* New York: McGraw-Hill, 2008: 101.)

▶ **Case 16**

A 6-month-old baby girl is brought to the pediatrician because she has been feeding poorly and has been lethargic for the past several months. The baby has also started breathing more rapidly than normal, and recently had a seizure. Laboratory studies reveal a serum pH of 7.20, an anion gap of 19, elevated levels of pyruvate and alanine, and decreased levels of citrate.

■ What is the most likely diagnosis?	Pyruvate dehydrogenase deficiency.
■ What is the pathophysiology of this condition?	Glycolysis is the pathway that converts one molecule of glucose into two molecules of pyruvate. Pyruvate dehydrogenase then converts pyruvate to acetyl-CoA, which can enter the tricarboxylic acid (TCA) cycle. (see Figure 2-11). Without this enzyme, the cells derive much less adenosine triphosphate (ATP) from each molecule of glucose, and rely more heavily on glycolysis alone. As pyruvate accumulates, some of it is converted to lactate in order to regenerate oxidized nicotinamide adenine dinucleotide (NAD^+). The elevated lactate level is responsible for the acidemia and anion gap observed in this baby.
■ Why are alanine levels high and citrate levels low in this condition?	Alanine levels are high because much of the excess pyruvate is converted to alanine in a reversible reaction by alanine aminotransferase. Citrate levels are low because there is little acetyl-CoA to combine with oxaloacetate to form citrate
■ What is the most appropriate treatment for this condition?	Treatment involves increased intake of ketogenic nutrients (foods with high fat content). The breakdown of fatty acids involves reduction of flavin adenine dinucleotide (FAD) and NAD, and produces one molecule of acetyl-CoA for every two carbon atoms in the fatty acid chain. The $FADH_2$ (1-5-dihydro-FAD) and NADH (reduced NADH oxidase) can be used by the electron transport chain to produce ATP, while the acetyl-CoA can enter the TCA cycle. Oral citrate is also helpful for replenishing the substrates of the citric acid cycle.
■ Which are the only purely ketogenic amino acids?	Leucine and lysine are the only purely ketogenic amino acids.

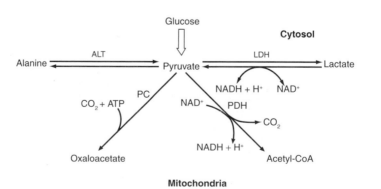

FIGURE 2-11. Pyruvate metabolism. (Reproduced, with permission, from Le T, Bhushan V, Rao DA. *First Aid for the USMLE Step 1: 2008.* New York: McGraw-Hill, 2008: 96.)

▶ **Case 17**

A 5-month-old girl is brought to her pediatrician by her parents, both of whom are Jewish. Although the baby girl was developing normally for the first 4 months of her life, she can no longer roll over by herself. In addition, while she often smiled at 3 months of age, she no longer does so. Funduscopic examination reveals a cherry-red spot on her macula.

▪ What is the most likely diagnosis?	Tay-Sachs disease.
▪ What is the biochemical defect in this condition?	This disease, one of the sphingolipidoses, is caused by a deficiency of **hexosaminidase A**. This enzyme is present within the lysosomes of central nervous system cells and helps degrade a lipid called GM2 ganglioside. GM2 ganglioside accumulation within the neurons leads to progressive neurodegeneration. Children become blind and deaf before paralysis ultimately sets in. Children with Tay-Sachs disease usually die by age 3 years.
▪ How is the gene responsible for this condition inherited?	Tay-Sachs disease is inherited in an autosomal recessive fashion. Fabry's disease is the only one of the sphingolipidoses that is inherited differently; it is X-linked.
▪ What other conditions present with similar findings on physical examination?	**Niemann-Pick disease**, which is caused by a deficiency of sphingomyelinase, also presents with a cherry-red spot in the macula in about 50% of cases. These patients often present with anemia, fever, and neurologic deterioration. The prognosis of Niemann-Pick disease is poor as well, with most patients dying by age 3 years.
▪ Which of the other sphingolipidoses also has a higher prevalence among Ashkenazi Jews?	**Gaucher's disease**, which is caused by a deficiency of β-glucocerebrosidase, also has a much higher incidence in this population.

► **Case 18**

A 36-year-old homeless man presents to a community health clinic complaining of increasing shortness of breath. On questioning, the man admits to an extensive history of alcoholism. A review of systems reveals he has also experienced tingling and burning in his legs for the past several weeks. Physical examination reveals that he is tachycardic (heart rate 122/min), has rales bilaterally, and has bilateral pitting edema. He also has decreased sensation in his feet and is hyporeflexive in his lower extremities. An x-ray of the chest shows an enlarged cardiac silhouette and bilateral pulmonary congestion.

■ What is the most likely diagnosis?	Vitamin B$_1$ (thiamine) deficiency.
■ What clinical manifestations are commonly present in this condition?	This patient has the symptoms of both wet and dry beriberi. Patients with **wet beriberi** present with high-output congestive heart failure and dilated cardiomyopathy. Patients with **dry beriberi** present with peripheral neuropathy consisting of muscular atrophy and diminished sensation and reflexes.
■ The deficient factor in this condition serves as a cofactor for which enzymes?	Thiamine is part of thiamine pyrophosphate (TPP). TPP acts as a cofactor for transketolase (an enzyme in the hexose monophosphate [HMP] shunt) (see Figure 2-12A), pyruvate decarboxylase (a component of the pyruvate dehydrogenase complex), and α-ketoglutarate decarboxylase (a component of the α-ketoglutarate dehydrogenase complex) (see Figure 2-12B).
■ What other pathologies are commonly seen with this vitamin deficiency?	**Wernicke's encephalopathy** is the central nervous system manifestation of thiamine deficiency. This disease classically consists of nystagmus, ophthalmoplegia, and cerebellar ataxia. When the additional symptoms of confusion/psychosis and confabulation are seen, the disease is known as **Wernicke-Korsakoff syndrome**.
■ What are the most likely findings on MRI?	Although degenerative changes are often seen in the cerebellum, brain stem, and diencephalon, atrophy of the mammillary bodies is most commonly noted.

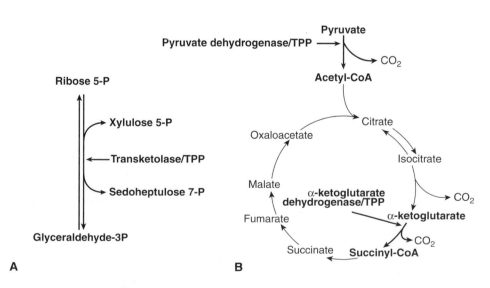

FIGURE 2-12. **(A) Thiamine in the HMP shunt. (B) Thiamine in the TCA cycle.**

▶ **Case 19**

A 6-month-old girl is brought to her pediatrician because of a 5-month history of restlessness, vomiting, and sweating. Her parents brought her in today after she had a seizure. On questioning, the parents note that the infant's symptoms most commonly occur between meals and subside after feeding. On physical examination, the baby is determined to be small for her age with a protuberant abdomen and xanthomas on the buttocks. Ultrasound shows hepatomegaly and bilaterally enlarged kidneys. Relevant laboratory values are serum glucose 20 mg/dL, anion gap 35, and lactic acid 9 mg/dL.

▪ What is the most likely diagnosis?	von Gierke's disease (type I glycogen storage disease).
▪ What is the biochemical defect in this condition?	This is a glycogen storage disease resulting from glucose-6-phosphatase deficiency. While the liver is able to create and break down glycogen, it is unable to release glucose into the blood, because glucose-6-phosphatase (which catalyzes the final step of this process) is deficient (see Figure 2-13). The result is poor glucose control and marked fasting hypoglycemia.
▪ What are the most likely findings on liver biopsy?	Glycogen lipid droplets and significant steatosis are most likely to be found on microscopy.
▪ What complications are commonly associated with this condition?	▪ Gout can develop as a result of hyperuricemia. ▪ Hyperlipidemia—especially hypertriglyceridemia—is also common and can lead to xanthoma formation and pancreatitis. ▪ Platelet dysfunction is common as well and presents as easy bruising and epistaxis. ▪ Over time, patients may develop liver adenomas that occasionally undergo malignant transformation. ▪ Nephropathy often develops from the accumulation of glycogen in the kidney.
▪ What is the most appropriate treatment for this condition?	The most appropriate treatment consists of frequent meals to prevent hypoglycemia. Some patients make cornstarch a central part of their diet because it is absorbed slowly and provides a steady glucose supply. Allopurinol is often used for gout. Liver transplantation is curative.

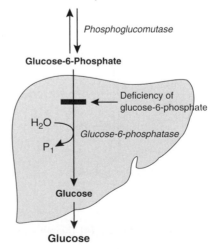

FIGURE 2-13. Glucose-6-phosphatase deficiency.

Microbiology and Immunology

Case 1	45
Case 2	46
Case 3	47
Case 4	48
Case 5	49
Case 6	50
Case 7	51
Case 8	52
Case 9	53
Case 10	54
Case 11	55
Case 12	56
Case 13	57
Case 14	58
Case 15	59
Case 16	60
Case 17	62
Case 18	63
Case 19	64
Case 20	65
Case 21	66
Case 22	68
Case 23	69
Case 24	70
Case 25	72

Case 26   73

Case 27   74

Case 28   76

Case 29   77

Case 30   78

Case 31   80

Case 32   82

Case 33   83

Case 34   84

Case 35   86

Case 36   87

Case 37   88

Case 38   89

Case 39   90

Case 40   91

Case 41   92

Case 42   93

Case 43   94

Case 44   95

Case 45   96

Case 46   97

Case 47   98

Case 48   99

Case 49   100

Case 50   101

Case 51   102

Case 52   103

Case 53   104

Case 54   105

Case 55   107

Case 56   108

Case 57   109

Case 58   111

Case 59   112

Case 60   113

Case 61   114

► **Case 1**

A 20-year-old college student has been pulling all-nighters for his upcoming exams. While trying to study, he often finds himself falling asleep fully dressed with his contacts still in. As finals week draws to a close, he begins to scratch his eyes because they feel dry and painful, as if there are foreign bodies in them. He also notices that his eyes are red and that he tears up frequently.

■ **What is the most likely diagnosis?**	Keratitis caused by the free-living amoeba *Acanthamoeba* is the most likely diagnosis. The differential would include herpes simplex or herpes zoster virus infection, and bacterial or fungal infection.
■ **What are the risk factors for developing this condition?**	In general, 1 in 20 contact lens wearers develop some sort of complication from their lenses annually. The number one risk factor for *Acanthamoeba* infection is **extended wearing of contact lenses**. Inadequate disinfection of the lenses with homemade saline solution, and wearing lenses while swimming and showering can also predispose one to this infection. *Acanthamoeba* organisms can live in soil, air, or water, and are resistant to chlorine.
■ **What are other symptoms and complications of this condition?**	Unlike bacterial keratitis, keratitis from *Acanthamoeba* takes days or weeks to cause symptoms. The initial symptoms are usually redness and a feeling of a foreign body in the eye. There may also be some blurring of vision. Over time, this progresses to pain, lid edema, and conjunctival injection. If untreated, there can be increased intraocular pressure, development of cataracts, and even loss of vision.
■ **How is this condition diagnosed and what is the treatment?**	The diagnosis is made by **slit-lamp examination** of the eye. There will be a thickened epithelium and rough corneal nerves. There is also a characteristic ring on the cornea seen with *Acanthamoeba* infection that appears about 6 weeks into the infection. Corneal scraping or biopsy will reveal irregular polygonal cysts that are also diagnostic. If caught early enough, treatment consists of topical antimicrobials such as miconazole and neomycin. Treatment usually lasts several months. If the infection has gone untreated (i.e., at the corneal ring stage), surgery such as corneal debridement is usually required.
■ **What other populations are at risk for this condition and how does it present in those populations?**	Other populations at risk for this are chronic disease patients, such as those with lymphoproliferative disorders, those on chronic steroids, those receiving chemotherapy, and AIDS patients. In these patients, the infection is usually not of the eye, but rather of the central nervous system. These patients present with changes in mental status, headache, and stiff neck. They can also develop cranial nerve palsies, ataxia, and hemiparesis. This is termed *granulomatous amebic encephalitis* (GAE). Treatment is urgent in such cases.

GENERAL PRINCIPLES

MICROBIOLOGY & IMMUNOLOGY

▶ **Case 2**

A pathologist is sent a poorly labeled sample; it resembles some kind of fluid, but the source is unknown. Gram staining reveals that the microorganism in the fluid is a filamentous, gram-positive rod forming long, branching filaments, resembling fungi.

■ What are the two most likely causative bacterial microorganisms?	*Actinomyces* and *Nocardia* would both fit this description. Although they resemble fungi on Gram stain, they are both actually bacteria, not fungi. They appear as characteristic gram-positive rods with long, branching filaments.
■ How are these two microorganisms differentiated?	When viewed under the microscope, a slide of *Actinomyces israelii* is non–acid-fast and will have "sulfur granules" (as shown on the gross specimen in Figure 3-1). *Nocardia*, on the other hand, is weakly acid-fast. Additionally, while *Actinomyces* is anaerobic, *Nocardia* is an aerobic microorganism.
■ After paging the intern, the pathologist discovers the sample provided was drained from an oral abscess. Now which of these two microorganisms is more likely?	*Actinomyces*, because it is part of the **normal oral flora** and can cause abscesses in the mouth or gastrointestinal tract after trauma. *Nocardia* is most often found in **lung abscesses** and in patients presenting with symptoms resembling pneumonia. It can also cause brain abscesses.
■ If this microorganism were found in a sputum sample that stained weakly acid-fast, what would this indicate about the patient's immune status?	This description fits *Nocardia*, and *Nocardia* is most often found in immunocompromised patients. Note the presentation is clinically similar to that of tuberculosis in this high-risk group, and this is a common misdiagnosis in these patients.
■ What is the most appropriate treatment for each of these microorganisms?	*Nocardia* should be treated with trimethoprim-sulfamethoxazole. *Actinomyces* is best treated with penicillin G.

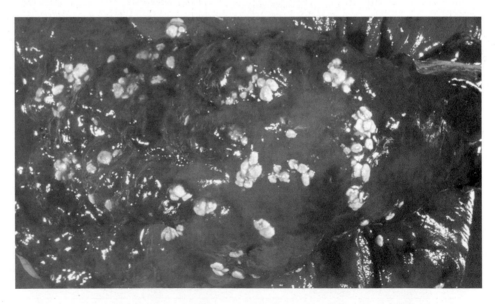

FIGURE 3-1. Gross specimen of *Actinomyces israelii* showing sulfur granules. (Reproduced, with permission, from the Pathology Education Instructional Resource Digital Library [http://peir.net] at the University of Alabama, Birmingham.)

▶ **Case 3**

A local craftsman who makes garments from the hides of goats visits his physician because over the past few days, he has developed several black lesions on his hands and arms (see Figure 3-2). The lesions are not painful, but he was alarmed by their appearance. He is afebrile and his physical examination is unremarkable.

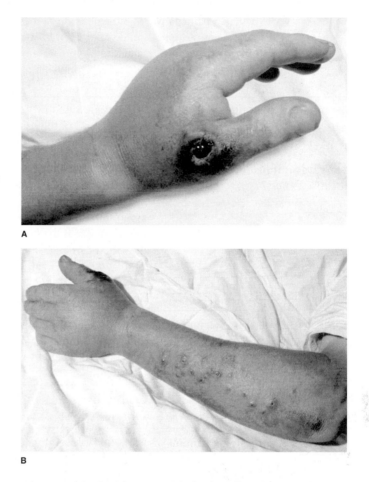

A

B

FIGURE 3-2. (Reproduced, with permission, from Wolff K, Johnson RA, Suurmond D. *Fitzpatrick's Color Atlas & Synopsis of Clinical Dermatology*, 5th ed. New York: McGraw-Hill, 2005: 631.)

▪ **What is the most likely diagnosis?**	Cutaneous anthrax, caused by *Bacillus anthracis*.
▪ **How would the causative microorganism appear on Gram staining?**	*B. anthracis* is a gram-positive rod.
▪ **Describe the capsule of this microorganism.**	*B. anthracis* is the only bacterium with a protein capsule. The capsule is composed of poly-D-glutamic acid.
▪ **What property of this microorganism makes it a feared bioterrorism agent?**	This microorganism forms spores that are resistant to many chemical disinfectants, heat, ultraviolet light, and drying.
▪ **What is the other main manifestation of this infection?**	Lung disease: inhaled anthrax spores reach the alveoli, are taken up by macrophages, and are carried to mediastinal lymph nodes, where they cause hemorrhage (**woolsorter's disease**). This is not a true pneumonia but is due to mediastinal hemorrhage and can also cause a bloody pleural effusion.

► **Case 4**

A 48-year-old woman from Alabama presents with diffuse, colicky abdominal pain in addition to sharp, intermittent, right upper quadrant pain and decreased frequency of bowel movements. She has noticed a weight loss of about 4.5 kg (10 lb) over the past month, without any change in her diet or behavior. She has not experienced fever, nausea, or vomiting. She had a screening colonoscopy 3 months prior to presentation, which was negative. CT of the abdomen reveals an inflamed gallbladder. A complete blood count demonstrates mild anemia and increased eosinophils. Liver function tests are significant for an alkaline phosphatase level of 150 U/L and a total bilirubin level of 4 mg/dL. A stool sample reveals rough-surfaced eggs.

■ What is the most likely diagnosis?	Ascariasis, caused by *Ascaris lumbricoides*, a nematode (roundworm) found in the southern United States as well as tropical climates. It is the most common helminthic infection worldwide.
■ How is this organism transmitted, and how does it cause illness?	Fecal-oral transmission allows the eggs to hatch in the small intestine. Hatched larvae pass through the intestinal wall to enter the bloodstream. They settle in the lungs by entering alveoli and ascending the respiratory tree, causing inflammation and possibly pneumonitis. If the larvae pass from the trachea to the pharynx, they then can enter the gastrointestinal (GI) tract and mature. From the GI tract, adult worms grow in size and length and can then migrate into the bile ducts and pancreas, causing obstruction.
■ What signs and symptoms are associated with this condition?	Infection can be asymptomatic, but it can also cause pneumonia and malnutrition. Complications of infection include intestinal obstruction caused by several worms grouped together and biliary obstruction caused by one worm traveling up the biliary tree.
■ What tests can be used to confirm the diagnosis?	Analysis of a stool sample will show eggs with a knobby, rough surface.
■ What are the most appropriate treatments for this condition?	Mebendazole or albendazole is the primary drug, although pyrantel pamoate may also be used.

► **Case 5**

A 54-year-old man with a history of tobacco use and chronic obstructive pulmonary disease (COPD) presents to the emergency department because of severe shortness of breath. The patient had a COPD exacerbation 3 weeks prior to admission and began taking oral corticosteroids at that time. His symptoms resolved and he had returned to his usual state of health until 1.5 weeks later, when he again began experiencing cough and shortness of breath. He developed hemoptysis 1 week prior to admission. The patient was started on prophylactic antibiotics and underwent bronchoalveolar lavage, which revealed the presence of 45°-branching septate hyphae (see Figure 3-3).

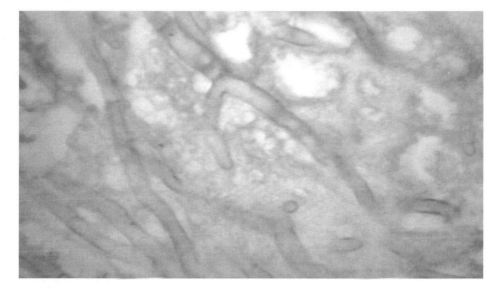

FIGURE 3-3. (Reproduced, with permission, from the Pathology Education Instructional Resource Digital Library [http://pcir.net] at the University of Alabama, Birmingham.)

▪ What is the most likely diagnosis?	This presentation, plus findings on lavage, indicate *Aspergillus* infection. *Candida* should also be considered, but would appear microscopically as pseudohyphae and budding yeasts.
▪ What are the likely findings on x-ray of the chest?	*Aspergillus* can appear as a "fungus ball" within preexisting cavitary lesions in the lungs. This form of *Aspergillus* infection is called an **aspergilloma**.
▪ The patient is treated with amphotericin B. What is the drug's mechanism of action and adverse effects?	Amphotericin B works by binding to ergosterol, a key component specific to fungal membranes, thereby disrupting the integrity of the cell membrane. Its side effects include fever, chills, kidney damage, hypotension, and arrhythmias.
▪ The patient's symptoms improve, and he is discharged several days later. However, he returns to the hospital 3 months later with worsened respiratory function, chest pain, and decreased urine output. Could these symptoms be sequelae of the condition that caused his previous admission?	The patient could be suffering from **invasive aspergillosis**, which is the result of hematogenous spread of his infection to his kidneys, pericardium, and elsewhere, causing these diffuse symptoms.
▪ Why is this patient particularly prone to these complications?	The corticosteroids that the patient takes for his COPD render his immune system less effective at fighting the infection, despite treatment with amphotericin B. Patients with <500 neutrophils/mm^3 (e.g., transplant recipients and patients with leukemia) are especially susceptible to invasive aspergillosis.

► **Case 6**

A patient presents complaining of nausea, vomiting, and blurred vision. He says the symptoms started rather suddenly. He also complains of weakness. On physical examination, he has fixed, dilated pupils and a decreased gag reflex. When asked, he admits that he often eats food that he has canned himself. The patient is admitted to the hospital for further monitoring.

■ What is the most likely diagnosis? What is the pathophysiology?	Botulism, resulting from ingestion of the botulinum toxin made by the bacteria *Clostridium botulinum*. The toxin acts by binding presynaptically and preventing the release of acetylcholine. The binding is irreversible and it takes about 6 months for new synapses to form.
■ What is the typical course seen in patients with this condition?	Usually in patients who ingest the botulinum toxin, symptoms present within 12–36 hours of ingestion of the contaminated food. The first symptoms seen involve gastrointestinal (GI) distress (i.e., cramps and nausea), followed by neurologic symptoms. The first nerves affected are the cranial nerves, with blurred vision, decreased eye movements, and a decreased gag reflex. The paralysis is symmetric and descending. Autonomic nerves can also be affected, resulting in such complications as ileus, urinary retention, and orthostatic hypotension. In addition, respiratory muscles can be affected, which results in the need for ventilator support.
■ What is the differential diagnosis for this presentation?	The differential includes Guillain-Barré, myasthenia gravis, Lambert-Eaton syndrome, tick paralysis, stroke, and poliomyelitis. Notably, the paralysis seen in Guillain-Barré is usually ascending.
■ How can this toxicity be acquired?	Most commonly, exposure to the toxin in adults occurs via ingestion of preformed toxin from contaminated canned foods (usually home canned). In infants, ingestion of bacterial spores can result in toxicity referred to as "**floppy baby syndrome.**" The spores germinate in the GI tract and then express the toxin. Traditionally, these spores are found in honey. The third exposure route is via wound infection. The bacterium itself is anaerobic and can thrive in devitalized tissue and release the toxin. Classically, wounds resulting from a traumatic injury that is contaminated with soil, from intravenous (IV) drug use, or from a contaminated cesarean section are associated with this infection.
■ How is the diagnosis made and what is the treatment?	The diagnosis is made by identifying the toxin. In addition, nerve conduction testing will be normal, but electromyography will show a decreased amplitude of muscle action potentials. The treatment in cases of ingestion is supportive care with airway management. There is also a trivalent antibody to the toxin available that will neutralize free-circulating toxin. In cases of wound infection, the bacteria expressing the toxin must also be killed, so antibiotic therapy is given. The choice is usually high-dose IV penicillins.

► **Case 7**   A patient with diabetes presents to her physician with an adherent white, flaky substance on the skin under her breasts. Another patient, a woman who has just completed a course of oral antibiotics, presents with itching and a copious vaginal discharge that resembles "cottage cheese." A third patient, with acquired immunodeficiency syndrome (AIDS), presents with a white exudate on his oral mucosa and soft palate. The physician diagnoses the same causative microorganism for all three cases.

▪ **What is the most likely diagnosis?**

The fungus *Candida albicans* can result in systemic or superficial fungal infection (candidiasis). Oral thrush, vaginitis (yeast infection), and diaper rash are common manifestations of local candidiasis.

▪ **Where is the microorganism that causes this condition normally found?**

C. albicans is part of the normal flora of mucous membranes of the gastrointestinal tract, respiratory tract, and female genital tract. Overgrowth, especially in warm, moist areas such as the skin under the breasts, causes candidiasis.

▪ **What laboratory tests can help confirm the diagnosis?**

A potassium hydroxide preparation (**KOH mount**) is used for skin or tissue scrapings. **Pseudohyphae** and **budding yeast** (see Figure 3-4) are observed in the tissues. Pseudohyphae are seen in culture at 20°C, and germ tube formation is seen at 37°C. For systemic disease (rare), blood cultures are positive for the fungus.

▪ **What are the most appropriate treatments for this condition?**

Fluconazole or nystatin is used for superficial infections, and amphotericin B or fluconazole can be used for systemic infections.

▪ **What populations are most at risk for this condition?**

Immunocompromised hosts are at highest risk: neonates, patients taking steroids, those with diabetes, and those with AIDS. These patients are also at higher risk for developing more serious forms of candidal infection such as esophagitis and systemic infection. **Intravenous drug users** are at higher risk for candidal endocarditis. Women who have just completed a course of **antibiotics** are at higher risk for vaginitis.

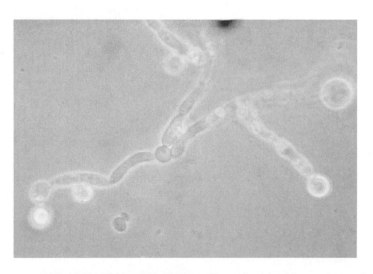

FIGURE 3-4. KOH mount of *Candida albicans*. (Reproduced, with permission, from Wolff K, Johnson RA, Suurmond D. *Fitzpatrick's Color Atlas & Synopsis of Clinical Dermatology*, 5th ed. New York: McGraw-Hill, 2005: 717.)

▶ **Case 8**

A 49-year-old woman who recently immigrated to the United States from Nicaragua presents to the clinic with difficulty swallowing, constipation, and abdominal pain. She says she has gone more than a week without having a bowel movement. Physical examination reveals she is tachycardic and her abdomen is distended. An electrocardiogram shows Mobitz type I heart block.

■ What is the most likely diagnosis?	Chagas' disease, or American trypanosomiasis, caused by the protozoan *Trypanosoma cruzi*.
■ What is the vector of the responsible protozoan?	The reduviid bug, also known as the "kissing bug."
■ Where in the world is this condition found?	Southern United States, Mexico, Central and South America (i.e., only in the Western hemisphere).
■ What is the pathophysiology of this condition?	This woman is experiencing chronic Chagas' disease, most often characterized by heart block, ventricular tachycardia, and dilated cardiomyopathy. Dilatation of the esophagus and colon (toxic megacolon) can cause the presentation outlined above. The acute phase of the disease can be characterized by a hard red area called a **chagoma** at the parasite's site of entry into the host, fever, and meningoencephalitis. In endemic areas, the acute phase is seen more frequently in children.
■ What is the most appropriate treatment for this condition?	Nifurtimox and benznidazole are used to treat acute cases. However, there is no effective treatment for chronic Chagas' disease. For chronic heart disease, supportive measures for congestive heart failure, antiarrhythmics to prevent recurrent ventricular tachycardia, and pacemaker implantation for heart block are used. For gastrointestinal disease, dilation of the esophageal sphincter, changes in diet, the use of laxatives and/or enemas, and in some cases eventual resection of the megacolon are used.

A 24-year-old American man is traveling in rural India during the monsoon season. During the course of a few hours, he develops severe watery diarrhea. Over the course of 30 hours he has approximately one episode per hour of liquid stools that appear clear with little white flecks of mucus. In addition, he has occasional episodes of vomiting. He quickly becomes very lethargic and generally ill and complains of crampy abdominal pain, but is afebrile. He attempts to rehydrate himself during the course of the illness, and the symptoms resolve within approximately 48 hours.

■ **What is the most likely diagnosis?**	This patient has cholera, caused by *Vibrio cholerae*. This microorganism is a gram-negative, curved, motile rod that resembles "shooting stars" on Gram stain. Symptomatic cholera usually manifests in epidemics, and it is endemic to developing countries such as Africa, Asia, South and Latin America, and recently the Middle East.
■ **How does the microorganism exert its effect on the gastrointestinal tract?**	Cholera is ingested through fecally contaminated water. It secretes an exotoxin (cholera toxin) that binds to the surface of intestinal epithelium. This toxin increases cyclic adenosine monophosphate within the intestinal mucosa, which causes increased chloride secretion and decreased sodium absorption. This leads to a massive loss of fluids and electrolytes.
■ **What are the clinical manifestations of this condition?**	The hallmark of cholera is **rice-water stools**, so described because the little white flecks of mucus look like rice. The onset of this diarrhea typically occurs from 1–3 days after infection. Many *V. cholerae* infections are asymptomatic, but severe cholera can lead to extreme dehydration that can result in death within hours. Vomiting and abdominal cramping are common, while fever (cholera is not invasive) and abdominal pain are rare.
■ **What are some of the severe potential consequences of this condition?**	The consequences of cholera result from extreme volume loss as well as the excretion of large amounts of sodium, potassium, chloride, and bicarbonate. The volume depletion can lead to renal failure, and the potassium loss can lead to hypokalemia, which in turn can cause arrhythmias, ileus, and cramps. The bicarbonate loss can lead to a metabolic acidosis. Left untreated, symptomatic cholera leads to death in 50%–70% of cases, and children are 10 times more likely to die than adults.
■ **What is the most appropriate treatment for this condition?**	The mainstay of cholera treatment is administration of **oral rehydration solution** (ORS), which has reduced mortality rates from 50% to <1%. ORS takes advantage of the fact that glucose facilitates sodium absorption from the gut, which allows for the concurrent absorption of water. A typical preparation of ORS contains glucose, potassium chloride, sodium chloride, and sodium bicarbonate. If patients become so ill they cannot drink, **intravenous fluid replacement** can be used. Antibiotics are of limited use in stopping the diarrhea, although early use of doxycycline has been shown to reduce the volume of diarrhea and decrease the duration of bacteria excretion by 1 day.

► **Case 10**

A 3-year-old boy is brought to his pediatrician with a fever, tachypnea, and a cough productive of rusty sputum. He has a history of recurrent lung and skin infections. He has had several fungal infections of his skin, as well as an abscess that formed where he had scraped his arm. An x-ray of the chest shows a normal thymic shadow but some hilar lymphadenopathy. Further questioning of the parents reveals that there is a maternal cousin who died at age 5 years of severe pneumonia, as well as a maternal uncle who has had two surgeries for intracranial fungal infections.

■ What is the most likely diagnosis?	This patient has an immunodeficiency that predisposes him to bacterial and fungal infections. The fact that his thymic shadow is normal suggests his problem is less likely to be caused by severe combined immunodeficiency (SCID) or DiGeorge syndrome. The strong family history on the patient's mother's side suggests the patient has a hereditary condition. The most likely diagnosis is chronic granulomatous disease (CGD), which is most frequently inherited in an X-linked fashion.
■ Infections with which organisms could be particularly severe and problematic in this patient?	Patients with CGD are at risk of serious infections with *Staphylococcus aureus*, *Aspergillus* species, and *Burkholderia cepacia*.
■ A deficiency of which protein is responsible for this disease?	Reduced nicotinamide adenine dinucleotide phosphate (NADPH) oxidase is deficient in patients with CGD. It is required for production of reactive oxygen species. The radicals are used by neutrophils during the oxidative burst to kill engulfed organisms. Many bacterial species make free radicals as by-products of their metabolism. These free radicals contribute to the toxic environment in the neutrophil lysosomes. However, catalase-positive bacteria such as *S. aureus* can neutralize these free radicals, and therefore frequently give rise to serious infections in patients with CGD.
■ What laboratory testing could be done to confirm this diagnosis?	The nitroblue tetrazolium test can be used to detect the presence of a respiratory burst in neutrophils.
■ What medical treatments are available for this condition?	Infections must be treated aggressively with appropriate antimicrobials. Trimethoprim-sulfamethoxazole can be used as long-term prophylaxis. In addition, interferon-α (IFN-α), an immunomodulator, is used in patients with CGD.
■ What therapy or procedure provides a definitive cure for this patient?	A bone marrow transplant provides a source of neutrophils with a functioning myeloperoxidase system.

An 85-year-old man is hospitalized for community-acquired pneumonia. He is treated with penicillin, and over the next week he feels that he is slowly recovering. On hospital day 10, he develops a low-grade fever, watery diarrhea, and lower abdominal pain.

▪ **What is the most likely diagnosis?**	Antibiotic-associated colitis or pseudomembranous colitis caused by ***Clostridium difficile*** superinfection (or overgrowth). *C. difficile* is a gram-positive, spore-forming anaerobe. It should be noted that most antibiotic-associated diarrhea (without fever) is osmotic, resulting from decreased carbohydrate digestion secondary to a loss of gut flora.
▪ **What is the differential diagnosis?**	The differential includes *Klebsiella oxytoca, Staphylococcus aureus*, and postinfectious irritable bowel syndrome.
▪ **What are the different manifestations of this condition?**	About 20% of hospitalized patients are colonized with *Clostridium difficile* and have no symptoms, but can act as carriers. Those with symptoms upon colonization usually present with a low-grade fever, watery diarrhea, lower abdominal pain, leukocytosis, and a recent history (within 10 weeks) of antibiotic use. In more severe cases, there are peritoneal findings (i.e., rebound tenderness). On colonoscopy, these patients would likely have **pseudomembranes** on the colon, which are raised yellowish-white plaques. These patients are also at risk for developing ileus and toxic megacolon, which can perforate and result in death.
▪ **Who is susceptible to this condition and what is the pathogenesis?**	Infection is most often seen in elderly hospitalized patients. *C. difficile* produces resistant spores, which are commonly found on objects in the hospital and the hands of health care workers. Common alcohol-based hand sanitizers are ineffective at eliminating *C. difficile* spores. This bacterium colonizes the gastrointestinal (GI) tract (usually the colon) after the normal gut flora is killed or altered by antibiotics. The antibiotics most commonly associated with this disease are the penicillins, cephalosporins, and clindamycin. Once it has colonized the GI tract, it releases toxins (toxins A and B) that target gut cells. There is a new, more virulent strain of this bacterium that produces a binary toxin. Infection by this strain is associated with the use of fluoroquinolones.
▪ **How is this condition diagnosed and treated?**	Definitive diagnosis can be made with a cytotoxicity assay, an enzyme-linked immunosorbent assay for *C. difficile* toxin A, or polymerase chain reaction. First-line treatment is with oral metronidazole or vancomycin.

► **Case 12**

A 5-year-old girl is brought to the clinic with a 3-month history of worsening vision and behavioral difficulty in school. She emigrated with her mother and a younger sibling 2 years previously from Guatemala. Her mother received no prenatal care and, through a translator, reports that the patient was delivered without complication at home. As an infant, the girl had a "wartlike" maculopapular rash around her mucous membranes, and three or four recurrent right-sided ear infections. Physical examination reveals the girl is in the 30th percentile for weight and 35th percentile for height. Also, the fundi were notable for nummular keratitis, and there was prominent notching of her upper two incisors and molars, as well as outward bowing of the tibia bilaterally.

■ What is the most likely diagnosis?	Congenital syphilis. This infection is one of the so-called **ToRCHeS** infections (**T**oxoplasmosis, **R**ubella, **C**ytomegalovirus, **H**erpes, **S**yphilis), the most common causes of congenital infection.
■ What is the causative microorganism in this condition?	*Treponema pallidum.*
■ What symptoms are commonly found in patients with this condition?	■ Bone abnormalities (osteochondritis and periostitis) ■ Eczematoid skin rash ■ Fissures (lips, nares) and mucous patches ■ Frontal bossing (i.e., a prominent forehead) ■ Hemolytic anemia ■ Hepatosplenomegaly ■ Interstitial keratitis ■ Jaundice ■ Pigmented retinopathy ■ Snuffles (nasal discharge, often bloody) ■ Tooth abnormalities (Hutchinson incisors, mulberry molars)
■ In the newborn, what tests can help confirm the diagnosis?	■ **Serum rapid plasma reagin (RPR) test:** Umbilical cord blood may show false-positive results due to maternal titers. ■ **Radiography of long bones:** Very poor sensitivity, difficult to obtain in the newborn. ■ **Lumbar puncture to attain cerebrospinal fluid samples for Venereal Disease Research Laboratory (VDRL) testing:** Pleocytosis and elevated protein level suggest infection.
■ What tests can be used to detect infection in the patient's mother?	■ Serologic testing ■ VDRL and RPR for screening ■ Positive results on fluorescent treponemal antigen-antibody absorption (FTA-ABS) test
■ What are the most appropriate treatments for this condition?	Benzathine penicillin G for 10–14 days. Because of the signs of tertiary involvement, congenital infection is highly likely; however, a social worker should be involved in case there is a question of sexual abuse as a possible route of transmission. The mother and younger sibling should both receive testing and/or treatment as well. Additionally, long-bone radiographs of the patient should be taken, and MRI can rule out neurologic involvement. A cerebrospinal fluid sample should be obtained for measuring cell counts and protein content and for VDRL testing. Also, the patient's auditory, visual, and dental issues need evaluation.

► **Case 13**   A pathologist is performing an autopsy on a 56-year-old male university professor who suffered a rapid demise from an undiagnosed neurologic disease. Approximately 1 year previously, the patient presented to a psychiatrist with symptoms of psychosis. Shortly thereafter, his symptoms advanced to include unsteadiness and involuntary movements, and the patient ultimately became immobile and unable to speak. A sample of brain tissue shows many vacuoles in the gray matter and a great deal of neuronal loss (see Figure 3-5).

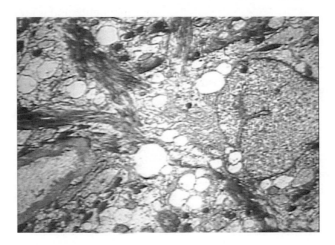

FIGURE 3-5. (Reproduced, with permission, from the Pathology Education Instructional Resource Digital Library [http://peir.net] at the University of Alabama, Birmingham.)

▪ What is the most likely diagnosis?	Creutzfeldt-Jakob disease (CJD) .
▪ How does the causative microorganism in this condition differ from other pathogens?	Prions do not contain RNA or DNA; they are composed only of protein.
▪ How is this condition transmitted?	Disease can be transmitted by central nervous system (CNS) tissue containing prions (transmission has been seen secondary to corneal transplants). Prion disease can also be inherited.
▪ What other condition is associated with this type of pathogen?	Prions cause two degenerative CNS diseases in humans: CJD and **kuru**, a slowly progressive, fatal disease found among tribes in Papua, New Guinea, who practice cannibalism.
▪ How does the structure of normal prions differ from that of pathologic prions?	Normal prions have α-helix conformations, while pathologic prions are composed of an abnormal isoform of β-pleated sheets.
▪ What treatment is most appropriate for this condition?	Unfortunately, there is no known treatment for CJD.
▪ What diseases are caused by so-called "slow viruses"?	**Slow virus** refers to the tempo of disease progression, not the growth rate of the virus. The slow viruses exist in patients for months to years before causing disease. For example, the **measles** virus can cause subacute sclerosing panencephalitis, which is a progressive demyelinating CNS disease most often seen in young people, who present with seizure, ataxia, and focal neurological symptoms. Reactivation of the **JC virus**, which causes disease in immunocompromised hosts, can cause progressive multifocal leukoencephalopathy. This is the result of progressive demyelination of oligodendrocytes.

► **Case 14**

A 32-year-old man with acquired immunodeficiency syndrome (AIDS) presents to the emergency department with complaints of worsening headache, fever, and a stiff neck. Lumbar puncture is performed, and analysis reveals an elevated opening pressure, increased protein level, and decreased glucose level. Special staining of the spinal fluid reveals budding yeast.

▪ What is the most likely diagnosis?	Cryptococcal meningitis is the most common fungal cause of meningitis and is prevalent among patients with AIDS.
▪ What microorganism causes this disease, and what is its morphology?	*Cryptococcus neoformans* is a heavily encapsulated yeast. It is found only as a yeast; it is not a dimorphic microorganism.
▪ How is the microorganism transmitted, and how does it cause illness?	*C. neoformans* is found in pigeon droppings, and is also found in soil. When inhaled, the yeast causes local infection in the lung that can be asymptomatic or result in pneumonia. Hematogenous spread to the central nervous system can result in meningitis and brain abscesses.
▪ What laboratory tests can help confirm the diagnosis?	**India ink** will stain the heavy polysaccharide capsule and reveal budding yeast (see Figure 3-6). **Serology** is most commonly used: latex agglutination detects polysaccharide capsular antigen. The microorganism can also be cultured on **Sabouraud's agar**.
▪ What is the most appropriate treatment for this condition?	Patients who are not immunocompromised can be treated sufficiently with amphotericin B and flucytosine for the meningitis. Patients with AIDS require lifetime suppression with fluconazole after induction with amphotericin B and flucytosine, without which the illness will relapse.

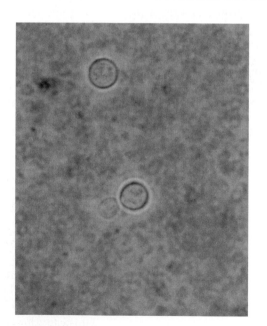

FIGURE 3-6. *Cryptococcus neoformans.*

A 42-year-old woman who works in a pork processing plant presents to her physician with new-onset seizures and bilateral lower extremity weakness. CT of the head reveals several calcified regions, but no mass lesion or evidence of bleeding. A complete blood count reveals mild anemia and a white blood cell (WBC) count of 78,000/mm^3, with 12% eosinophils.

■ What is the most likely diagnosis?	Cysticercosis, caused by *Taenia solium* (pork tapeworm), which is a cestode (tapeworm).
■ How is this organism transmitted, and how does it cause illness?	Ingestion of undercooked pork allows for introduction of larvae from pig muscle into the human gastrointestinal (GI) system. These larvae mature in the small intestine. Eggs from the adult worms are released into the feces. Ingestion of these eggs via the fecal-oral route allows eggs to enter the GI tract, where they develop into larvae. The larvae then penetrate the intestinal wall and migrate into the blood and tissues. Because humans are not a natural host for this stage of the organism, the larvae encyst into whichever organs they end up in (i.e., the brain, potentially causing seizures). When this happens, it is termed cysticercosis.
■ What signs and symptoms are associated with this condition?	Infection can be asymptomatic, or cause malnutrition and abdominal discomfort. Cysticercosis can be found anywhere in the body, including the brain and eye, leading to seizures, focal neurological symptoms, and blindness.
■ What tests can help confirm the diagnosis?	Intestinal infection is revealed by eggs in stool. Calcified cysticerci can be observed on CT when cysticercosis occurs in the brain (see arrow in Figure 3-7). X-ray films may reveal calcified cysticerci in other parts of the body, such as muscle.
■ What are the most appropriate treatments for this condition?	Praziquantel or albendazole is used for cysticercosis. In addition, steroids and anticonvulsants may be given for neurocysticercosis. Asymptomatic patients are rarely treated.

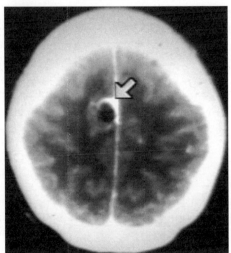

FIGURE 3-7. Cysticercosis. (Reproduced, with permission, from the Pathology Education Instructional Resource Digital Library [http://peir.net] at the University of Alabama, Birmingham.)

▶ **Case 16**

A 12-year-old girl presents to clinic with a sore throat and fever. She says she feels very tired. On physical examination, there is notable cervical lymphadenopathy, but the spleen is not palpable. A heterophile agglutinin test is negative. On histology, the image shown in Figure 3-8 is seen.

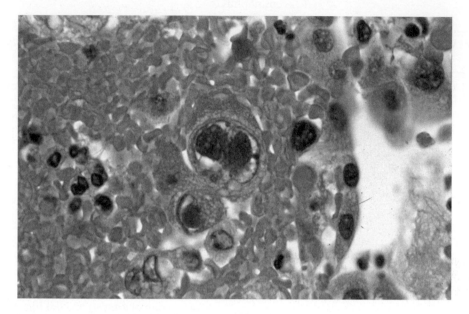

FIGURE 3-8. (Reproduced, with permission, from Pathology Education Instructional Resource Digital Library [http://peir.net] at the University of Alabama, Birmingham.)

■ **What is the most likely diagnosis and what are the characteristics of this pathogen?**	Infectious mononucleosis syndrome resulting from cytomegalovirus (CMV) infection. CMV is a double-stranded linear virus in the family Herpesviridae. Infected cells have intranuclear inclusions, and on histology have an "**owl's-eye**" appearance, as indicated by the arrow in Figure 3-8.
■ **How does this infection usually present and how is it transmitted?**	In the majority of people, CMV infection is asymptomatic. In those with symptoms, it usually presents with a mononucleosis syndrome, which includes pharyngitis, cervical lymphadenopathy, fever, lethargy, and sometimes splenomegaly. Unlike the mononucleosis syndrome seen with Epstein-Barr virus, the **heterophile agglutinin test** (monospot test) would be negative. CMV can be transmitted by direct contact, blood transfusions, organ transplantation, breast milk, sexual contact, and vertically (i.e., mother to fetus). It is one of the **TORCH** infections (Toxoplasmosis, Other infections, Rubella, Cytomegalovirus infection, and Herpes simplex).
■ **What populations are at risk for complications of this infection and how do they present?**	The populations most at risk are those with decreased cellular immunity, such as patients with AIDS and organ transplants (especially bone marrow and lung transplant patients). The main complication in the transplant population is CMV pneumonia. The main complication in the AIDS population is CMV retinitis, which usually presents when the CD4$^+$ count goes below 50 cells/mm^3. In both populations, prophylactic ganciclovir can be given.

- **How does this condition present in those infected congenitally?**

In those congenitally infected with CMV, the complications include petechiae, jaundice, microcephaly, being small for gestational age, retinitis, neurologic abnormalities, and deafness. The fetuses at risk are those whose mothers have a primary infection, which would be seen in a mother with high IgM levels (the IgG levels could be low or high). Mothers with low IgM levels and high IgG levels likely have a secondary infection, and are more likely to be able to prevent the virus from being transmitted to their fetus.

- **What is the treatment for this condition?**

Though most patients will not need treatment, the treatment is ganciclovir, a nucleoside analog. This drug acts when viral kinase phosphorylates the drug and allows it to inhibit CMV DNA polymerase. Acyclovir is not effective against CMV.

► **Case 17**

A woman who has recently returned from a city in Southeast Asia presents to her physician with sudden-onset fever and pain that occurs when she moves her eyes. She also complains of severe muscle pain in her back and extremities as well as recent joint pain in her knees. Examination reveals an erythematous rash that covers her face and body along with generalized lymphadenopathy.

▪ **What is the most likely diagnosis?**	This woman is likely experiencing "breakbone fever," also known as dengue fever.
▪ **What is the vector for this disease?**	The vector is the *Aedes aegypti* mosquito. These mosquitos are diurnal and live near cities. They are most commonly found in pools of stagnant water, such as those in old tires. This distinguishes them from malaria-carrying *Anopheles* mosquitoes, which are nocturnal and are less populous near urban areas. Once a rare disease in the United States, dengue fever began to reappear in the 1970s, when bans on pesticides such as DDT allowed these mosquitoes to once again thrive. The same vector can also carry yellow fever and chikungunya.
▪ **Which microorganism causes this infection?**	Dengue fever is caused by the positive, single-stranded RNA dengue fever virus of the Flavivirus family. This family also includes St. Louis encephalitis virus, Japanese encephalitis virus, hepatitis C virus, and West Nile virus.
▪ **After recovering from her infection, will the patient be immune to this condition in the future?**	The dengue fever virus has four different serotypes. Thus, the patient will develop lasting immunity to the serotype of the virus with which she was infected, but she will not be immune to the remaining three serotypes. This means that she could contract dengue fever four times in all.
▪ **Reinfection with a different serotype poses what potential complications?**	The most serious complications of dengue fever are dengue hemorrhagic fever (DHF) and dengue shock syndrome (DSS), both of which can be fatal. These conditions are characterized by bleeding (often from the gastrointestinal tract or from mucosa); petechiae, ecchymoses, or purpura; thrombocytopenia; fluid leakage (manifested as pleural effusions, ascites, or hemoconcentration); and shock. Such complications most frequently occur in patients who have already been infected with a different serotype of the virus. One theory underlying this phenomenon, termed **antibody-dependent enhancement**, proposes that antibodies from previous infections actually allow for increased viral replication upon reinfection with a different serotype. The fact that reinfection with different serotypes can result in complications such as DHF has hindered the development of a vaccine, since the vaccine must provide adequate protection against all four serotypes or it could put the patient at risk for DHF/DSS.

► **Case 18**

A 7-year-old girl is brought to her primary care physician because of a sore throat and fever of 38.3°C (101°F). Physical examination reveals a grayish membrane covering her pharynx, as well as cervical lymphadenopathy. The child was born in Africa and did not receive all of her childhood vaccinations.

▪ What is the most likely diagnosis?	The child most likely has diphtheria caused by *Corynebacterium diphtheriae*.
▪ How does this microorganism cause this presentation?	Exotoxin A is an enzyme that blocks protein synthesis by inactivating elongation factor EF-2 by ribosylating adenosine phosphate. This results in decreased mRNA translation and protein synthesis. Note that *Pseudomonas* toxin has a similar mechanism.
▪ What growth media are used to identify this microorganism, and how does it appear on culture?	Potassium tellurite agar and Loeffler's coagulated blood serum media are the media to use for isolating this microorganism. *C. diphtheriae* is a gram-positive rod. In culture, it often appears in clumps described as "**Chinese characters.**"
▪ Which vaccine would have prevented this child's illness?	The inactivated form, or toxoid, is a component of the DPT vaccine (**D**iphtheria, **P**ertussis, **T**etanus).
▪ What is the most appropriate treatment for this condition?	Antitoxin can inactivate circulating toxin that has not yet reached its target tissue. Penicillin or erythromycin can be given to prevent further bacterial growth and exotoxin release, thus making the patient noncontagious. The patient also needs cardiac monitoring with electrocardiography and telemetry to monitor for myocarditis; treatment of any heart failure or arrhythmias; monitoring of neurologic function for motor deficits; and supportive care to ensure a secure airway and to avoid aspiration pneumonia.

► **Case 19**

A 32-year-old man presents with extreme swelling of his legs (see Figure 3-9) and scrotum. The skin associated with the swollen areas is thick and scaly. The patient admits to an episode of fever associated with enlarged inguinal lymph nodes some time ago, but did not think much of it. His travel history is significant for spending 9 months in the tropics approximately 2 years prior to presentation.

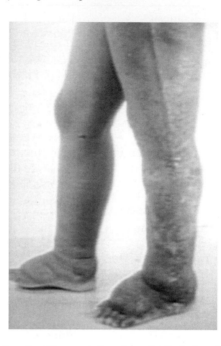

FIGURE 3-9. (Reproduced, with permission, from the Pathology Education Instructional Resource Digital Library [http://peir.net] at the University of Alabama, Birmingham.)

■ What is the most likely diagnosis?	Elephantiasis, caused by the nematode (roundworm) *Wuchereria bancrofti*.
■ How is this organism transmitted, and how does it cause illness?	The organism is transmitted by the bite of a female mosquito.
	Larvae are released into the bloodstream and travel to the lymphatics of the lower extremities and genitals, where they mature. Approximately 1 year later, adult worms, which reside in lymph nodes, trigger an inflammatory response.
■ What signs and symptoms are associated with this condition?	Inflammation resulting from the presence of adult worms causes fever and swelling of lymph nodes. Repeated infections cause repeated bouts of inflammation, resulting in fibrosis around the dead adult worms in the lymph nodes. This fibrosis can obstruct lymphatic drainage and lead to edema and scaly skin.
■ What test can be used to confirm the diagnosis?	Blood smears reveal larvae (**microfilariae**). As larvae usually emerge at night, drawing blood in the evening is preferred.
■ What is the most appropriate treatment for this condition?	Diethylcarbamazine is effective in killing the larvae, but is not effective against the adult worms.

> **Case 20**   A previously healthy 24-year-old man goes to see his doctor with complaints of significant weight loss, flatulence, and foul-smelling stools. He reports feeling fatigued since his return from Peru 3 months previously, and has suffered abdominal cramping and intermittent loose, nonbloody stools since then. The patient's stool ova and parasite studies demonstrated characteristic trophozoites on two separate occasions (see Figure 3-10). He was prescribed a course of drug therapy and warned that consumption of alcohol during treatment could lead to nausea and vomiting.

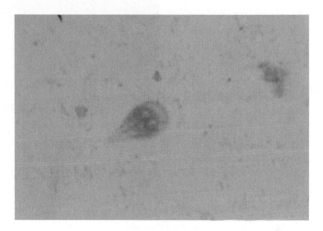

FIGURE 3-10. (Reproduced, with permission, from Le T, Bhushan V, Rao DA. *First Aid for the USMLE Step 1: 2008.* New York: McGraw-Hill, 2008: Color Image 5.)

■ What is the most likely diagnosis?	Giardiasis due to *Giardia lamblia* infection. *Giardia* appear as both a flagellated, motile, dinucleated trophozoite and as a round cyst.
■ What is another less likely infecting microorganism?	*Entamoeba histolytica* can also cause a similar spectrum of symptoms, although there is debate over whether *E. histolytica* can in fact cause nondysenteric diarrhea. Amebic dysentery would present with bloody diarrhea in addition to the above clinical spectrum.
■ What is the most appropriate treatment for this condition?	Metronidazole. The described effects of concurrent alcohol use with metronidazole is a "disulfiram-like effect," in reference to the use of disulfiram to discourage alcohol consumption in situations of alcohol addiction. Metronidazole interferes with the action of aldehyde dehydrogenase in ethanol metabolism, which increases serum acetaldehyde levels and thus leads to nausea, vomiting, flushing, thirst, palpitations, vertigo, and chest pain.
■ What is the mechanism of action of this antibiotic?	Metronidazole is effective specifically against anaerobic microorganisms. It diffuses across the cell membrane of microorganisms and is reduced in the mitochondria of obligate anaerobes to cytotoxic intermediates. These intermediates cause DNA strand breakage and generate free radicals to consequently damage the cell. Furthermore, the reduction of metronidazole creates a concentration gradient that leads to further uptake of the drug.
■ What are other uses of this antibiotic?	Metronidazole is used to treat *Clostridium difficile* infection in pseudomembranous colitis, amebic dysentery, bacterial vaginitis, and *Trichomonas* vaginitis, and as a component of triple therapy for *Helicobacter pylori* eradication. Broadly, it is effective against most anaerobic bacteria as well as various protozoa.

► **Case 21**

A 23-year-old sexually active woman presents to her physician because of a painful left knee and pain with urination. Physical examination reveals a swollen, tender, erythematous left knee with decreased range of motion. Examination of her skin reveals small papules with an erythematous base on her arms. Pelvic examination is notable for purulent endocervical discharge (see Figure 3-11).

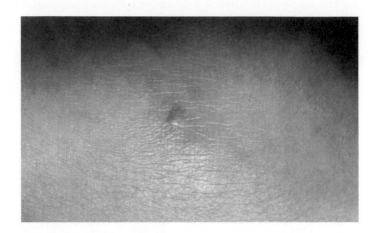

FIGURE 3-11. **Pustular skin lesion with peripheral erythema.** (Reproduced, with permission, from Tintinalli JE, Kelen GD, Stapczynski JS. *Tintinalli's Emergency Medicine: A Comprehensive Study Guide*, 6th ed. New York: McGraw-Hill, 2004: 1518.)

▪ **What is the likely causative organism?**	This patient most likely became infected with *Neisseria gonorrhoeae* through sexual contact with an infected partner. The vaginal infection can cause discharge and dysuria. If the bacteria disseminate, the patient can develop skin lesions, tenosynovitis, or septic arthritis. Septic arthritis is a serious condition that must be treated aggressively to prevent permanent damage to the joint. Surgical drainage is often required, in addition to medical treatment with antibiotics.
▪ **What would a Gram stain of a cervical swab show?**	A stain would show gram-negative kidney-shaped cocci in pairs. Though gonococci are not obligate intracellular organisms, they are often found inside macrophages and neutrophils. However, the endocervical Gram stain in women is a poor test, both insensitive and nonspecific. Gonorrhea in women is best diagnosed by nucleic acid testing (NAT).
▪ **What laboratory technique could be used to distinguish between this organism and meningococci?**	*N. gonorrhoeae* and *N. meningitidis* have many similarities. One way to distinguish them is by the fact that while they both ferment glucose, only *N. meningitidis* is capable of fermenting maltose.
▪ **What antibiotic is recommended for treatment of this condition?**	Ceftriaxone is a first-line treatment for gonococcal infections, particularly if disseminated.
▪ **What other antibiotic should be empirically used to treat a likely coinfection?**	Patients with gonorrhea have a high risk of concurrent infection with *Chlamydia trachomatis*. Therefore, patients are empirically treated for both infections with doxycycline and ceftriaxone.

■ **If not treated early, what is a serious potential gynecologic complication of this infection?**

If the infection persists, it can develop into pelvic inflammatory disease (PID). The bacteria can ascend to the uterus, uterine tubes, and ovaries. This can cause endometritis, salpingitis, oophoritis, and tubo-ovarian abscesses. The infection and subsequent scarring can reduce the patient's fertility, as oocytes are unable to travel through the scarred uterine tubes. In addition, it increases the risk of ectopic tubular pregnancy.

▶ **Case 22**

A 22-year-old woman presents to the emergency department in labor. This is her first pregnancy, and she has received no prenatal care. At the clinic she has a normal spontaneous vaginal delivery of a boy. The baby appears normal at birth. However, 12 hours later he begins to show signs of lethargy. He becomes tachypneic, his blood pressure drops, and his hands and feet begin to feel cold.

▪ What infectious agents are most frequently responsible for neonatal sepsis?	Group B streptococci (GBS), *Escherichia coli*, and *Listeria monocytogenes* are common causes of sepsis, pneumonia, and meningitis in newborns.
▪ What tests could be performed to characterize the causative agent?	Depending on the extent of the infection, blood and cerebrospinal fluid (CSF) smears may demonstrate bacteria on Gram staining. Cultures could be performed to further identify the organism. GBS would appear as gram-positive cocci. *E. coli* and *L. monocytogenes* are both gram-negative rods.
▪ How did the infant become infected?	These bacteria can spread through the placenta, or can be acquired from the birth canal during delivery. The mother may be infected or colonized but have no symptoms. However, pregnant and postpartum women are at risk for GBS urinary tract infection or chorioamnionitis.
▪ What testing is routinely performed prenatally to reduce the risk of infection of the infant in the birth canal?	Between 35 and 37 weeks of gestation, cultures of the mother's vagina and rectum are performed to determine whether she is colonized with GBS.
▪ What treatment is initiated if the testing mentioned above is positive?	Treatment of GBS in infected mothers or newborns involves the use of antepartum antibiotics such as penicillin. In mothers who are colonized vaginally or rectally, but who are not actively infected, intrapartum antibiotics are recommended.
▪ If the baby develops meningitis from this organism, what CSF findings would be expected?	In bacterial meningitis, the CSF may show bacteria on Gram stain. In addition, the WBC count is elevated with primarily neutrophils, the protein level is elevated, and the glucose level is reduced.

► **Case 23**

A 3-year-old boy is brought to the pediatrician by his mother. The mother states that 2 days ago, the child started refusing solid foods, preferring his bottle and applesauce. Today, the mother noticed a rash on her son's hands and feet (see Figure 3-12), and found that he was also running a low-grade fever, which prompted her to bring him to the doctor.

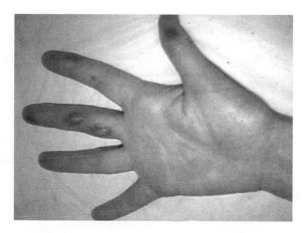

FIGURE 3-12. (Reproduced, with permission, from the Pathology Education Instructional Resource Digital Library [http://peir.net] at the University of Alabama, Birmingham.)

■ **What is the most likely diagnosis?**	This is a case of hand, foot, and mouth syndrome, caused by coxsackie A virus (a picornavirus). This syndrome presents with a tender rash on the palms, soles, and often the buttocks, in addition to painful vesicles on the oral mucosa. This patient's avoidance of solid food strongly suggests involvement of the oral mucosa.
■ **What other microorganisms are included in this family, and what are their characteristics?**	The picornavirus family are enteroviruses (they infect intestinal epithelia and lymphoid cells), and include: ■ Poliovirus ■ Echovirus ■ Hepatitis A virus ■ Coxsackie viruses ■ Rhinovirus The pico**RNA**viruses all have a single-stranded, positive polarity, linear, **RNA** genome in a nonenveloped icosahedral capsid.
■ **What other illnesses can this particular microorganism cause?**	Coxsackie A virus may also cause **herpangina**, which presents with sore throat, red vesicles on the back of the throat, pain with swallowing, and fever. Herpangina is a mild, self-limited disease that presents in children and usually results in complete recovery. Less commonly, coxsackie A virus can cause petechial and purpuric rashes, which may also have a hemorrhagic component.
■ **What illnesses may be caused by the group B coxsackie viruses?**	The coxsackie B virus may cause aseptic meningitis, myocarditis, pericarditis, orchitis, and epidemic pleurodynia (fever, headache, spasms of the chest wall muscles, and pleuritic pain). Nephritic syndrome may also occur after a coxsackie B virus infection.
■ **What type of immune response would this infection elicit?**	Because this is a viral infection, it will elicit a cell-mediated and antibody-mediated immune response. As the virus infects cells, viral particles will be presented by class I major histocompatibility complex (MHC), activating CD4$^+$ cells. These cells will release cytokines that subsequently activate both cytotoxic T cells (CD8$^+$) and B cells, which will synthesize immunoglobulin.

► **Case 24**

An 18-year-old woman presents to clinic with a fever and headache. She also complains of vaginal itching and dysuria. When asked, she says that she recently became sexually active. On physical examination, there is tender inguinal lymphadenopathy. There are also red, pustular, painful vesicles on her labia majora (see Figure 3-13).

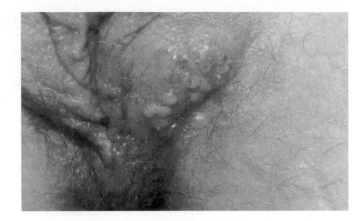

FIGURE 3-13. (Reproduced, with permission, from Klausner JD, Hook EW III. *Current Diagnosis & Treatment of Sexually Transmitted Diseases.* New York: McGraw-Hill, 2007: 86.)

■ **What is the most likely diagnosis?**	Herpes simplex virus type 2 (HSV-2).
■ **What are the characteristics of this pathogen?**	HSV-2 is a member of the herpesvirus family, which also includes herpes simplex virus type 1 (HSV-1), varicella-zoster virus (VZV), Epstein-Barr virus (EBV), cytomegalovirus, human herpesvirus-6, and human herpesvirus-8. This family of viruses has linear double-stranded DNA and is enveloped. HSV-1, HSV-2, and VZV can be recognized by multinucleated giant cells on Tzanck smear, and by eosinophilic intranuclear inclusions.
■ **What is the typical course of this infection?**	HSV-2 is transmitted by direct contact of the virus with mucosal surfaces or open skin surfaces. It can also be transmitted from a mother to her newborn during delivery. Eighty percent of those infected are asymptomatic. The primary infection often presents with constitutional symptoms such as fever, headache, malaise, and myalgia. Later, genital vesicles may appear, which can rupture and leave behind painful ulcers. Other genital symptoms include itching and tender inguinal lymphadenopathy. Like other viruses in the family, HSV-2 becomes latent and can be reactivated. Triggers for reactivation include fever, trauma, emotional stress, sunlight, and menstruation. Upon reactivation, there is often a viral prodrome that involves tenderness, pain, and burning at the future site of vesicle eruption. The lesions last 4–15 days before crusting over and reepithelializing.

- **What populations are most at risk for complications of this infection?**

  The populations most at risk for complications are those deficient in cell-mediated immunity, which is needed to keep the virus under control. Encephalitis resulting from HSV-2 is usually seen only in those infected at birth. Unlike encephalitis from HSV-1, which is localized to the temporal and occipital lobes, encephalitis from HSV-2 is a diffuse brain process.

- **What is the treatment for this condition?**

  The treatment for HSV-2 is acyclovir, a nucleoside analog that acts by inhibiting viral DNA polymerase when it is phosphorylated by viral thymidine kinase. It can also be used to treat VZV and HSV-1.

► **Case 25**

A 9-year-old girl is brought to a public clinic by her mother. The family immigrated from Guatemala 3 years previously. Her mother reports the girl seems very small for her age and has been continually lethargic for quite some time. Physical examination reveals a small girl with a thin, scaphoid abdomen. Relevant laboratory findings are as follows:

Hematocrit: 36%
Mean corpuscular volume: 83 fL
WBC count: 11,000/mm^3
Differential: 35% segmented cells, 1% bands, 33% lymphocytes, 21% eosinophils

■ What is the most likely diagnosis, and what test can be used to confirm this?	The patient's eosinophilia points to a possible parasitic infection, therefore, a stool ova and parasite study should be the next step. The patient's immigration from Guatemala increases the risk of a parasitic infection.
■ The test demonstrates the patient is infected with the hookworm *Ancylostoma duodenale*. What are the characteristic findings of this infection?	*A. duodenale* presents as characteristic small, round eggs and occasional worms approximately 1 cm in size. The ova and parasite examination can differentiate among the helminthic causes of eosinophilia. The stool exam is useful only in chronic hookworm infections.
■ How does this infection cause disease in humans?	Percutaneous infection occurs most commonly through the soles of the feet. The larvae pass into the lungs, and 8–21 days later they cross the pulmonary vasculature and enter the airways. They ascend to the pharynx and are swallowed. By the time they reach the small intestine, the larvae have become adult worms. The adults attach to the mucosa and feed with the help of an orally secreted factor X inhibitor. The females produce eggs that are passed through the stool and deposited in the soil.
■ What are the signs of both acute and chronic infection?	**Acute symptoms:** ■ Cutaneous tracks of larval migration under the skin (less common) ■ Diarrhea ■ Flatulence ■ Nausea ■ Postprandial abdominal pain ■ Pruritic maculopapular eruption at the site of entry (less common) ■ Vomiting **Chronic hookworm infection:** ■ Failure to thrive ■ Iron deficiency anemia This patient has symptoms of chronic hookworm infection. Chronic hookworm infection leads to the high morbidity of the disease in countries where hookworm infection is prevalent.
■ What are the most appropriate treatments for this condition?	Mebendazole. Alternatively, pyrantel pamoate and albendazole can be used.

A 46-year-old woman visits her physician complaining of "feeling poorly," with fever, chills, muscle aches, dry cough, and sore throat. She has had these symptoms for several days with no significant improvement. She works as a secretary and says these symptoms have been "going around the office." Physical examination reveals small, tender cervical lymphadenopathy, swollen nasal mucosa, and an erythematous pharynx.

■ **What is the most likely diagnosis?**	Infection with influenza virus.
■ **What are the defining structural features of this class of microorganisms?**	Orthomyxoviruses are helical, enveloped, negative, single-stranded RNA viruses.
■ **Even though the patient has had a similar infection, why isn't her immune system protecting her from this illness?**	Because of a phenomenon known as **antigenic drift**. This is the result of random small mutations causing changes in the antigenic structure of the virus. These mutations result in antigen structures that are only partially recognized by the host immune system.
■ **What characteristic of this microorganism's genome makes deadly epidemics possible?**	Influenza A virus infects diverse species including birds, horses, and swine; in contrast, influenza B and C infect only man. With its segmented genome, influenza A can swap segments of RNA between animal and human strains, leading to new human strains with novel surface antigens not recognized by the immune system. This type of change is termed **antigenic shift**.
■ **What pharmacologic agents can be used as prophylaxis against this infection?**	Amantadine and rimantadine can be used to treat the symptoms of influenza A infection. However, these are rarely used nowadays due to high levels of resistance to them. Zanamivir and oseltamivir can be used to treat both influenza A and B infections of these, oseltamivir is easier to administer). These need to be started in the first 2 days of symptom onset to be most effective. The vaccine should be given in October or November, prior to the start of flu season. It takes about 2 weeks for the body to make antibodies to the viruses.

► **Case 27**

A 25-year-old man is brought to the emergency department by ambulance after a motor vehicle collision. He is lucid but suffered severe bleeding from his leg. His wife is with him, and she provides the history. The patient has generally been healthy, although he had several bouts of "lung infections" and "ear infections" as a child. He also has a history of milk allergy and periodically suffers from diarrhea. In the emergency department he is given 1 unit of type-matched red blood cells (RBCs) and soon afterwards develops a severe reaction. He develops a red, itchy rash over most of his body (see Figure 3-14) and begins to have difficulty breathing. His blood pressure begins to drop in spite of continuous fluid infusion.

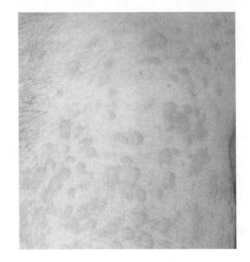

FIGURE 3-14. This image shows erythematous papules and plaques typical of urticaria. (Reproduced, with permission from, Kasper DL, Braunwald E, Fauci AS, Hauser SL, Longo DL, Jameson NL, Isselbacher KJ [eds]. *Harrison's Principles of Internal Medicine*, 16th ed. New York: McGraw-Hill, 2005: 287.)

■ **What is the likely underlying cause of this patient's repeated infections and the allergic reaction to the blood transfusion?**	This patient is having an anaphylactic reaction. He most likely has hereditary deficiency of IgA, and is reacting to the IgA in the transfused blood product. He is particularly susceptible to gastrointestinal infections, for which secretory IgA plays an important protective role. IgA deficiency can occur as an isolated syndrome, or may involve concurrent IgG deficiency, which increases the risk of sinopulmonary infections.
■ **What is the cause of the patient's milk allergy?**	In the absence of intestinal IgA, large proteins are more likely to enter the bloodstream whole. An IgG antibody reaction to these proteins can then cause an allergic reaction. (Remember, this is different from lactose intolerance, which is not a true allergy and involves a deficiency of lactase.) For the same reasons, patients with IgA deficiency are at increased risk of developing antibodies against wheat proteins and celiac disease.
■ **What accounts for the anaphylactic reaction to the transfusion?**	Patients with IgA deficiency may develop IgG antibodies that can bind to IgA (anti-IgA IgG antibodies). They can develop even without prior exposure to exogenous IgA.

- Describe the stages in B-cell development that lead up to IgA secretion.

Pluripotent stem cells first differentiate into lymphoid stem cells, then to pro-B cells, followed by formation of pre-B cells. Pre-B cells contain the IgM (mu) heavy chains intracellularly, but no surface IgM. The next step is formation of immature or naïve B cells that express surface IgM. After stimulation by antigen, the immature cells can mature into IgM-secreting cells, or with CD4+ T-cell stimulation can class-switch. They can also undergo affinity maturation to select for antibodies with higher binding affinities for the antigen. After class-switching the cells first express surface IgG, IgA, or IgE, and then can form plasma cells that secrete the antibodies.

- At what stage in activation would a defect give rise to agammaglobulinemia and B cells that do not express surface antibody?

Bruton's agammaglobulinemia is caused by a failure of pre-B cells to develop into immature B cells. The cells are arrested at the pre-B stage and contain intracellular mu heavy chain protein. This is an X-linked disease, and so is found most frequently in males.

- Deficiency of which component would give rise to hyper-IgM syndrome?

A defect of the CD40L protein on the surface of CD4+ T-helper cells causes this syndrome. Without the CD40L interaction with CD40 on B cells, the B cells cannot undergo class switching. Therefore, IgM can be generated, but production of other classes of antibodies is defective. Patients with this syndrome are at risk for severe pyogenic infections.

▶ **Case 28**

A 43-year-old man with human immunodeficiency virus (HIV) infection presents to the HIV clinic with multiple, reddish-purple plaques, in addition to a few papules of the same color, distributed across the skin (see Figure 3-15). The patient says he feels fine, and denies fever, chills, malaise, or headache. A complete blood count reveals his CD4+ T cell count is 350 cells/L.

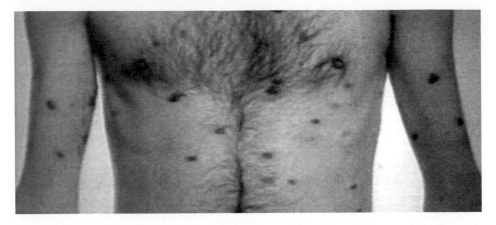

FIGURE 3-15. (Reproduced, with permission, from the Pathology Education Instructional Resource Digital Library [http://peir.net] at the University of Alabama, Birmingham.)

■ What is the most likely diagnosis? What important alternative diagnosis must be ruled out?

This is Kaposi's sarcoma, a neoplasm prevalent in HIV-positive patients. Kaposi's sarcoma is caused by human herpesvirus-8 (HHV-8), a member of the herpesvirus family. Members of the herpes family are DNA viruses with a double-stranded, linear genome in an enveloped, icosahedral capsid. An important alternative diagnosis for such skin lesions is bacillary angiomatosis (BA), which typically presents with systemic symptoms such as fever, chills, and malaise. Because BA is caused by *Bartonella* bacteria, however, it can readily be treated with antibiotics.

■ How does the microorganism cause the characteristic discolored skin lesions?

HHV-8 has a tropism for endothelium cells, and is thought to induce vascular endothelial growth factor (VEGF), which causes irregular vascular channels to develop in the skin. Red blood cells extravasate into these spaces, causing the characteristic purple-red skin lesions as seen in Figure 3-15.

■ What other diseases are associated with this microorganism?

Kaposi's sarcoma is not limited to the skin; the gastrointestinal tract, oral mucosa, lungs, lymph nodes, and other visceral organs may be infected. HHV-8 also infects B lymphocytes, and has been linked to **body-cavity B-cell lymphoma** (a non-Hodgkin's lymphoma subtype) and to **Castleman's disease** (a lymphoproliferative disorder that may progress to lymphoma).

■ What other patient population is at increased risk for developing this infection?

Transplant patients, who, like patients with HIV, are chronically immunosuppressed have a higher incidence of infection than the general public.

■ What are the most appropriate treatments for this condition?

Daunorubicin and doxorubicin. Both drugs cause DNA breaks by two mechanisms: (1) intercalating into the DNA double helix, and (2) creating oxygen free radicals that damage DNA. A major adverse effect of their use, however, is cardiotoxicity. In HIV-positive patients, the first goal is to boost immunity by starting highly active antiretroviral therapy, which often leads to improvement of the disease.

A 17-year-old boy who recently immigrated from India presents to the emergency department with complaints of spiking fevers, weight loss, and lethargy. On examination he is cachectic with a gray skin tone, and he is found to have pronounced splenomegaly and mild hepatomegaly. Laboratory tests reveal pancytopenia. Microscopic examination of a bone marrow aspirate from this patient revealed parasites in the histiocytes.

■ **What is the most likely diagnosis?**	This patient is suffering from kala azar, or visceral leishmaniasis. The form found in the human host is the amastigote, which is small and round, and has a flagellum that is difficult to visualize. The prominently flagellated form of the parasite is found in the insect vector and is known as the promastigote.
■ **What is the vector of this pathogen?**	Humans are infected with *Leishmania donovani* through the bite of a sandfly. It can also be transmitted by intravenous drug use or blood transfusion.
■ **On the blood smear, some macrophages are noted that contain basophilic inclusions (Figure 3-17). What are these inclusions?**	These inclusions are called Donovan bodies and consist of the amastigote form of the parasite.
■ **What treatment is used for this infection?**	Treatment is with sodium stibogluconate or pentamidine.
■ **What diseases are caused by other blood-borne flagellates?**	Trypanosomes are another flagellated parasite that can be found in the blood. *Trypanosoma cruzi* is transmitted by the reduviid bug and is found in South America and causes Chagas' disease. *T. gambiense* and *T. rhodesiense* are transmitted by the tsetse fly and are the cause of African sleeping sickness.

▶ **Case 30**

A 64-year-old man with a past history of smoking and well-controlled diabetes mellitus presents to the emergency department with a 3-day history of low-grade fevers, mild diarrhea, and nonproductive cough. He works as a maintenance worker in a local apartment complex. Workup includes a Gram stain of sputum, which shows prominent polymorphonuclear leukocytes, but no microorganisms. X-ray of the chest reveals diffuse, patchy bilateral infiltrates (see Figure 3-16). Relevant laboratory findings are as follows:

Hemoglobin: 14 g/mL
Hematocrit: 40%
Platelets: 200,000/mm^3
WBCs: 15,000/mm^3
Blood urea nitrogen: 16 mg/dL
Creatinine: 1.2 mg/dL
Urinalysis: 2+ proteinuria;
  no glucose, ketones, or blood

Sodium: 128 mEq/L
Chloride: 90 mEq/L
Potassium: 4.2 mEq/L
Bicarbonate: 17 mEq/L
Glucose: 110 mg/dL

The patient is treated empirically with a β-lactam antibiotic, with no clinical improvement.

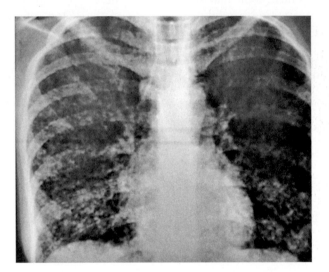

FIGURE 3-16. (Reproduced, with permission, from Le T, Bhushan V, Rao DA. *First Aid for the USMLE Step 1: 2008.* New York: McGraw-Hill, 2008: Image 126A.)

■ **What are the abnormal laboratory findings? Based on all the data, what is the most likely diagnosis?**

The patient's laboratory studies reveal hyponatremia, a low bicarbonate level, and leukocytosis.

Diarrhea, when prolonged and severe, can cause hyponatremia. *Legionella* infection, a common source of community-acquired pneumonia (CAP), is also associated with hyponatremia. The leukocytosis suggests an immune response to some type of pathogen. The patient's subacute clinical presentation, relatively benign chest x-ray findings, and laboratory abnormalities suggest an atypical CAP such as that caused by *Mycoplasma*, *Chlamydia*, or *Legionella*.

■ **An astute intern orders a commonly used urinary antigen test for CAP, which comes back positive. What does this test measure, and can it explain the patient's symptoms?**

The urinary antigen test described is likely a *Legionella* antigen test, which measures *Legionella* serotype 1. *Legionella*, as discussed above, is a possible source of the patient's symptoms.

- **What risk factors does the patient have for developing this condition?**

The patient's history of diabetes and smoking predisposes him to *Legionella* infection. Given his occupation as a maintenance man, he may work with air conditioning systems. As this microorganism grows in infected water sources, the patient's occupation places him at risk.

- **What is the best way to Gram stain and culture this microorganism? Why does it not show up when traditional Gram staining methods are used?**

Legionella is a gram-negative rod that can be identified using a silver stain. *Legionella* is primarily intracellular, which explains its poor staining characteristics. It is cultured on charcoal yeast extract agar, supplemented with iron and cysteine.

- **What are the most appropriate treatments for this condition?**

Legionella responds best to antibiotics that can achieve a high intracellular concentration, such as the newer macrolides (examples include erythromycin, clarithromycin, and azithromycin), quinolones, and tetracyclines. *Legionella* produces β-lactamase, and therefore cephalosporins and penicillins are ineffective.

► **Case 31**

A 41-year-old woman who is a recent immigrant from Mexico presents to a local clinic complaining of "white spots" on her body. The woman says she first noticed the lesions about 1 month ago and thought they were from the sun, but they have gradually increased in number and did not seem to improve despite her new job indoors. Physical examination reveals multiple, asymmetrically distributed, circular, hypopigmented lesions on the patient's arms, abdomen, and back (see Figure 3-18). The lesions are sharply demarcated, with raised, erythematous borders and atrophic, scaly centers. The lesions are anesthetic, and there is no hair growth within any of the hypopigmented areas. Biopsy of the lesions demonstrates granuloma formation within the dermal nerves of the forearm.

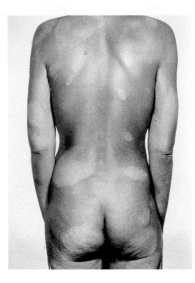

FIGURE 3-18. (Reproduced, with permission, from Wolff K, Johnson RA, Suurmond D. *Fitzpatrick's Color Atlas & Synopsis of Clinical Dermatology*, 5th ed. New York: McGraw-Hill, 2005: 657.)

■ **What is the most likely diagnosis?**	The lesions described are characteristic for tuberculoid leprosy. Lesions in this disease typically evolve from hypopigmented, well-demarcated macules to fully developed lesions that are anesthetic and devoid of hair follicles or sweat glands.
■ **What conditions should be included in the differential diagnosis of these lesions?**	■ Leishmaniasis ■ Lupus vulgaris ■ Lymphoma ■ Sarcoidosis ■ Syphilis ■ Yaws However, the biopsy findings here are pathognomonic for leprosy. Sarcoidosis causes granuloma formation around peripheral nerves, but the finding here of granulomas within the nerves is diagnostic of leprosy.
■ **Under what conditions does this microorganism grow?**	Both lepromatous and tuberculoid leprosy are caused by *Mycobacterium leprae*, an acid-fast bacillus that cannot be grown in vitro. *M. leprae* is an obligate intracellular bacillus that, like other mycobacteria, contains mycolic acid in its cell wall. *M. leprae* grows best in cooler temperatures (skin, peripheral nerves, testes, upper respiratory tract).

- **How does this patient's condition differ from the more severe form?**

Tuberculoid leprosy is a disease largely confined to the skin (hypopigmented macules) and peripheral nerves. Cell-mediated immunity is intact, and patients' T cells recognize *M. leprae* (positive lepromin skin test). Lepromatous leprosy holds a much worse prognosis because patients have ineffective cell-mediated immunity (negative lepromin skin test). Skin lesions and nerve involvement are much more extensive than in the tuberculoid form, and there may be involvement of the testes, upper respiratory tract, and anterior chamber of the eye.

- **What is the most appropriate treatment for this condition?**

Both tuberculoid and lepromatous leprosy can be treated with a course of oral dapsone. The tuberculoid form is reliably cured by a short course of this medication. Patients with lepromatous leprosy have an exceptionally high bacterial load and may require an extended or even lifelong course of chemotherapy. Alternate therapies for leprosy include rifampin or a combination of clofazimine and dapsone.

▶ **Case 32**

The mother of a 1-week-old female infant calls her pediatrician because the infant has been fussy all morning. The infant's temperature is 39°C (102.2°F), and the mother is asked to bring the infant to the hospital for further workup and treatment. The workup includes cerebrospinal fluid (CSF) analysis, hematology studies, and cultures. Empiric antibiotic therapy is initiated. Later, upon microscopic examination of the CSF, microorganisms with tumbling end-over-end motility are visualized.

■ What is the most likely diagnosis?

Meningitis due to *Listeria* infection. This microorganism, identifiable by its classical tumbling motility, is a gram-positive rod.

■ What findings are most likely on laboratory testing?

The white blood cell (WBC) count would likely be elevated. The WBC differential would show predominantly neutrophils and/or monocytes. Protein levels may be elevated, and glucose levels should be normal or decreased. The microorganisms visualized in the CSF are bacteria. Compare this CSF profile to CSF profiles seen in fungal or viral CSF infections (see Table 3-1).

■ What microorganisms should empiric antibiotic therapy target?

Group B streptococcus, *Escherichia coli*, and *Listeria monocytogenes* are the most common causes of sepsis and bacterial meningitis in infants <1 month old. Other notable causes of sepsis/meningitis in this age group include *Streptococcus pneumoniae*, *Haemophilus influenzae*, *Staphylococcus aureus*, *Neisseria meningitidis*, and *Salmonella*.

■ How does this microorganism evade the host immune response?

L. monocytogenes is a facultative intracellular bacterium able to survive in the macrophages of neonates and immunosuppressed patients. In an immunocompetent host, activation of macrophages will destroy phagocytosed *Listeria*.

■ What is the most appropriate treatment for this condition?

Ampicillin and gentamicin, which act together as synergists. Ampicillin disrupts cell wall synthesis, resulting in increased uptake of gentamicin into bacterial cells.

TABLE 3-1. CSF Findings in Meningitis

	PRESSURE	CELL TYPE	PROTEIN	GLUCOSE
Bacterial	↑	↑ PMNs	↑	↓
Fungal/TB	↑	↑ lymphocytes	↑	↓
Viral	Normal/↑	↑ lymphocytes	Normal	Normal

PMN, polymorphonuclear neutrophil; TB, tuberculosis (Reproduced, with permission, from Le T, Bhushan V, Rao DA. *First Aid for the USMLE Step 1: 2008.* New York: McGraw-Hill, 2008: 172.)

► **Case 33**

A 30-year-old woman presents to clinic with abdominal pain, a low-grade fever, and a sensation of abdominal fullness. She says the symptoms have been going on for some time and have been gradually worsening. On physical examination she appears somewhat jaundiced with notable scleral icterus. She says she is originally from South America. A CT scan of the abdomen is shown in Figure 3-19.

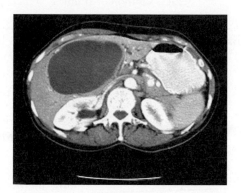

FIGURE 3-19. (Reproduced, with permission, from the Pathology Education Instructional Resource Digital Library [http://peir.net] at the University of Alabama, Birmingham.)

■ **What is the most likely diagnosis?**	The patient most likely has a liver cyst from *Echinococcus* infection.
■ **How is this infection transmitted?**	*Echinococcus* is a tapeworm that is transmitted by food or water contaminated with feces containing eggs from the tapeworm. Infection is not endemic to the United States, and so is most commonly seen in immigrants or those with a travel history to endemic areas.
■ **What is the typical presentation of this infection?**	*Echinococcus* causes slow-growing cysts in the liver. As a result, symptoms are often gradual in onset and include abdominal pain, cough, low-grade fever, a sense of abdominal fullness, hepatomegaly, and obstructive jaundice. Leakage of cysts can cause flushing and urticaria, while rupture can cause anaphylaxis and death. The other organs that can be involved include the lungs and the brain. In the lungs, the presentation includes chronic cough, dyspnea, hemoptysis, and pleuritic chest pain. In the brain, presentation includes headache, dizziness, increased intracranial pressure, and hydrocephalus.
■ **How is the diagnosis of this condition made?**	Usually, the diagnosis cannot be made with radiology alone, and so is usually made with an enzyme-linked immunosorbent assay. In addition, 25% of patients have eosinophilia and on x-ray there is often a rim of calcification around the cyst, which distinguishes it from amebic and pyogenic cysts.
■ **What is the treatment for this condition?**	The treatment for *Echinococcus* is usually surgical and involves aspiration of cyst contents followed by excision. In some cases, therapy with a combination of albendazole and mebendazole is sufficient. A third method involves aspiration of cyst contents, injection of a scolicide (i.e., formalin), and reaspiration.

▶ **Case 34**

While doing a rotation in Ghana, a medical student encounters a patient who has been having nearly continuous high-grade fevers with occasional chills and sweats. Physical examination reveals a palpable spleen. A drop of the patient's blood placed in a copper sulfate solution reveals the patient is anemic. Over the next few days, while waiting for medication to arrive, the patient's level of consciousness waxes and wanes, and the patient is somnolent at times.

■ **What is the most likely diagnosis?**

Malaria, most likely due to *Plasmodium falciparum*. The symptoms give a clue as to the species. The patient's altered mental status is consistent with a diagnosis of *P. falciparum* malaria, since this is the only strain that commonly has cerebral involvement. This patient's continuous fever and irregular chills and sweats are also characteristic of *P. falciparum* malaria. While early in infection, irregular fevers are common in all types of malaria, the fever can become periodic in well-established cases of non-*falciparum* disease. For example, *P. vivax* and *P. ovale* cause episodes of fever, chills, and sweats every 48 hours. With *P. malariae*, these episodes occur every 72 hours.

■ **What phase of the microorganism's life cycle results in the development of anemia?**

Red blood cell (RBC) lysis occurs during the erythrocytic cycle, when the products of asexual replication inside the RBCs (the **merozoite** form) are released. The immune response to the merozoites, and resultant cytokine release, is responsible for the fever, chills, and sweats.

■ **What are the likely findings on peripheral blood smear (PBS)?**

A PBS is likely to show ring-shaped trophozoites inside the RBCs (see Figure 3-20), and there may be several trophozoites per RBC. **Schizonts**, the large, multinucleated cells formed from the trophozoite by multiple cycles of nuclear division, may be visible in the erythrocytes in non-*falciparum* malaria, but are very rarely seen in *falciparum* disease. Outside the RBCs, oblong **gametocytes**, diagnostic for *P. falciparum*, may also be visible.

■ **In an area without drug-resistant microorganisms, what is the drug of choice for treating this condition?**

Chloroquine is the drug of choice in the few areas where there is no resistance. Its major mode of action against *Plasmodium* is inhibition of the enzyme responsible for polymerizing heme. This results in the accumulation of free heme, which is toxic to the protozoan.

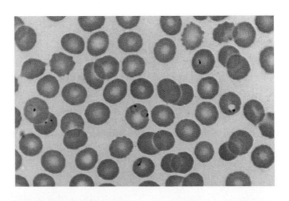

FIGURE 3-20. Malaria. *Plasmodium vivax*. Blood film. Trophozoites (ring forms) in red cells. (Reproduced, with permission from Lichtman MA, Shafer MS, Felgar, Wang N: *Lichtman's Atlas of Hematology*, New York McGraw-Hill, 2007. Figure III.A.21.)

■ **In areas where drug resistance is high, what are the drugs of choice for treating this condition?**

Quinidine in combination with doxycycline or pyrimethamine/sulfadoxine is commonly used as first-line treatment for chloroquine-resistant *P. falciparum*. Other effective drugs include mefloquine and atovaquone-proguanil. Artemesinins are being widely used in Africa and Asia, and are the treatment of choice for chloroquine-resistant *P. falciparum* in many areas. However, they are not currently available in the United States.

▶ **Case 35**

A 49-year-old man comes to the clinic complaining of vertigo and fatigue for the past day. He has no chronic health condition and enjoys walking several miles a day in the park for exercise. Physical examination reveals a bull's-eye-shaped rash on the patient's left shoulder, as depicted in Figure 3-21.

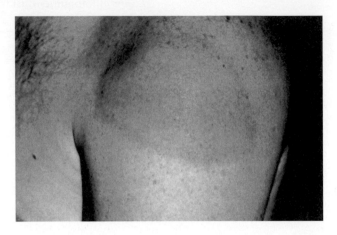

FIGURE 3-21. (Reproduced, with permission, from Wolff K, Johnson RA, Suurmond D. *Fitzpatrick's Color Atlas & Synopsis of Clinical Dermatology*, 5th ed. New York: McGraw-Hill, 2005: 679.)

▪ What is the most likely diagnosis?	Lyme disease. This disease is caused by *Borrelia burgdorferi*, a spirochete that is a gram-negative, corkscrew-shaped bacterium too small to be visualized under light microscopy. They are better visualized using **darkfield microscopy**, immunologic staining, or silver stains.
▪ How are human beings infected?	The *Ixodes* **tick** can transmit *B. burgdorferi* from white-footed mice, other small rodents, and white-tailed deer to man by attaching to a person **for at least 24 hours (and needing up to 72 hours to transmit the bacteria)**. Checking for ticks at least once a day can prevent infection resulting from a tick bite.
▪ What is the name for the rash on the patient's shoulder?	**Erythema chronicum migrans.** This name describes the ring of erythema that migrates outward (over time) from the site of the tick bite.
▪ What organs are affected in the early disseminated stage of infection?	▪ Heart (heart block, myocarditis) ▪ Musculoskeletal system (arthritis) ▪ Nervous system (encephalitis, Bell's palsy, peripheral neuropathy) ▪ Skin (erythema chronicum migrans)
▪ In the detection of anti–*B. burgdorferi* antibodies, some protocols recommend using enzyme-linked immunosorbent assays (ELISA) first. If anti–*B. burgdorferi* antibodies are found using ELISA, then a Western blot is performed. What can be inferred about the sensitivity and specificity of these two tests?	Since ELISA is used as a screening test, it must be a relatively sensitive test, identifying most disease but with a higher false-positive rate. However, Western blots must be more specific, with a low false-positive rate, since it is used to confirm the presence of the antibody in question.
▪ What is the most appropriate treatment for this condition?	Doxycycline or amoxicillin is used for primary infection. For disseminated infection (i.e., cardiac or central nervous system involvement), ceftriaxone is preferred. Doxycycline or azithromycin is used for arthritis.

► **Case 36**

A 4-year-old girl is brought to her pediatrician by her mother because she has been experiencing flulike symptoms. The child is pale and febrile, and her respiratory rate is 25/min. Her buccal mucosa has multiple blue-gray spots, and she has a maculopapular rash. Upon questioning, the mother admits the child's immunizations are not up to date. The physician orders that the girl stay home from preschool and avoid all unvaccinated contacts in the family.

▪ **What is the most likely diagnosis?**	Measles, one of the most transmissible viral infections.
▪ **What microorganism causes this condition, and how does it cause illness?**	Measles is caused by an RNA virus that is a member of the genus *Morbillivirus* and the family Paramyxoviridae. Transmission is through respiratory droplets, and the virus is able to traverse the respiratory epithelium and spread hematogenously. Spread of the virus to the mucosa, dermis, respiratory tract, and brain causes illness.
▪ **What signs and symptoms are associated with this condition?**	Clinical presentation includes flulike symptoms, **Koplik's spots** (bluish-gray spots on the buccal mucosa), and a maculopapular rash that starts at the head and moves to the feet (as shown in an older patient in Figure 3-22). Respiratory tract involvement causes rhinorrhea and cough. Involvement of the brain can result in meningitis or encephalitis. A variant form of measles called subacute sclerosing panencephalitis (SSPE) causes slowly progressive neurologic disease, which eventually leads to death.
▪ **What tests can help confirm the diagnosis, and which clinical findings are pathognomonic for the condition?**	Diagnosis can be confirmed by isolating virus from nasopharyngeal secretions, blood, or urine. Koplik's spots on the mucosa and/or **Warthin-Finkeldey cells** (multinucleated giant cells with inclusion bodies in the nucleus and cytoplasm) in the respiratory secretions are pathognomonic.
▪ **What is the most appropriate treatment for this condition?**	No treatment is available for active infection. Vaccination with the live attenuated measles virus in the MMR (measles-mumps-rubella) vaccine is available.

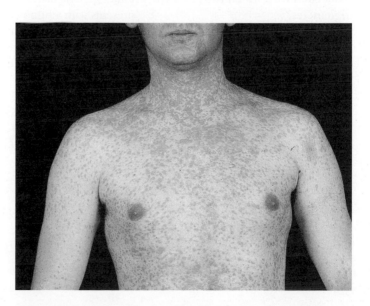

FIGURE 3-22. Measles rash. (Reproduced, with permission, from Wolff K, Johnson RA, Suurmond D. *Fitzpatrick's Color Atlas & Synopsis of Clinical Dermatology*, 5th ed. New York: McGraw-Hill, 2005: 788.)

► **Case 37**

A 19-year-old college sophomore comes to the university health clinic complaining of a worsening sore throat, headache, and fatigue of 1 week's duration. The young man has a slightly elevated temperature of 37.7°C (99.9°F). Physical examination reveals enlarged, tender cervical lymph nodes and a palpable spleen. His throat is notable for a gray-green tonsillar exudate.

■ What is the most likely diagnosis?	Infectious mononucleosis, most frequently caused by Epstein-Barr virus (EBV).
■ To confirm the clinical diagnosis, a Monospot test is performed. What is the basis of this test?	When infected with EBV, many people synthesize antibody that is cross-reactive with a surface antigen on sheep red blood cells (RBCs) (**heterophile antibodies**). The Monospot test uses serum from the patient added to sheep RBCs. A positive test results in agglutination of the RBCs. This test provides rapid diagnosis of active EBV infection. Other serological tests may be used to de termine EBV immune status, or to diagnose acute EBV infection in the minority of patients (<5%, and usually under 5 years old) who are heterophile antibody negative.
■ What are the likely findings on peripheral blood smear (PBS)?	**Atypical lymphocytes** are the hallmark finding on PBS during acute infectious mononucleosis (see Figure 3-23). These cells are activated T lymphocytes with a large amount of cytoplasm. However, it should be noted that atypical lymphocytes may also be found with other infections (e.g., cytomegalovirus, rubella, and toxoplasmosis), some malignancies, and as a result of drug reactions.
■ What are the defining structural features of this microorganism?	EBV is an enveloped, double-stranded, linear DNA virus (like cytomegalovirus, varicella zoster, and herpes simplex virus). EBV preferentially infects B lymphocytes—the virus adheres to the C3d complement receptor found on the surface of B cells.
■ Infection with this microorganism has been associated with which two major malignancies?	■ **Burkitt's lymphoma** is endemic to Africa, and primarily affects children. The disease is a B-cell lymphoma and often presents with a tumor of the jaw. ■ **Nasopharyngeal carcinoma** is one of the most common cancers in southern China, where evidence supports EBV as the primary causative agent in this neoplasm.

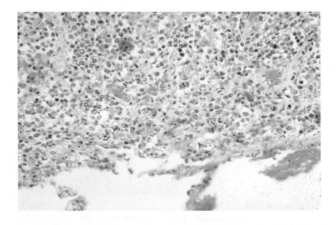

FIGURE 3-23. Atypical lymphocytes in acute infectious mononucleosis. (Reproduced, with permission, from the Pathology Education Instructional Resource Digital Library [http://peir.net] at the University of Alabama, Birmingham.)

A 55-year-old woman who was diagnosed with type 1 diabetes at 12 years of age is brought to the emergency department with a fever and in a state of confusion. She had been working long hours and had not been monitoring her glucose well. On admission she is found to be tachypneic and tachycardic, and her breath has a fruity smell. She is treated for diabetic ketoacidosis, and her symptoms begin to improve. However, 4 days after admission she develops a thick nasal discharge and swelling around her left eye (see Figure 3-24). She is treated with antibiotics but fails to improve.

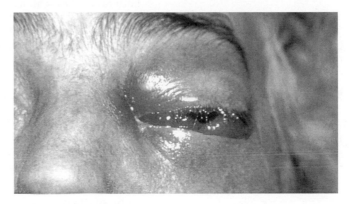

FIGURE 3-24. **Periorbital swelling of the left eye as seen with this infection.** (Reproduced from the Center for Disease Control Public Health Image Library, [http://phil.cdc.gov],)

■ What is the most likely infectious agent responsible for this patient's symptoms?	One of the zygomycetes is most likely responsible. These fungi cause the disease known as zygomycosis or mucormycosis. The clinically significant genera of zygomycetes include *Mucor*, *Rhizopus*, *Rhizomucor*, and *Absidia* species, as well as others less commonly associated with human disease.
■ What does this organism look like at the microscopic level?	The zygomycetes are nonseptate, branching fungi, with wide (>90°) branch angles and large hyphae.
■ What patients are at increased risk of infection with this agent?	Mucormycosis is usually seen in diabetic patients with poor glucose control or those with acidosis, neutropenic patients, burn victims, and patients treated with iron-chelating drugs.
■ How did this organism spread within this patient's body?	The fungi grow along blood vessels, and the presence of the hyphae causes thrombosis and therefore necrosis of the tissue fed by the vessel. The necrotic tissue then serves as nutrient for continued fungal growth. There can be necrotic destruction of the bony walls of the sinuses and the cribiform plate, with spread through the paranasal sinuses and into the orbit as well as into the brain. This is the rhinocephalic form of the infection. Other forms include pulmonary, gastrointestinal, cutaneous, and disseminated.
■ What is the most appropriate management for this condition?	Surgical debridement of infected and necrotic tissue is essential. Reversal of the underlying condition; diabetic acidosis or neutropenia, also improves outcomes. Antifungal therapy with amphotericin B is also employed. Mucormycosis carries a significant mortality even with optimal management.
■ This organism is one of the few that can spread through the cribiform plate and infect the CNS. What is another organism that can spread in this way?	*Naegleria fowleri* is a protozoan that can spread through the cribiform plate. It is acquired from swimming and diving in freshwater lakes. It causes a meningoencephalitis that is typically rapidly fatal and has no effective treatment, though a variety of therapies have shown modest success in isolated cases.

▶ **Case 39**

A 21-year-old man from Guatemala presents to the physician with a 2-day history of painful unilateral testicular swelling. The patient admits to minimal fever and myalgias about a week earlier. Physical examination reveals the parotid glands are swollen and painful. No vaccination history is available, but the patient does not believe that he received any shots when he was younger.

▪ **What is the most likely diagnosis?**	Mumps. In rare instances, the orchitis described above can affect both testes. This can lead to sterility.
▪ **What microorganism causes this condition, and how does it cause illness?**	The mumps virus is a member of the Paramyxoviridae family of single-stranded RNA viruses. The virus has a 2- to 3-week incubation period, after which the infection results in painful enlargement (inflammation and edema) of glandular tissues including the parotid gland, testes, and ovaries.
▪ **What other clinical syndrome can result from infection with this microorganism?**	If the viral infection spreads to the meninges, **aseptic meningitis** may develop. This virus, along with coxsackievirus and echovirus, is one of the three most common causes of aseptic meningitis worldwide. However, as a result of the mumps vaccination program in the United States, coxsackievirus and other enteroviridiae cause substantially more cases of aseptic meningitis than does the mumps virus.
▪ **In what bodily fluids can the virus be detected?**	The virus can be detected in the saliva, serum, urine, or cerebrospinal fluid.
▪ **What is the most appropriate treatment for this condition?**	The treatment is supportive and directed at reducing pain. Analgesics and compression of the parotid gland can be useful. Vaccination with live attenuated mumps virus as part of the measles-mumps-rubella vaccine is used to prevent disease.

An 18-year-old college freshman is brought to the university health center by his dormitory roommate. The patient complains of 2 days of fever, several episodes of vomiting, and joint and muscle pain. His temperature is 38.9°C (102°F). Physical examination reveals nuchal rigidity, a petechial rash on the lower extremities, and photophobia.

■ What is the most likely diagnosis?	*Neisseria meningitidis* meningitis.
■ What test can confirm the diagnosis?	Lumbar puncture would show gram-negative, bean-shaped diplococci, an elevated white blood cell count (with mainly polymorphonuclear cells), decreased glucose levels, and normal to high protein levels.
■ What laboratory test can confirm the pathogen involved?	Culture of meningococcus from cerebrospinal fluid or blood on Thayer-Martin media (chocolate agar with antibiotics to kill competing bacteria) and additional identification procedures can positively identify N. *meningitidis*. N. *meningitidis* is oxidase positive and ferments both maltose and glucose.
■ What are some of the most important virulence factors and toxins of this microorganism?	■ **Pili:** These are thin protrusions from the bacterium that assist in attachment to nasopharyngeal epithelial cells. ■ **IgA protease:** This cleaves lysosome-associated membrane protein 1, which promotes survival within epithelial cells. ■ **Capsule:** The polyanionic polysaccharides that serve as physical protection from host defense factors such as complement and phagocytosis. Serogrouping is possible based on immunochemical differences in the capsule. ■ **Endotoxin:** Lipopolysaccharide in the cell wall of this gram-negative bacterium induces sepsis and hemorrhage. This causes the characteristic petechial rash seen in meningococcemia. ■ No exotoxins!
■ What is the most appropriate treatment for this condition?	Penicillin G or ceftriaxone. Contacts of the index case may be given rifampin as prophylaxis.

▶ **Case 41**

A 35-year-old woman is seen in a clinic in a riverside village in central Africa. She complains of itchy, hyperpigmented skin. She also has several nodules on her hips and legs. Visual testing reveals she has decreased visual acuity of her right eye.

▪ **What is the most likely diagnosis?**	Onchocerciasis (river blindness), which is caused by *Onchocerca volvulus*. This organism is a nematode (roundworm) and is found near rivers.
▪ **How is this organism transmitted, and how does it cause illness?**	The bite of a female black fly transmits larvae (microfilariae) into the host's skin. The larvae become adults, and subsequent fibrosis around the adult worms results in subcutaneous nodules. From within the nodule, mating and release of new larvae can occur. The movement of larvae through subcutaneous tissue induces an inflammatory response.
▪ **What signs and symptoms are associated with this condition?**	Inflammation of subcutaneous tissue causes itching, thickening, and hyperpigmentation of the skin. If the larvae reach the eye, the inflammation can cause blindness.
▪ **What tests can help confirm the diagnosis?**	A skin biopsy reveals larvae. Nodules will contain the adult filaria.
▪ **What are the most appropriate treatments for this condition?**	Ivermectin is effective against the larvae (microfiliariae). The subcutaneous nodules containing adult worms can be surgically removed.

A 30-year-old man presents to the emergency department with complaints of extreme throbbing pain in his right shin, in addition to chills and myalgias. He was previously healthy but underwent surgery to the knee 3 weeks prior. His temperature is 40°C (104°F), blood pressure is 130/80 mm Hg, and heart rate is 80/min. Physical examination reveals that his right leg is red, tender, warm, and swollen over the right anterior tibia just below the knee. X-ray of the extremity demonstrates periosteal elevation and changes consistent with soft tissue swelling adjacent to the tibia. The patient is admitted, and blood and bone biopsy cultures are pending.

■ **What is the most likely diagnosis?**	Osteomyelitis. *Staphylococcus aureus* is responsible for about 90% of pyogenic osteomyelitis. *S. aureus* expresses receptors for the bone matrix, thus allowing it to adhere to bone and produce a focus of infection. Many affected adults have a previous history of a compound fracture or surgery. Children may develop osteomyelitis secondary to hematogenous spread.
■ **If this man has a history of intravenous drug use, which pathogen should be considered?**	Osteomyelitis in the context of intravenous drug use is often caused by *Pseudomonas* infection, but *S. aureus* is still more common in this population.
■ **How does a subperiosteal abscess lead to accelerated bone necrosis?**	A subperiosteal abscess separates the bone from its blood supply in the periosteum, thus leading to ischemic injury and necrosis.
■ **A history of sickle cell disease would place this patient at increased risk of infection from which pathogen?**	Patients with sickle cell disease have an increased risk of developing *Salmonella* osteomyelitis.
■ **What are the typical findings on imaging?**	Periosteal elevation is often found on radiography. This finding, however, can lag behind the onset of the infection by days to weeks.

► **Case 43**

A 4-year-old boy is brought to the pediatrician because of perianal itching, which is worse at night. He attends preschool during the day, where he shares toys and play areas with other children. The patient's mother recalls her son playing with another child who had been "scratching his backside" and wonders if there is a connection.

▪ What is the most likely diagnosis?	Pinworm infection caused by *Enterobius vermicularis*, a nematode (roundworm).
▪ How is this organism transmitted, and how does it cause illness?	Fecal-oral transmission allows eggs to hatch in the small intestine. Adults mature in the ileum and large intestine and mate in the colon. Females exit the rectum at night to lay eggs in the perianal area.
▪ What symptom is commonly associated with this condition?	Perianal itching is the primary symptom. It is often worst at night, when the worm exits the anus to lay its eggs.
▪ What test can help confirm the diagnosis?	**Scotch tape test:** The physician places adhesive tape over the perianal area and then removes and examines the tape. The presence of eggs under light microscopy is indicative of pinworm infection (see Figure 3-25).
▪ What are the most appropriate treatments for this condition?	Mebendazole or albendazole is first-line therapy. Pyrantel pamoate can also be helpful.

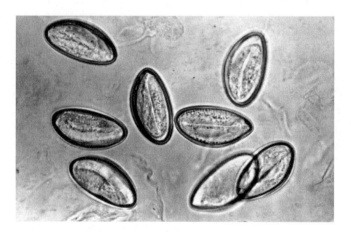

FIGURE 3-25. **Eggs acquired from the perianal area of an infected individual.** (Reproduced from the Center for Disease Control Public Health Image Library, [http://phil.cdc.gov].)

▶ **Case 44**

A 52-year-old woman with acquired immunodeficiency syndrome (AIDS) presents to her physician with difficulty breathing. She has experienced slowly worsening dry cough and dyspnea for about 1 week prior to presentation. Her most recent CD4⁺ T-cell count is 175 cells/μL. In the office, her oxygen saturation is 92%. The patient relates that she is not currently taking any medications because she is "tired of taking pills."

▪ What is the most likely diagnosis?	*Pneumocystis jiroveci* (formerly *carinii*) pneumonia. *P. jiroveci* causes interstitial pneumonia in certain patient populations. Once thought to be a protozoan, it is now recognized to be a fungus (yeast).
▪ What patients are most at risk for developing clinical infection with this microorganism?	Most individuals are exposed to *P. jiroveci* during childhood, but develop no symptoms. However, immunocompromised patients (including patients with AIDS who have low CD4⁺ cell counts) and malnourished infants may develop severe clinical disease. *Pneumocystis* pneumonia in steroid-treated immunocompromised patients is most often seen as steroids are being withdrawn.
▪ What are the likely findings on x-ray of the chest?	"Ground-glass" bilateral infiltrates are commonly seen on x-ray of the chest (see Figure 3-26). In these patients, hypoxia (characterized by decreased arterial oxygen pressure) is often out of proportion to the radiographic findings.
▪ What tests can help confirm the diagnosis?	Sputum samples, bronchoalveolar lavage, or lung biopsy treated with **silver stain** will demonstrate cysts and dark oval bodies contained within the cyst (**sporozoites**).
▪ What is the most appropriate treatment for this condition?	Treatment is with trimethoprim-sulfamethoxazole, pentamidine, or clindamycin-primaquine. In immunocompromised patients, trimethoprim-sulfamethoxazole or dapsone may be used as prophylaxis when CD4⁺ cell counts fall below 200 cells/μL. In severely ill patients (HIV patients with severe PCP as defined by a room air arterial oxygen pressure <70 mm Hg or arterial-alveolar O_2 gradient >35 mm Hg), steroids should be given as adjunctive therapy to prevent worsening respiratory status due to the inflammatory response induced by treatment.

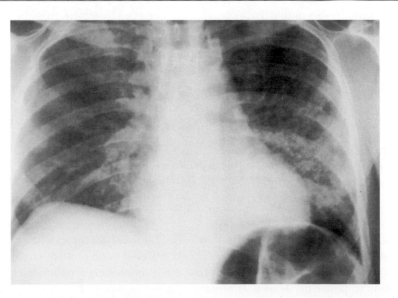

FIGURE 3-26. *Pneumocystis jiroveci* **pneumonia.** (Reproduced, with permission, from Kasper DL, Braunwald E, Fauci AS, Hauser SL, Longo DL, Jameson LJ, Isselbacher KJ [eds]. *Harrison's Principles of Internal Medicine*, 16th ed. New York: McGraw-Hill, 2005: 1195.)

▶ **Case 45**

A 20-year-old woman returns from a day hike in a densely wooded area and develops a rash that evening. The next day she presents to her physician. The patient has never had a similar rash, and the area is one that she has hiked in several times before. Physical examination reveals that the rash (see Figure 3-27) is mostly on the legs, arms, and hands, areas the patient says "were not covered by clothing." The patient has no significant past medical history. She is afebrile.

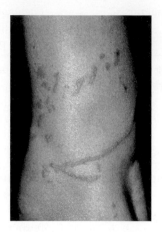

FIGURE 3-27. (Reproduced, with permission, from Wolff K, Johnson RA, Suurmond D. *Fitzpatrick's Color Atlas & Synopsis of Clinical Dermatology*, 5th ed. New York: McGraw-Hill, 2005: 29.)

■ What is the most likely diagnosis?	Poison ivy. This rash is characterized by vesicles, fluid-filled domes <5 mm in diameter. The leaves of poison ivy brush across the skin in a linear path; thus, the typical poison ivy rash consists of lines of vesicles, as seen in the image shown.
■ What are the four types of hypersensitivity reactions?	■ **Type I:** Anaphylactic and atopic ■ **Type II:** Cytotoxic ■ **Type III:** Immune complex/serum sickness/Arthus reaction ■ **Type IV:** Delayed/cell-mediated
■ Which type of hypersensitivity reaction is occurring in this patient?	Type IV hypersensitivity (delayed or cell-mediated) includes contact hypersensitivity from poison ivy, transplant rejection, hypersensitivity pneumonitis, granulomatous hypersensitivity reactions, and the tuberculosis skin test. Type IV reactions are also important in the control of mycobacterial and fungal infections.
■ Which cells mediate the immune response in this condition?	**Type 1 T-helper cells** and **CD8+** cytotoxic T cells are the mediators of this immune response.
■ Why is this rash occurring now, when she has hiked the area several times previously without developing this rash?	A key feature of type IV hypersensitivity is that the patient must be sensitized to the antigen prior to development of hypersensitivity on subsequent exposure. The tuberculin skin test, another example of type IV hypersensitivity, relies on the principle of prior sensitization to assess for previous exposure to tuberculosis.
■ The oil that causes the skin reaction in this patient's condition (urushiol or pentadecacatechol) can bind to antibodies, but cannot elicit an adaptive immune response on its own. It must be linked to a protein to elicit an adaptive immune response. What term describes this type of molecule?	A **hapten** is a small molecule that is not immunogenic by itself, but can become so when attached to a carrier protein. Only proteins and protein-bound substances can be presented on the major histocompatibility complexes.

A 27-year-old graduate student who recently returned from working in sub-Saharan Africa presents to the clinic complaining of paralysis of his lower extremities. He says he had a mild fever about 2 weeks previously, then several days ago the fever recurred and he experienced nuchal rigidity followed by paralysis of both legs. The student was not born in the United States and his vaccination history is unknown. Physical examination demonstrates 0/5 strength and hyporeflexia (without sensory loss) of the lower extremities.

■ **What is the most likely diagnosis?**	Poliovirus can cause subclinical infection, aseptic meningitis, or poliomyelitis. **Poliomyelitis** results in the classic flaccid paralysis secondary to destruction of anterior horn cells of the spinal cord.
■ **Of which family is this infectious agent a member?**	Poliovirus is a member of the Picornavirus family. Other members include the enteroviruses, rhinovirus, coxsackievirus, and hepatitis A virus.
■ **Describe the morphology of this microorganism.**	Poliovirus is a single-stranded, positive-sense RNA virus. Its coat has icosahedral symmetry, and it is not enveloped.
■ **How is this condition transmitted?**	Poliovirus is spread by the fecal-oral route. The virus can attach to and infect host cells in the pharynx and ileum. It can then disseminate hematogenously to lymphoid tissue during a primary "minor" viremia, which is typically asymptomatic. In a minority of patients, there is a secondary or "major" viremia that is likely responsible for allowing spread of the virus to the central nervous system (CNS). During the second viremia patients experience mild symptoms and low-grade fever. Subsequent CNS disease typically occurs 11 to 17 days after exposure.
■ **What treatments are available to prevent this condition, and how do they differ?**	■ **Salk vaccine:** Formalin-killed virus leads to an IgG response. This is the form used in the United States. ■ **Sabin vaccine:** Oral attenuated poliovirus leads to an IgG response as well as an IgA response in the gastrointestinal tract. This vaccine should not be given to immunocompromised individuals.

GENERAL PRINCIPLES

MICROBIOLOGY & IMMUNOLOGY

▶ **Case 47**

An 18-year-old man with cystic fibrosis and a history of multiple respiratory infections is brought to the emergency department after recent onset of cough productive of purulent sputum, dyspnea, and chills. His mother reports he has been lethargic, and recorded his temperature at 39°C (102.2°F). Physical examination reveals a poorly responsive man in moderate respiratory distress. Laboratory studies are notable for a white blood cell count of 17,000/mm^3, with a left shift on the differential. Sputum culture yields gram-negative, non–lactose-fermenting bacilli.

■ **What is the most likely diagnosis?**

Pseudomonas aeruginosa infection. This bacterium is an opportunistic pathogen and causes infection in patients with impaired defense mechanisms, especially immunocompromised individuals and burn victims. It commonly lives in water or wet environments and can be particularly problematic for patients on ventilators. Additionally, it is a major cause of respiratory failure in patients with cystic fibrosis.

■ **What are some common consequences of infection with this microorganism?**

Community-acquired infections:
■ Otitis externa ("swimmer's ear")
■ Endocarditis (in intravenous drug users)
■ Osteomyelitis
■ Pneumonia (especially in patients with human immunodeficiency virus infection or cystic fibrosis)

Nosocomial *Pseudomonas* infections:
■ Bacteremia in neutropenic patients
■ Burn sepsis
■ Neonatal sepsis
■ Lung infection associated with ventilator use
■ Urinary tract infection from indwelling Foley catheters

■ **What is the pathology of chronic respiratory infection with this microorganism in patients with cystic fibrosis?**

Pseudomonas can colonize the lungs of patients with cystic fibrosis. The patient's immune response causes a chronic inflammatory state that eventually results in progressive loss of pulmonary function.

■ **What virulence factors contribute to acute infection with this microorganism?**

Pseudomonas has a host of virulence factors that contribute to pathology in acute infection. These include pili and a flagellum for host invasion; lipopolysaccharide (endotoxin); exotoxins A, S, and U; elastase; and various cytotoxins.

■ **What are the most appropriate treatments for this condition?**

Pseudomonas is frequently resistant to multiple drug regimens, so therapy guided by antimicrobial susceptibility testing is essential. In addition to its intrinsic resistance to many antibiotics, it is able to acquire resistance rapidly during treatment. Potentially useful antibiotics include ceftazidime, cefepime, ciprofloxacin, aztreonam, imipenem, piperacillin-tazobactam, and the aminoglycosides. These drugs are usually employed in combinations of two drugs of different classes. Topical (e.g., inhaled) as well as systemic antibiotic therapy is employed in CF patients. Colistin is a drug of last resort for severe cases of multidrug-resistant *Pseudomonas* infection.

A 15-year-old boy is camping with his family in the Adirondack Mountains when he is bitten on the leg by a raccoon. His family cuts the vacation short and brings the boy to the nearest emergency department.

■ **What condition is this boy at risk of contracting?**	Rabies. If left untreated, rabies results in a nearly 100% mortality rate. It causes, at most, a few deaths per year in the United States, but is a much bigger concern in countries with unvaccinated animals. (In India, rabies-infected dog bites cause tens of thousands of deaths each year.)
■ **What microorganism is the cause of this condition, and what are its characteristics?**	Rhabdoviridae are single-stranded RNA viruses enveloped by a bullet-shaped capsid, which is covered by glycoprotein "spikes." The spikes bind to acetylcholine receptors, a property that may contribute to virulence.
■ **How is this microorganism transmitted, and how does it cause illness?**	Animals transfer the virus to humans via bites. The virus remains local for a period of days to months, then binds to acetylcholine receptors on neurons and travels to the central nervous system (CNS). In the CNS, the virus infects neurons, including Ammon's horn cells of the hippocampus. Rabies carries a significant person-to-person transmission risk via bites or mucous membrane exposure. Immunoprophylaxis is indicated for close contacts of infected patients.
■ **What signs and symptoms are commonly associated with this condition?**	Spasms of the pharyngeal muscles cause dysphagia, which leads to painful swallowing and hydrophobia. There is also excess autonomic stimulation that can cause hypersalivation. The buildup of saliva accounts for the apparent "foaming at the mouth." As rabies travels via axons to various organs and multiplies in the CNS, many symptoms result: confusion, agitation, hallucinations, sensitivity to bright light, and focal neurologic deficits such as cranial nerve palsies. Encephalitis can give rise to seizures and eventually leads to coma, then death.
■ **How is the condition diagnosed, and what kinds of treatment are available?**	Identification of cytoplasmic inclusions called **Negri bodies** in infected cells, polymerase chain reaction for viral RNA, and serology are diagnostic. Treatment includes washing the wound and administering **human diploid cell vaccine**, a live, attenuated virus that is used after a bite. **Human rabies immune globulin** is used to confer passive immunity, and immunization of domesticated animals is used to prevent the disease. Unfortunately, once symptoms appear, there is no effective treatment.

▶ **Case 49**

A 30-year-old man who recently joined a gym complains of itching between his toes. Physical examination reveals pustules on the fingers of both hands, and white macerated tissue between the toes (see Figure 3-28). The patient says the pustules have been quite itchy, and appeared about a week after the itching between the toes began.

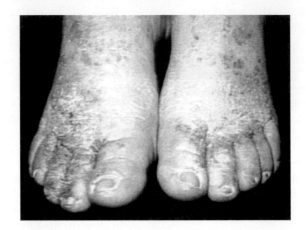

FIGURE 3-28. (Reproduced, with permission, from the Pathology Education Instructional Resource Digital Library [http://peir.net] at the University of Alabama, Birmingham.)

■ **What is the most likely diagnosis?**	Ringworm (tinea pedis) infection. Each dermatophytosis is named after the region of the body that it infects: tinea cruris (perineum and creases of inner thigh; "jock itch"), tinea pedis ("athlete's foot"), tinea capitis (scalp), tinea unguium (nails), and tinea corporis (body).
■ **What are the three microorganisms that are often responsible for this presentation?**	*Microsporum*, *Trichophyton*, and *Epidermophyton* are three filamentous fungi that cause dermatophytosis.
■ **How is the microorganism transmitted, and how does it cause illness?**	After contact with an infected host, the keratinized epithelium of warm, moist skin is colonized. The infection expands radially, and is characterized by curvy (wormlike) circular borders. Thus, it is termed "ringworm," despite the fact that the causative microorganism is actually a fungus.
■ **What tests can help confirm the diagnosis?**	Branched hyphae are observed on potassium hydroxide preparation (**KOH mount**). This fungus is not dimorphic. A sample from the lesions on the patient's feet will likely demonstrate the organism.
■ **What is the most appropriate treatment for this condition?**	Topical azoles (e.g., fluconazole), butenafine, terbinafine, or griseofulvin are used for treatment.

► **Case 50**

A 4-year-old boy, who had been camping in the Appalachians with his family, was brought to the emergency department because of a headache, rash, and the abrupt onset of a high fever. The rash had begun on his palms and soles, but had spread up his ankles and arms (see Figure 3-29). On examination he was found to have palpable purpura on his wrists and lower legs.

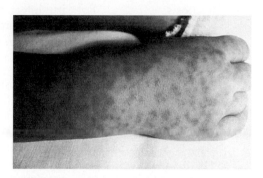

FIGURE 3-29. Rash on the right hand and wrist in a patient with this infection. (Reproduced from the Center for Disease Control Public Health Image Library, [http://phil.cdc.gov].)

■ **What infections frequently give rise to a rash on the palms and soles?**	Infections with *Rickettsia rickettsii*, *Treponema pallidum*, and coxsackievirus A can all cause a rash in this distribution.
■ **What is the most likely infectious agent in this case?**	This patient is most likely infected with *R. rickettsii*. The clinical course is typical for Rocky Mountain spotted fever (RMSF). It is characterized by fever with abrupt onset, and a rash that spreads from the extremities toward the trunk. Palpable purpura is a poor prognostic sign, as it indicates active vasculitis and leakage of blood into the skin. The rash in syphilis and coxsackievirus is typically more gradual in onset.
■ **How is this pathogen transmitted to humans?**	*R. rickettsii* is acquired from *Dermacentor* tick bites.
■ **What other bacteria are in the same class as the one infecting this patient?**	Other rickettsial organisms and the diseases they cause include: ■ *Rickettsia typhi*: Endemic typhus ■ *Rickettsia prowazekii*: Epidemic typhus ■ *Rickettsia akari*: Rickettsial pox ■ *Bartonella henselae*: Cat scratch fever ■ *Ehrlichia chaffeensis*: Human monocytic ehrlichiosis ■ *Anaplasma phagocytophila*: Human granulocytic anaplasmosis ■ *Coxiella burnetii*: Q fever (*Coxiella* is unusual in that it is acquired through inhalation rather than through an arthropod vector.)
■ **What laboratory technique can be used to identify the cause of this patient's illness?**	Direct fluorescent antibody or PCR testing of a skin biopsy of one of the petechial lesions is the test of choice, but is performed only in reference laboratories and may not be available rapidly enough to guide clinical decision-making. RMSF antibody testing can be used to confirm the diagnosis after recovery.
■ **What is the treatment of choice for organisms of this class?**	Tetracyclines are most frequently used in rickettsial infections. *Rickettsia* are obligate intracellular organisms, as they require coenzyme A (CoA) and nicotinamide adenine dinucleotide (NAD) from the host cell; they also lack the peptidoglycan cell wall targeted by many antibiotic classes. Tetracyclines can enter cells and act on ribosomal targets.

► **Case 51**

In the month of January, a 2-year-old girl is brought to her pediatrician by her parents because of a 3-day history of watery, nonbloody diarrhea, nausea, vomiting, and abdominal pain. Physical examination reveals the child is slightly tachycardic, with sunken eyes and poor skin turgor.

▪ **What is the most likely diagnosis?**	Rotavirus infection is the most common infectious cause of diarrhea in infants and young children, and it is a major cause of acute diarrhea in the United States during the winter. It is also the most important cause of gastroenteritis in infants globally.
▪ **How does the infectious agent cause illness?**	Rotavirus is transmitted via the fecal-oral route and infects villus cells of the proximal small intestine. The virus replicates intracellularly and eventually causes host cell lysis. Cell destruction results in decreased absorption from the intestinal lumen, thus causing watery diarrhea. Rotavirus does not cause inflammation, so the stool is nonbloody.
▪ **What are the defining structural features of this class of organisms?**	Rotavirus belongs to the Reoviridae family, which also contains the reoviruses and orbiviruses. These nonenveloped (naked) viruses are the only RNA viruses that are double stranded (think: "repeato"-viridae). The viruses contain 10 or 11 segments of dsRNA, allowing for frequent gene reassortment.
▪ **How is this condition diagnosed and treated?**	Viral antigens can be detected by enzyme-linked immunosorbent assay (ELISA) of a stool specimen. Treatment is supportive via rehydration.
▪ **In what age group is this condition usually seen?**	Infection is not commonly seen before 6 months of age, as the child has passive immunity from IgA passed from the mother's breast milk. By age 3 years, most individuals worldwide have developed lifelong immunity from prior infection. Therefore, it is most common between these two ages.

► **Case 52**

A 21-year-old woman presents to the clinic with fever, hives, headache, weight loss, and cough. She reports doing field research in Egypt with a professor from her university over the summer. When the patient is asked about previous fresh water exposure, she recalls an intense itching reaction within minutes of wading into a river while she was in Africa. Physical examination reveals lymphadenopathy and hepatosplenomegaly.

■ **What is the most likely diagnosis?**	Schistosomiasis, caused by a type of trematode (fluke), likely acquired from contact with contaminated water. The three main flukes are *Schistosoma japonicum* (in East Asia), *S. mansoni* (in South America and Africa), and *S. haematobium* (in Africa).
■ **What is the intermediate host of this organism, and what are the reservoirs?**	Snails are the intermediate host for all trematodes. Reservoirs include primates (*S. mansoni* and *S. haematobium*) and domesticated animals (*S. japonicum*).
■ **In which human organs are the organisms found?**	*S. japonicum* and *S. mansoni* reside in the intestines, where organisms mate in the mesenteric veins and release eggs into the feces as well as the portal circulation. *S. haematobium* resides in the bladder, where organisms mate in the vesicular (bladder) veins and release eggs into the urine.
■ **How is this condition diagnosed?**	Examination of the urine (*S. haematobium*) and stool (all three species), or rectal biopsy, will reveal eggs.
■ **What are the acute and chronic manifestations of this condition?**	An immediate manifestation of schistosomiasis is **swimmer's itch**, a dermatitis that occurs as the organism initially penetrates the skin. Manifestations 4–8 weeks after infection include **Katayama fever**, which occurs as the adult organisms lay eggs. Chronic manifestations include granulomas, fibrosis, and inflammation at the sites of egg deposition. For example, eggs that pass into the portal system become foci for granulomatous inflammation of the liver, eventually leading to fibrosis. Complications include portal hypertension (*S. japonicum* and *S. mansoni*), pulmonary artery hypertension, chronic abdominal pain, and central nervous system injury. *S. haematobium* can increase the risk for developing squamous cell bladder cancer.
■ **What is the most appropriate treatment for this condition?**	Praziquantel is the treatment of choice.

► **Case 53**

A 9-year-old boy is brought to the emergency department with a 5-day history of abdominal pain and diarrhea. One day prior to admission he noticed that his stool appeared bloody. He is admitted to the hospital for intravenous fluid replacement and further workup. His stool is found to be positive for Shiga-like toxin. After 4 days his abdominal pain begins to subside but he notices that his urine is grossly bloody. A blood smear is shown in Figure 3-30A. A biopsy of his kidney is shown in Figure 3-30B.

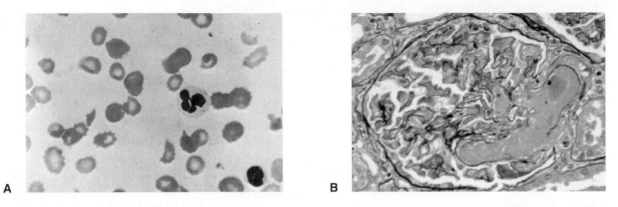

A   B

FIGURE 3-30. **A. Peripheral blood smear showing fragmented red blood cells. B. Biopsy of the kidney, showing fibrin thrombi within the glomerular vessels typical of patients with this syndrome.** (Figure A reproduced, with permission, from Lichtman MA, Beutler E, Kipps TJ, Seligsohn U, Kaushansky K, Prchal JT. *Williams Hematology*, 7th ed. New York: McGraw-Hill, 2006: Figure 35-2.; Figure B reproduced, with permission, from Fauci AS, Kasper DL, Braunwald E, Hauser SL, Longo DL, Jameson JL, Loscalzo J [eds.]. *Harrison's Principles of Internal Medicine*, 17th ed. New York: McGraw-Hill, 2008: Figure e9-21.)

■ What is the most likely causative organism?	Enterohemorrhagic *Escherichia coli* (EHEC) serotype O157:H7. Infection with this organism most commonly occurs through consumption of undercooked meat or contaminated vegetables.
■ What is the mechanism of action of Shiga toxin and Shiga-like toxin?	These toxins are very similar. One is produced by *Shigella* and the other by *E. coli* O157:H7. They act by binding to host ribosomes and cleaving a particular glycosidic bond. This inhibits ribosome function. The reduction in cellular translation triggers events that lead to apoptosis.
■ What is the cause of the blood in the patient's urine?	The patient has developed hemolytic-uremic syndrome (HUS). This is a complication of infection with *Shigella* and EHEC in which the toxin damages the renal vascular endothelium, compromising vascular integrity.
■ What is the classic triad of findings associated with this condition?	In HUS the triad of findings includes: renal damage, hemolytic anemia, and thrombocytopenia.
■ What are the most likely findings on a peripheral blood smear?	Damage to the renal blood vessels leads to microangiopathic hemolysis of the RBCs, leaving schistocytes, which are fragmented and distorted RBCs. HUS has a presentation similar to that of thrombotic thrombocytopenic purpura.
■ What serum markers should be measured to follow the progression or recovery of this patient?	The platelet count is a useful marker for this syndrome. In addition, the blood urea nitrogen and creatinine levels should be measured to follow renal recovery. The hemoglobin and hematocrit should be followed to assess the need for transfusion.

▶ **Case 54**

A 59-year-old woman complains of fatigue and a "burning" pain on her scalp for the previous 2 days. Her temperature is 38°C (100.4°F). Physical examination indicates her pain is localized to the left parietal-occipital scalp, and extends down to include the skin of the left side of her neck. She denies any recent rash in the area, headaches, mental status changes, or recent infections.

■ Which sensory nerve root is implicated in this patient's condition?	Nerves from the right C2 root innervate the parietal-occipital scalp. C3 innervates the neck, and C4 innervates the superior surface of the shoulder.
■ What infectious agent may be responsible for this woman's pain?	This woman is suffering from herpes zoster, or "shingles," a late complication of prior infection with varicella zoster-virus (VZV), one of the herpesviruses.
■ What laboratory test can be used to detect the presence of the suspected pathogen's genome in a sample?	Polymerase chain reaction (PCR) can be used to amplify and aid in the detection of viral nucleic acid (double-stranded DNA in the case of herpesviruses). Key steps in PCR include: 1. **Denaturing** the DNA with heat to separate complementary paired strands. 2. Cooling to allow DNA primers to **anneal** to denatured strands of DNA. 3. Extending the DNA sequence from the DNA primers by heat-stable **DNA polymerase**. 4. Repeating steps 1–3 to achieve the desired level of amplification. In addition to molecular testing, direct fluorescent antibody testing (DFA) can be used to detect VZV antigen in skin lesions.
■ Four days later, the patient develops an erythematous vesicular rash in the same area (see Figure 3-31). What are the likely findings on histologic examination of these vesicles?	A **Tzanck smear** may demonstrate multinucleate giant cells, which are typical for infection with varicella and herpes simplex viruses. This test is rarely used for diagnosis, having been superseded by more specific DFA and molecular tests.

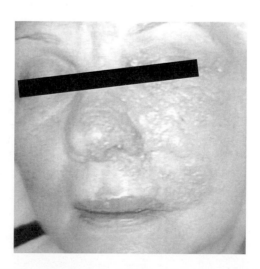

FIGURE 3-31. Shingles. (Reproduced, with permission, from the Pathology Education Instructional Resource Digital Library [http://peir.net] at the University of Alabama, Birmingham.)

- **What are the most appropriate treatments for this condition?**

  Acyclovir is activated by viral thymidine kinase to inhibit viral DNA polymerase. Valacyclovir and famciclovir have a similar mechanism and longer half-lives. These drugs target herpesviruses and may provide relief, speed recovery, and prevent postherpetic neuralgia.

- **What type of vaccine is the varicella vaccine, and what branches of the immune system does it stimulate?**

  A live attenuated vaccine is used for prevention of initial varicella infection (chickenpox). Live attenuated vaccines induce both humoral and cell-mediated immunity.

A 36-year-old woman from Georgia presents with abdominal pain and diarrhea of 3 days' duration. She does not complain of nausea, vomiting, or fever. She has no sick contacts or significant travel history. A complete blood count is performed, and results are normal except for elevated eosinophils at 13%. A stool sample is obtained, which reveals larvae. Further questioning reveals that the woman frequently gardens in her backyard while barefoot.

■ **What is the most likely diagnosis?**	Strongyloidiasis, caused by *Strongyloides stercoralis*, a nematode (roundworm).
■ **How is this agent transmitted, and how does it cause illness?**	Larvae in the soil penetrate the skin, usually the sole of the foot (fecal-cutaneous transmission). Local itching at the entry site promotes scratching, which aids larval entry into the bloodstream. Once in the blood, the larvae settle in the respiratory tree and can make their way up the trachea into the pharynx to be swallowed. They enter the small intestine, where the larvae mature into adults. Female adults invade the intestinal wall and lay eggs. During passage through the gastrointestinal tract, the eggs hatch into larvae. Most of these larvae pass with the stool and can continue the life cycle in the soil; some, however, directly penetrate the colonic wall or perianal skin and continue the life cycle within the original host. These continually migrating parasites are responsible for the eosinophilia commonly seen in chronic *Strongyloides* infections.
■ **What other two organisms demonstrate the same route of transmission in humans?**	*Necator americanus* (New World hookworm), and *Ancylostoma duodenale* (Old World hookworm).
■ **What signs and symptoms are commonly associated with this condition?**	Disease can range from asymptomatic to mild pneumonitis, to gastroenteritis with malabsorption. Infection/inflammation in the intestinal wall causes pain and diarrhea. Exit of feces in diarrhea facilitates release of larvae into the soil/environment. The **hyperinfection syndrome**, caused by uncontrolled autoinfection, can result in increased parasitic burden and widely disseminated disease. This is more common in individuals with defective eosinophil function, such as patients treated with steroids or cytotoxic chemotherapeutic agents that cause granulocytopenia.
■ **What tests can help confirm the diagnosis?**	A stool sample would reveal larvae (not eggs as in hookworm infection). Blood samples will reveal eosinophilia. *Strongyloides* antibody testing can also be valuable in patients with unexplained eosinophilia, as larvae are not always detectable in the stool.
■ **What are the most appropriate treatments for this condition?**	Ivermectin or thiabendazole.

A 52-year-old man from Ohio presents with worsening cough, fever, chills, and pleuritic chest pain. He has also noted multiple ulcerated sores on his skin, which began as pimple-like lesions. X-ray of the chest reveals segmental consolidation. Biopsy of a skin lesion reveals big, broad-based, budding yeasts.

■ What is the most likely diagnosis?	Blastomycosis, one of the systemic mycoses.
■ To what areas are the systemic mycoses endemic?	■ **Coccidioidomycosis** (also called desert bumps, San Joaquin Valley bumps, or "valley fever") is specific to the southwestern United States. ■ **Histoplasmosis** is endemic to the Mississippi and Ohio River valleys, and is found in bird and bat droppings. ■ **Blastomycosis** is found east of the Mississippi River (and in Central America). ■ **Paracoccidioidomycosis** is found in rural Latin America.
■ What tests can help confirm the diagnosis?	Culture on **Sabouraud's agar** at multiple temperatures. Systemic mycoses are caused by dimorphic fungi, which grow as mold in the cold (e.g., in the soil) and as yeast at higher temperatures (e.g., in tissues at 37°C). The exception is coccidioidomycosis, which is a spherule in tissue. In addition, a tissue biopsy revealing broad-based budding yeast is diagnostic for blastomycosis. Tissue biopsy demonstrating yeast cells within macrophages is diagnostic of histoplasmosis. A biopsy showing "captain's wheel" morphology of budding yeast is diagnostic of paracoccidioidomycosis. Serologic testing for antifungal antibodies is also useful in some patients, and a histoplasma antigen test is the diagnostic test of choice for systemic (but not localized) *Histoplasma* infections.
■ What are the typical findings on x-ray of the chest?	These diseases can mimic tuberculosis, forming **granulomas**, which appear as small calcium deposits on x-ray films.
■ What is the most appropriate treatment for this condition?	Systemic infection is treated with itraconazole or amphotericin B.

► Case 57

A 13-year-old girl is brought into the physician's office by her mother. Her mother says the girl had a sudden onset of fever, with a temperature of 39.4°C (103°F), lightheadedness, nausea, vomiting, and watery diarrhea. Physical examination reveals a desquamating rash of her palms and soles. She has no sick contacts, and there is no evidence of ingestion of unsafe food. Upon questioning, the patient says she began menstruating a little over a month ago.

■ What is the most likely diagnosis?	Toxic shock syndrome (TSS).
■ What microorganism is the most likely cause of this condition?	*Staphylococcus aureus* is the most common cause, although β-hemolytic group A streptococci can cause a similar presentation. The most common nidi of infection are tampons and cutaneous wounds.
■ What are the distinguishing characteristics of the responsible microorganism?	*S. aureus* is a gram-positive coccus. It is catalase- and coagulase-positive, and produces an enterotoxin. Figure 3-32 shows a useful laboratory algorithm for differentiating the gram-positive bacteria.

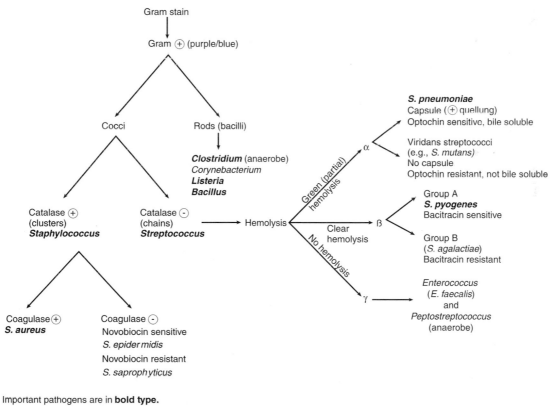

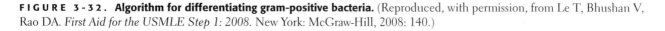

FIGURE 3-32. Algorithm for differentiating gram-positive bacteria. (Reproduced, with permission, from Le T, Bhushan V, Rao DA. *First Aid for the USMLE Step 1: 2008*. New York: McGraw-Hill, 2008: 140.)

■ **What is the pathophysiology of this condition?**	The exotoxin (TSST-1) acts as a "superantigen" and is responsible for this presentation. Superantigens activate large numbers of T cells at once by simultaneously binding directly to T-cell receptors and major histocompatibility complex (MHC) molecules, regardless of the peptide presented by MHC. Activated T cells then release large amounts of inflammatory cytokines, which are responsible for the manifestations of TSS.
■ **What other conditions should be considered in the differential diagnosis?**	■ Gram-negative sepsis (rare in healthy, nonhospitalized individuals) ■ Meningococcemia (associated with petechial rash) ■ Pneumococcal sepsis ■ Rocky Mountain spotted fever (associated with rash on palms and soles) ■ Staphylococcal scalded skin syndrome ■ Streptococcal scarlet fever ■ An allergic drug reaction
■ **What is the most appropriate treatment for this condition?**	Removal of the infected wound dressing or tampon is the first step, followed by supportive care. Antibiotics that cover both *Staphylococcus* and *Streptococcus* will kill these bacteria and stop the production of additional exotoxin. However, it is the toxin, not the bacteria, that is responsible for the symptoms. In severe cases, intravenous immunoglobulin is also given.

A 54-year-old man with human immunodeficiency virus (HIV) infection presents to the emergency department after suffering a grand mal seizure. He has no known personal or family history of seizures. He is afebrile and his vital signs are stable. Funduscopic examination reveals yellow cotton-like lesions on his retina. Findings on physical examination are otherwise unremarkable. A CT scan of the head demonstrates multiple ring-enhancing lesions in the cerebral cortex. Laboratory studies reveal a CD4+ cell count of 53 cells/μL.

■ What is the most likely cause of this patient's seizure?	*Toxoplasma gondii* infection.
■ How did this patient likely become infected with this microorganism?	It is likely that this man (like many individuals) has been latently infected with this protozoan for many years. However, his immunocompromised status has resulted in disease reactivation. Humans are most often infected by ingestion of cysts in undercooked meat, or by ingestion of food contaminated by cat feces.
■ In what other patient population is infection with this microorganism particularly dangerous?	Primary infection with *T. gondii* in a pregnant woman can result in parasites crossing the placenta. This leads to congenital problems in the newborn, including mental retardation, microcephaly, chorioretinitis, intracerebral calcifications, and blindness. It is one of the **TORCH** infections (**T**oxoplasmosis, **O**ther infections, **R**ubella, **C**ytomegalovirus, and **H**erpes simplex virus).
■ Given this patient's ring-enhancing lesions on CT, what other conditions should be included in the differential diagnosis?	This patient is also at an increased risk of lymphoma, cryptococcosis, and tuberculosis, all of which appear as ring-enhancing lesions on CT and can also cause seizures.
■ What is the most appropriate treatment for this condition?	First-line treatment is a regimen of pyrimethamine and sulfadiazine.

A 55-year-old male with end-stage renal disease is scheduled to undergo a kidney transplant operation.

■ **What tests should be performed prior to transplantation in order to prevent hyperacute rejection?**	Hyperacute rejection occurs within minutes of the transplant. It is due to preformed antibodies that recognize graft antigens. The patient's serum should be tested for antibodies that bind to a biopsy of the graft tissue.
■ **What histology would be evident on a kidney that had undergone hyperacute rejection?**	The kidney would show fibrinoid necrosis of the small vessels and thromboses.
■ **Acute rejection can occur from days to months after the operation. What is the immunologic mechanism of acute rejection?**	There are two mechanisms that can give rise to acute rejection. Host T cells can infiltrate the grafted organ and bind to donor major histocompatibility complex (MHC) surface proteins. They become activated and mount an immune response against the foreign tissue. Alternatively, donor antigen-presenting cells can migrate to the host lymph nodes and activate host T cells through the interaction between host T-cell receptors and graft MHC protein with a bound peptide.
■ **What histology would be evident in a kidney that had undergone acute rejection?**	Acute rejection is primarily cell mediated, although antibodies can also cause damage to graft tissue. A biopsy would reveal T-cell and macrophage infiltrates as well as blood vessel and parenchymal damage.
■ **This patient's transplant operation was successful, and he was maintained on immunosuppressive therapy with no major complications until 3 years later when his blood urea nitrogen and creatinine levels began to rise. What is the likely diagnosis?**	Chronic rejection is characterized by vascular damage. Damage to graft blood vessels can be due to antibody binding, complement activation, T-cell activation, and cytokines. The result is intimal proliferation, causing narrowing of the vessel lumen and tissue ischemia. Examination of the graft would show a small, scarred kidney.
■ **Patients who undergo bone marrow or hematopoietic cell transplantation are at risk of another potential complication, graft-versus-host disease (GVHD). What is the mechanism of GVHD, and what organs are affected most frequently?**	GVHD can occur when grafted T cells bind to host antigen and become activated. They can then cause damage to host tissue. The most frequent sites of injury are the skin, the liver, and the gastrointestinal tract.

A man visiting rural Argentina develops fever, headache, pain in his knees and back, and nausea and vomiting. After 3 days these symptoms resolve, and the man decides not to seek medical help. However, 2 days later, the symptoms return, and he develops epigastric pain and yellowing of his skin, and his vomitus becomes dark in color.

■ **What is the most likely diagnosis?**	Yellow fever, which is endemic in South America and parts of Africa. It is characterized by an initial febrile illness, during which time serum aspartate aminotransferase and alanine aminotransferase levels may begin to rise, followed by a remission of symptoms. About 15% of those infected will experience a return of symptoms 2–3 days later, developing further liver dysfunction (resulting in jaundice and coagulopathy), renal damage, and myocardial damage.
■ **What other infectious agents are in the same family as the one responsible for this patient's illness?**	The yellow fever virus is a Flavivirus, a family that also includes the following: ■ Dengue fever virus ■ St. Louis encephalitis virus ■ Japanese encephalitis virus ■ Hepatitis C virus ■ West Nile virus These viruses have positive, single-stranded RNA genomes in icosahedral, enveloped capsids.
■ **How do viruses with this type of genome replicate?**	Viruses with positive-stranded RNA genomes have genetic material that can be directly translated by the host ribosomes. Thus, after the viral particle contacts the surface of the host cell, enters the cell by endocytosis, and uncoats, the RNA is translated into structural proteins, and non-structural proteins, including an RNA-dependent RNA polymerase (RdRp). A (–) sense RNA transcript is made by the RdRp, using the (+) strand genome as a template. More (+) strand copies are then made using the (–) sense strand as a template. The newly synthesized (+) sense RNA can be used to translate more viral proteins, and can be packaged within virions as the viral genome. Once the virions are assembled, they are released and can infect other cells.
■ **What are the most likely findings on liver biopsy?**	The characteristic finding on liver biopsy is midzone hepatocellular death, with sparing of cells bordering the central vein and portal tracts. **Councilman bodies** are found in the affected hepatocytes. These are eosinophilic inclusions that represent condensed chromatin. Typically, there is no inflammatory response. Liver biopsies are usually not done in patients because of their concomitant coagulopathy.
■ **Enzyme-linked immunosorbent assay (ELISA) may be useful in confirming the diagnosis by detecting antibody to the virus. How does ELISA work?**	ELISA is a technique often used for serologic testing. It involves the coating of a surface with the desired antigen (in this case, yellow fever viral particles), then placing the patient's serum on the surface, followed by a secondary antibody (antihuman antibody) that is linked to an enzyme. If the patient's serum has antibody to the antigen, the secondary antibody will bind. The linked enzyme can be detected by a reaction that produces an alteration in color with a colorimetric agent. The color change can be quantified by spectroscopy. Detection of antibody to yellow fever virus in a patient with exposure can support a clinical diagnosis of the disease.

► **Case 61**

A 34-year-old nurse complains to her physician of occasional rust-colored sputum and fever of 6 months' duration. She also notes her clothes fit more loosely than they used to. Her only medication is an oral contraceptive. X-ray of the chest is shown in Figure 3-33.

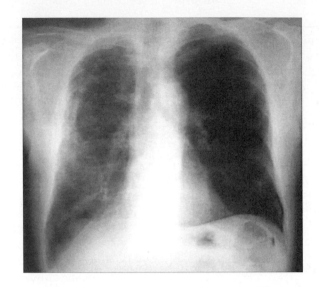

FIGURE 3-33. (Reproduced, with permission, from the Pathology Education Instructional Resource Digital Library [http://peir.net] at the University of Alabama, Birmingham.)

■ What is the most likely diagnosis?	Her symptoms and x-ray of the chest suggest tuberculosis (TB). Associated findings include a positive purified protein derivative (PPD) test, granulomatous inflammation in the upper lobes of the lung, positive culture, and/or positive acid-fast staining of bacteria from sputum samples.
■ Where are the lesions in this condition usually located?	Primary lesions are usually found in the lower lobes as Ghon foci. If there is lymph node involvement, the lesions are termed Ghon complexes. As seen in this chest x-ray, secondary, or reactivation TB lesions are usually seen in the apical and posterior portions of the upper lobes. The hilar lymph nodes may also be involved.
■ How is the microorganism that causes this condition cultured and stained?	*Mycoplasma tuberculosis* is cultured on **Lowenstein-Jensen agar**. It is an acid-fast bacterium, and therefore stains with **Ziehl-Neelsen stain**.
■ What is the most appropriate treatment for this condition?	The standard treatment lasts for 6 months. **R**ifampin, **I**soniazid, **P**yrazinamide, and **E**thambutol (**RIPE**) are used for the initial phase of therapy (usually 2 months), followed by rifampin and isoniazid for an additional 4 months. Susceptibility testing is necessary to guide the choice of agents. More drugs may need to be used in multidrug-resistant TB (MDR-TB). Prophylactic treatment is with isoniazid.

■ **What are the main adverse effects of treatment with these agents?**

■ Rifampin colors urine, feces, sweat, and tears a reddish-orange color. It also upregulates the cytochrome P450 isoenzyme system, increasing the metabolism of many drugs, including oral contraceptives. If the patient stays on her current dose of birth control pills and remains sexually active, she is more likely to become pregnant while taking rifampin.
■ Isoniazid causes peripheral neuropathies and hepatitis. It is given with vitamin B_6 to reduce these adverse events.
■ Pyrazinamide is associated with liver toxicity.
■ Ethambutol can cause impaired color vision.

Pharmacology

Case 1	118
Case 2	119
Case 3	120
Case 4	121
Case 5	122
Case 6	123
Case 7	124
Case 8	126
Case 9	128
Case 10	129
Case 11	130
Case 12	132
Case 13	133

▶ **Case 1**

A 20-year-old woman is brought to the emergency department by her roommate, who found the woman lethargic and covered in vomit. The roommate explains that the woman appeared normal the day before but adds that she had been depressed and had started a new antidepressant 1 week earlier. On examination, the patient is sweaty and lethargic with marked right upper quadrant tenderness. Her transaminase values are elevated, with an aspartate aminotransferase (AST) level of 1245 U/L. A urine toxicity screen is sent.

▪ **What is the most likely diagnosis?**	Acetaminophen overdose. At therapeutic doses, a small quantity of acetaminophen is metabolized by hepatic cytochrome P450 into a hepatotoxic intermediate, N-acetyl-p-benzoquinone imine (NAPQI) (see Figure 4-1A). Glutathione rapidly conjugates with NAPQI to form nontoxic compounds. At toxic doses, glutathione storage is depleted and hepatic damage ensues (see Figure 4-1B).
▪ **What is the antidote and its mechanism of action?**	N-acetylcysteine (NAC), the antidote, works via several pathways. In general, NAC enhances the conjugation of NAPQI into nontoxic compounds. Notably, NAC increases glutathione stores to allow for more conjugation and detoxification of NAPQI. NAC can also directly conjugate with, and detoxify, NAPQI. Other benefits of NAC include anti-inflammatory, antioxidant, and vasodilatory effects.
▪ **Why is it important to ask about this patient's history of alcohol use?**	Lower doses of acetaminophen may be toxic in a patient with a history of chronic alcohol use. Chronic alcohol exposure upregulates cytochrome P450, thereby speeding the production of NAPQI. Chronic alcohol ingestion can also lead to depletion of glutathione stores.
▪ **What changes in bilirubin levels are characteristic of this condition?**	Total bilirubin increases, primarily as a result of increased indirect (unconjugated) bilirubin levels and impaired conjugation of bilirubin in the liver.
▪ **What vital organs are directly damaged by this condition?**	The liver and the kidneys are both damaged by NAPQI by similar mechanisms. Indirect effects result from damage to these organs, including coagulation disorders and hepatic encephalitis.

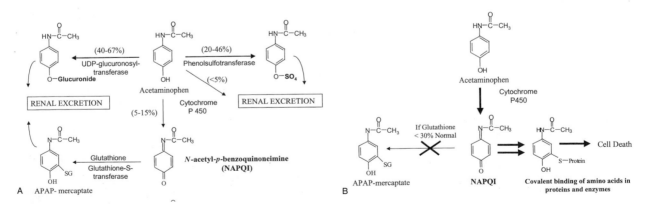

FIGURE 4-1. A and B: Acetaminophen metabolism. (Reproduced, with permission, from Tintinalli JE, Kelen GD, Stapczynski JS, Ma OH, Cline DM. *Tintinalli's Emergency Medicine: A Comprehensive Study Guide*, 6th ed. New York: McGraw-Hill, 2004: 1089.)

► **Case 2**

A 45-year-old woman is brought to the emergency department by the police for unusual and disruptive behavior. She is muttering to herself, does not make eye contact, and does not answer any of the physician's questions but is otherwise cooperative. The patient's temperature is 38°C (100.4°F). A throat examination yields the findings shown in Figure 4-2. Her urine screen is negative for drugs and alcohol, and she is found to be HIV-negative. Relevant laboratory findings are as follows:

WBC count: 2000/mm³   Hemoglobin: 12 g/dL
Neutrophils: 1%   Lymphocytes: 74%
Monocytes: 15%   Platelet count: 270,000/mm³
Eosinophils: 8%
Basophils: 2%

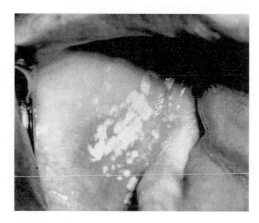

FIGURE 4-2. (Courtesy of James F. Steiner, DDS, as published in Knoop KJ. Stack LB, Storrow AB. *Atlas of Emergency Medicine*, 2nd ed. New York: McGraw-Hill, 2002: 177.)

■ **What is the most likely diagnosis given Figure 4-2?**	Oral candidiasis (thrush); Figure 4-2 shows the characteristic whitish plaques on the buccal mucosa. The lymphoreticular disorders in this patient suggest agranulocytosis.
■ **Given her laboratory functions, this patient is most susceptible to which types of pathogens?**	This can be determined by looking at her WBC differential, which shows neutropenia. Patients with neutropenia often present clinically with recurrent bacterial and fungal infections.
■ **Given this patient's presentation, what medication is she likely to be taking?**	She is likely taking clozapine. This patient is acutely psychotic and suffering from agranulocytosis. Clozapine, an antipsychotic, causes agranulocytosis in 1%–2% of patients.
■ **What treatment would help restore this patient's neutrophil count?**	Iatrogenic agranulocytosis usually resolves within 1 month after discontinuation of the offending drug.
■ **What is the most appropriate treatment for this patient's throat condition?**	Oral thrush is treated with nystatin "swish and swallow."
■ **What are two mechanisms by which drugs can lead to the development of this condition?**	■ **Direct toxicity:** Drugs can be directly toxic to granulocytic precursors and neutrophils (e.g., cyclophosphamide). ■ **Autoimmune destruction of neutrophils:** Drugs may lead to autoimmune destruction of neutrophils by binding to neutrophil membranes and acting as haptens.

A 37-year-old homeless man is brought to the emergency department by the police. He was seen yelling and stumbling over the furniture and says that he feels bugs crawling all over him. The man is taken to the psychiatric unit. On questioning, he claims that he has not had any alcohol in several days.

■ What is the most likely diagnosis and what is the appropriate treatment?	The patient is most likely suffering from alcohol withdrawal, also known as delirium tremens. He should be treated with benzodiazepines.
■ What are some other uses for the drug class of the agent administered, and what is its mechanism of action?	Benzodiazepines have many uses, including: anxiety, status epilepticus, night terrors, and somnambulism. Benzodiazepines act by increasing the **frequency** of GABA$_A$ chloride channel opening.
■ How do benzodiazepines differ from barbiturates?	Barbiturates increase GABA$_A$ signaling by increasing the **duration** of chloride channel opening, which causes a hyperpolarization. Barbiturates are contraindicated in porphyria and are used primarily for their sedative effects. Importantly, barbiturates have a greater risk of coma and respiratory depression than benzodiazepines. In clinical practice, benzodiazepines have largely replaced barbiturates.
■ What treatment is used for benzodiazepine and barbiturate overdose?	Benzodiazepine overdose can be treated with flumazenil, a competitive antagonist at the GABA receptor. Barbiturate overdose is more dangerous because there is no competitive agonist to displace the drug. Thus, symptomatic management and ventilator support are the only ways to treat barbiturate overdose.

► **Case 4**

A 36-year-old man is brought to the emergency department after his wife finds him in a confused and drowsy state. Questioning reveals he has a chronic anxiety disorder and has taken his entire anxiolytic prescription in a suicide attempt. He is found to have a decreased respiratory rate and his blood pressure is 100/65 mm Hg. He is ataxic and his speech is slurred.

■ **Which class of drug did this patient likely ingest?**	A benzodiazepine (e.g., lorazepam, alprazolam, diazepam).
■ **What is the mechanism of action of this class of drugs?**	Benzodiazepines bind to γ-aminobutyric acid (GABA) receptors of the central nervous system, enhancing the affinity of GABA for the receptor and thus increasing the conductance of the associated chloride channel. This results in hyperpolarization of the neuron and inhibition of firing (see Figure 4-3).
■ **What is the antidote and its mechanism of action?**	Flumazenil may be given in benzodiazepine overdose. Flumazenil acts as a competitive inhibitor at the GABA receptor, interrupting the GABA-benzodiazepine complex. Because the half-life of flumazenil is much shorter than that of benzodiazepines, flumenazil must be administered frequently. One must also be aware that flumazenil may decrease the seizure threshold by blocking GABA. If it is given to a patient who has ingested a substance that induces seizure activity, seizure activity may result.
■ **If the patient has been taking this anxiolytic for many years, what are some of the possible adverse effects of rapid reversal with this class of drugs?**	Abrupt discontinuation of benzodiazepines after chronic high doses can precipitate withdrawal symptoms, including confusion, agitation, gastrointestinal upset, and anxiety. If the benzodiazepine is being given for seizure control, flumazenil may precipitate seizure.
■ **For what other conditions is this class of drugs commonly used?**	■ **Panic disorders.** ■ **Status epilepticus:** Diazepam is the drug of choice. ■ **Sleep disorders,** including insomnia. ■ **Alcohol withdrawal:** Diazepam is the drug of choice.

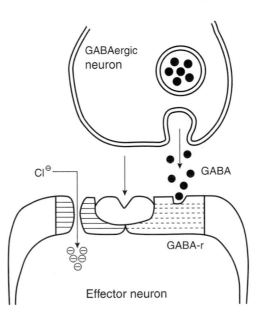

FIGURE 4-3. GABA receptors at work.

▶ **Case 5**

A 32-year-old woman with a history of asthma begins to have difficulty breathing. She has forgotten her inhaler and is brought to the emergency department, where she is noted to be in moderate respiratory distress. She is using her accessory muscles and her oxygen saturation is 96%. She is becoming anxious because it is becoming more and more difficult for her to breathe. She is immediately given an albuterol treatment.

▪ On what type of receptor does this drug act?	Albuterol is a β_2-adrenergic agonist that causes bronchodilation. Other β_2 agonists include terbutaline, metaproterenol, and ritodrine.
▪ In what other locations can this subset of receptors be found?	β_2 receptors are also found: ▪ On blood vessels, where they induce vasodilation. ▪ On bronchioles, where they facilitate bronchodilation. ▪ In pancreatic α cells, where they stimulate glucagon release. ▪ In the central nervous system. ▪ On parietal cells of the gastric mucosa, where they stimulate acid secretion. ▪ In the uterine myometrium, where they cause uterine relaxation.
▪ What second-messenger system does stimulation of these receptors activate?	All adrenergic receptors, including α- and β-adrenergic receptors (see Table 4-1), are G protein–linked receptors, and β_2 receptors are linked to the S class of G proteins.
▪ What is the mechanism of action for this subclass of G receptors?	The G_s protein activates adenyl cyclase, which converts adenosine triphosphate (ATP) to cyclic adenosine monophosphate (cAMP), which in turn activates protein kinase A (PKA). In uterine myometrial cells, the activated PKA phosphorylates other proteins; this leads to a reduction in intracellular Ca^{2+} concentration and hence to decreased activity of myosin light-chain kinase and diminished contractility of the uterine muscle cells.
▪ What other classes of receptors are linked to this particular subclass of G receptors?	Other receptors linked to G_s include β_1, D_1, H_2, and V_2 receptors. Activation of any of these receptors leads to activation of G_s and adenyl cyclase.

TABLE 4-1. G Protein–Linked Second Messengers

	G_i RECEPTOR	G_s RECEPTOR	G_q RECEPTOR
Action	Adenyl cyclase → $\downarrow$ cAMP → $\downarrow$ PKA	Adenyl cyclase → $\uparrow$ cAMP → $\uparrow$ PKA	PLC → PIP_2 → IP_3 → $\uparrow Ca^{2+}$
Types of receptors	α_2 M_2 D_2	β_1, β_2, β_3 H_2 D_1 V_2	α_1 M_1, M_3 H_1 V_1

► **Case 6**

A 30-year-old farmer is brought to the emergency department with severe diarrhea, shortness of breath, sweating, abdominal pain, and urinary incontinence. The patient appears confused and his speech is slurred. His brother reports having seen the farmer drink liquid from an unlabeled bottle approximately 1 hour earlier.

■ **What is the most likely diagnosis?**

Organophosphate ingestion. Organophosphates, which are cholinesterase suicide inhibitors commonly found in insecticides, cause an excess of acetylcholine in the synapse. Symptoms resulting from this parasympathetic excess can be summarized by the mnemonic **DUMBBELSS**: Diarrhea, Urinary incontinence, Miosis, Bronchospasm, Bradycardia, Excitation of skeletal muscle and central nervous system, Lacrimation, Sweating, and Salivation. Central nervous system effects, such as confusion or slurred speech, are common.

■ **What are the antidotes and their mechanism of action?**

Atropine and pralidoxime (2-PAM) can reverse organophosphate poisoning. Atropine works by inhibiting muscarinic receptors, thereby decreasing the effect of acetylcholine. 2-PAM works by inhibiting the binding of organophosphates to acetylcholinesterase. A schematic of neuromuscular blockade is shown in Figure 4-4.

■ **What adverse events are associated with this treatment?**

Atropine poisoning can lead to sympathomimetic adverse effects, including pupillary dilation, decreased gastrointestinal motility, increased body temperature, rapid heart rate, dry mouth, dry skin, constipation, and disorientation.

■ **If this patient had a thymectomy in the past, what other adverse events might be seen?**

Thymectomy can be therapeutic in myasthenia gravis. Anticholinesterases such as pyridostigmine and neostigmine are common treatments for myasthenia gravis. Toxic levels of these agents can also result in symptoms of parasympathomimetic excess.

GENERAL PRINCIPLES

PHARMACOLOGY

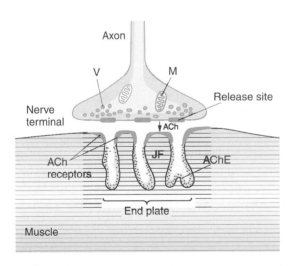

FIGURE 4-4. Neuromuscular blockade. (Modified, with permission, from Drachman DB. Myasthenia gravis. *N Engl J Med* 1978;298:135. Copyright © 1978 Massachusetts Medical Society. All rights reserved.)

A small biotechnology company has developed a new drug that holds promise for the treatment of osteoarthritis. Currently, it is being tested on a group of 100 patients with osteoarthritis, some of whom are receiving placebo.

■ **In which stage of testing is this drug?**	The drug is in **phase 2** of clinical testing. Phase 2 entails enrolling a small group of patients, usually between 100 and 300. These trials are usually single-blinded and compare the new product to placebo as well as to an older drug that has already been proven effective. However, they can also be double-blind and placebo-controlled only.
■ **What stages of testing has the drug already been through?**	Before a drug reaches clinical trials, it must first be extensively evaluated in animal models and in vitro systems such as cell and tissue cultures. Information about acute toxicity, chronic toxicity, teratogenicity, carcinogenicity, and mutagenicity must then be obtained from these trials before testing is conducted on humans. The first step of clinical testing, **phase 1**, involves nonblinded testing on a small group (20–30) of healthy volunteers (see Figure 4-5). The goals in this phase are to determine if humans have significantly different responses to the drug than do animals, as well as to determine the effects of the drug as a function of dose. Phase 2, discussed above, follows.
■ **What are the next stages of testing?**	**Phase 3** involves evaluating the drug in a large group of patients (between hundreds and thousands). The trial is usually double-blinded and aims to further show efficacy and safety. If phase 3 testing is successful, the company will submit a New Drug Application to the Food and Drug Administration (FDA), which will include preclinical and clinical data. The FDA will then review this material in a process that may take several years. If the drug is approved for market, phase 4 starts. **Phase 4** entails monitoring of the drug as it is used in real conditions with large numbers of patients. **This phase is important for discovering low-incidence toxicities that would not be uncovered in clinical trials.** Phase 4 continues indefinitely.
■ **What is a double-blind study, and why are such studies the gold standard for drug testing?**	A **double-blind** study means that neither the patients being treated nor the physicians administering the drug know who is receiving medication or who is receiving placebo. Masking this information eliminates both observer and subject bias.
■ **If this drug passes all stages of testing, when will a generic form become available?**	A drug patent lasts for 20–25 years, after which time generics become available. However, the evaluation of the new drug application by the FDA may take several years. Up to 5 years of the review time may be added back to the patent.

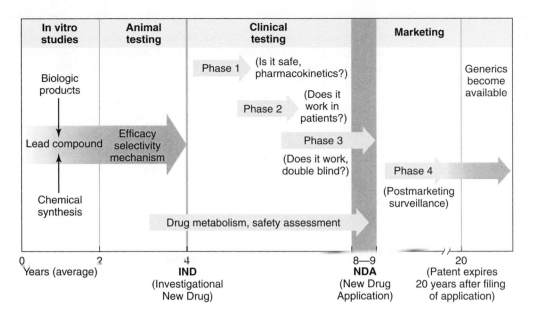

FIGURE 4-5. Phases of FDA review process. (Adapted, with permission, from Katzung BG, Trevor AJ. *Pharmacology: Examination & Board Review,* 5th ed. Stamford, CT: Appleton & Lange, 1998: 365. Copyright © The McGraw-Hill Companies, Inc.)

► **Case 8**

A 53-year-old woman presented to her primary care physician 3 months ago for a checkup, her first in 5 years. She is found to be hypertensive and was prescribed hydralazine, a β-blocker, and furosemide. The woman takes no additional prescription or over-the-counter medications. At the current follow-up visit, she complains of muscle aches, joint pain, and a rash. Physical examination reveals an erythematous, slightly scaly rash on her chest and back. The patient is febrile. The physician orders an autoantibody panel that yields the following results:

Antinuclear antibodies: Positive
Anti-RNP antibodies: Negative
Anti-Sm antibodies: Negative
Anti-DNA antibodies: Negative
Antihistone antibodies: Positive

■ **What is the most likely diagnosis?**

This is a case of drug-induced lupus, as suggested by the rash, arthralgias, and antihistone antibodies. Hydralazine is the causative agent in this case.

■ **What other medications might cause a similar presentation?**

Drugs known to induce lupus include procainamide, chlorpromazine, isoniazid, methyldopa, minocycline, penicillamine, and diltiazem.

■ **What underlying metabolic defect is likely contributing to the patient's reaction?**

Drug-induced lupus develops more frequently in people who have polymorphisms in the genes that participate in acetylation reactions of drug metabolism. In these individuals, acetylation occurs more slowly. Thus, drugs have a longer half-life during which time they may be converted to toxic metabolites. This in turn induces antibody formation and the lupus-like syndrome.

■ **How are lipid-soluble medications metabolized?**

Lipid-soluble medications are metabolized by the liver in phase I and phase II reactions (see Figure 4-6). **Phase I reactions** convert lipophilic drugs into more polar molecules, which may increase, decrease, or have no effect on the drug's activity. Many phase I reactions involve the P450 system; other reactions include amine oxidation, hydrolysis, and dehydrogenation. **Phase II reactions** are conjugation reactions that make the molecules even more water-soluble for excretion in the kidney. The drug may be conjugated to glucuronic acid, sulfuric acid, an amino acid, or an acetyl group, among others.

■ **What is the mechanism of action of the causative agent?**

Hydralazine is a direct vasodilator that acts on arteries and arterioles more than on venous circulation. One result of its vasodilating effects is reflex tachycardia and stimulation of the renin-angiotensin-aldosterone pathway. Thus, hydralazine is almost always administered with a β-blocker and a diuretic.

GENERAL PRINCIPLES

PHARMACOLOGY

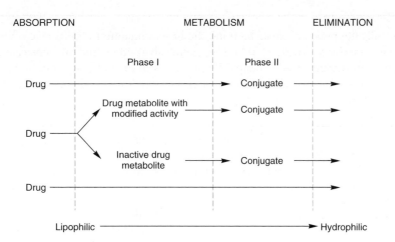

FIGURE 4-6. Phase I and phase II reactions. (Reproduced, with permission, from Katzung BG. *Basic & Clinical Pharmacology*, 9th ed. New York: McGraw-Hill, 2004: 52.)

▶ **Case 9**

A man calls the police because he thinks he hears someone in the garage of his house who may be trying to break in. When the police arrive, they find an intoxicated homeless man with slurred speech collapsed by a closet full of automotive fluids. The homeless man is immediately rushed to the emergency department. Blood tests show a large anion gap acidosis.

■ **What is the most likely diagnosis?**	The most likely diagnosis is poisoning with ethylene glycol, also known as antifreeze. It has a mildly sweet taste, which allows both unintentional consumption by children and adults often in large quantities.
■ **If this patient were not treated, what symptoms would likely occur?**	Ethylene glycol poisoning typically follows three stages. Stage 1 is pure intoxication with dizziness and slurred speech. Stage 2 is comprised of a metabolic acidosis, tachycardia, and hypertension due to the toxic metabolite, **oxalic acid**, formed by metabolism of ethylene glycol by alcohol dehydrogenase. Stage 3 is often kidney failure.
■ **Why might kidney failure occur if this patient is not treated?**	Alcohol dehydrogenase is an endogenous enzyme that can metabolize ethanol, methanol, and ethylene glycol to eventually produce acetate, formaldehyde, and oxalate, respectively. The calcium in the kidney can combine with the oxalate to produce calcium oxalate crystals in the kidney, which causes renal failure.
■ **What is the treatment for ethylene glycol poisoning?**	Treatment usually involves several elements. If discovered early enough, gastric lavage or nasogastric suction can be used to empty the stomach of any ethylene glycol that has not reached the duodenum. Also, intravenous fluid containing 5% dextrose and 5%–10% ethanol with water is given. The ethanol competes with the ethylene glycol for alcohol dehydrogenase allowing the ethylene glycol to be excreted prior to its conversion to oxalic acid. Furthermore, **fomepizole** can be used to inhibit alcohol dehydrogenase and allow ethylene glycol to be excreted unmetabolized.

A 5-year-old boy is brought to the emergency department by his grandmother. The grandmother states that she saw the boy playing with old paint cans in the basement and a few hours later heard the boy screaming in pain. When the physician asks the boy to describe his pain, the boy simply says his tummy hurts.

▪ **What is the most likely diagnosis?**	The most likely diagnosis is lead poisoning given the exposure to old paint cans. Furthermore, abdominal colic is one of the hallmark symptoms of lead poisoning and can be followed by bloody diarrhea.
▪ **If a smear of this patient's blood were examined microscopically, what signs would help confirm the diagnosis?**	Commonly, basophilic stippling of erythrocytes is seen with lead poisoning. In addition, lead poisoning may present in the form of sideroblastic anemia.
▪ **What neurologic complications can occur with the patient's diagnosis?**	Lead poisoning may present with neurologic symptoms such as wrist and foot drop, reflecting radial and common peroneal neuropathies, respectively. In addition, lead poisoning may cause encephalopathy.
▪ **If this patient's diagnosis were a chronic condition rather than acute, what additional radiographic finding may be present?**	After time, lead deposits can form in the epiphyses of long bones.
▪ **What is the treatment for this young patient? What would be the treatment if the patient were an adult?**	Succimer is used to treat children with lead poisoning. For adults, the first-line treatment is ethylenediaminetetraacetic acid (EDTA) and dimercaprol.

GENERAL PRINCIPLES

PHARMACOLOGY

► **Case 11**

Several new drugs are being tested for their effects on β_2-adrenergic receptors. The investigator plots an S-shaped curve of the activity of adenylate cyclase versus drug dose in response to drug A. When the response of drug D is similarly plotted, D is found to have a lower median effective dose (ED_{50}) and a lower maximal response than A. In the presence of drug A plus drug B, the curve has the same shape but is now shifted to the right. In the presence of drug A plus drug C, the curve is not shifted, but the maximal response is lower.

■ Which drug, A or D, is more efficacious?	**Efficacy** refers to the maximal response a drug elicits. Thus, drug A has a higher efficacy, since it produces a higher maximal response (see Figure 4-7).
■ Which drug is more potent?	Drug D is more potent (see Figure 4-7). **Potency** is the amount of drug required for a specified response. Typically, potency is measured by the ED_{50}, or the dose that gives 50% of the maximal response. The lower the ED_{50}, the more potent the drug.
■ What type of antagonist is drug B?	Drug B is a competitive antagonist—that is, it binds to the same site on the receptor as does drug A (see Figure 4-8A). It does not affect the maximal response the agonist can elicit, but it does increase the ED_{50}, requiring more agonist to achieve the same response.
■ What type of antagonist is drug C?	Drug C is a **noncompetitive antagonist** (see Figure 4-8B). These drugs act by binding irreversibly to a site on the receptor distinct from the site of agonist binding. Noncompetitive antagonists do not affect the ED_{50} but do affect the maximal response that the agonist can elicit.
■ How can the effect of drug B be overcome?	Since **competitive antagonists** bind at the same site as the agonist, their action can be overcome by increasing agonist dose.

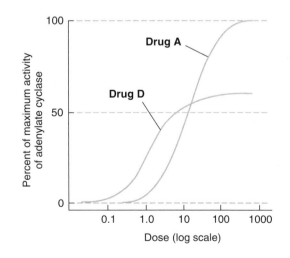

FIGURE 4-7. Dose-response curves comparing drug A and drug D.

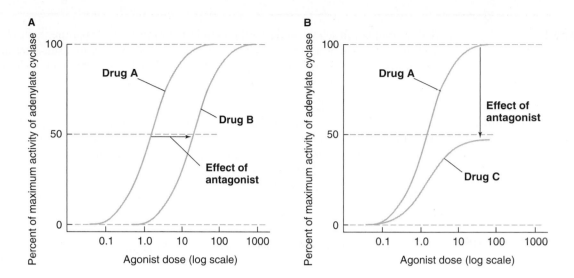

FIGURE 4-8. A and B: Dose-response curves showing drug A, drug B, and drug C.

A 17-year-old high school student is brought to the emergency department after feeling a tearing sensation in his knee when he was tackled while playing football. After the initial consult, it is determined that the boy will need surgery to reattach a torn ligament. During anesthesia, a neuromuscular blocking drug is given.

▪ What are neuromuscular blocking drugs used to treat? What are some examples of these drugs?	Neuromuscular blocking agents are used for muscle paralysis during surgery or mechanical ventilation. Examples of these agents include succinylcholine, tubocurarine, and most drugs that end with "–curium" or "–curonium."
▪ For what types of receptors is this class of drug selective?	Neuromuscular agents are specific for the motor nicotinic acetylcholine receptor present at the neuromuscular junction.
▪ What are the two types of neuromuscular blocking drugs?	There are depolarizing and nondepolarizing blocking agents.
▪ What is the mechanism of action of depolarizing blocking agents?	Depolarizing agents such as succinylcholine act in two phases. Phase I consists of active depolarization of sodium channels which can be potentiated by cholinesterase inhibitors. Phase II keeps sodium channels stuck in their depolarized state. Phase II can be **reversed** with cholinesterase inhibitors.
▪ What is the mechanism of action of nondepolarizing blocking agents?	These drugs are mostly close relatives of tubocurarine. They act by competing with acetylcholine for nicotinic motor receptors. These drugs can be reversed using cholinesterase inhibitors.
▪ What is an important potential risk of using succinylcholine?	The combination of inhalational anesthetics and succinylcholine may result in malignant hyperthermia due to the prevention of calcium release from the sarcoplasmic reticulum of skeletal muscle. This condition can be treated with dantrolene.

GENERAL PRINCIPLES

PHARMACOLOGY

The kinetics of a new pharmaceutical are being tested in an animal model. A dose of 50 mg of the substance is injected intravenously into a rat. The concentration of the substance in the animal's blood is measured every 30 minutes thereafter for the next 10 hours. The concentration of the drug plotted against time produces the graph shown in Figure 4–9A.

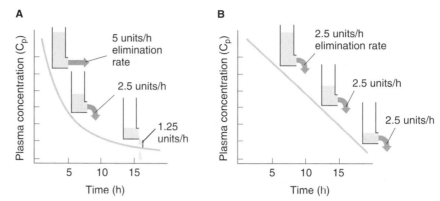

A

Plasma concentration (C_p)

5 units/h elimination rate

2.5 units/h

1.25 units/h

5 10 15

Time (h)

B

Plasma concentration (C_p)

2.5 units/h elimination rate

2.5 units/h

2.5 units/h

5 10 15

Time (h)

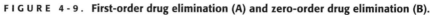

FIGURE 4-9. **First-order drug elimination (A) and zero-order drug elimination (B).**
(Reproduced, with permission, from Katzung BC, Trevor AJ. *Pharmacology: Examination & Board Review*, 5th ed. Stamford, CT: Appleton & Lange. Copyright by McGraw-Hill, 1998: 5.)

■ **Is this substance being metabolized by first-order or zero-order kinetics?**	The shape of the graph shows that the drug is being eliminated by **first-order kinetics** (see Figure 4-9A), meaning that a constant **fraction** of the substance is eliminated per unit of time. As a result, the rate of elimination is proportional to the concentration of the drug. In contrast, **zero-order kinetics** (see Figure 4-9B) result in a constant **amount** of the substance being cleared per unit of time; the elimination rate is constant regardless of the **plasma concentration** (C_p), and the plot of C_p versus time is a straight line.
■ **What is the half-life of this substance, and how does the half-life change if a dosage of 100 mg is administered?**	**Half-life** ($t_{1/2}$) is the time necessary to decrease the C_p of the drug by 50%. As shown in the graph below, at 5 hours the C_p of the drug is half of the initial concentration, and thus $t_{1/2}$ is 5 hours. Half-life does not depend on the size of the dose being eliminated.
■ **If renal clearance is determined to be 2 mL/min, what is the volume of distribution for this substance?**	**Volume of distribution** (V_d) is the amount of drug in the body divided by C_p. A useful equation is the following: $$t_{1/2} = (0.7 \times V_d)/\text{clearance}$$ From this equation, V_d = 857 mL. A large volume of distribution indicates that most of the drug is not in the plasma compartment.
■ **Why does the volume of distribution affect the half-life of a drug?**	As indicated by the equation above, $t_{1/2}$ is directly proportional to V_d. This is because the larger the V_d, the less drug is present in the plasma compartment, and therefore the less drug is circulated through the kidneys and liver for metabolism and excretion.
■ **How would the therapeutic index of this drug be determined, and why is this important?**	**Therapeutic index** is the ratio of a drug's toxic dose to the therapeutic dose. Safe drugs will have a high therapeutic index, indicating a large difference between the dose used to treat patients and the dose resulting in toxicity.

GENERAL PRINCIPLES

PHARMACOLOGY

SECTION II

Organ Systems

▶ Cardiovascular

▶ Endocrine

▶ Gastrointestinal

▶ Hematology and Oncology

▶ Musculoskeletal

▶ Neurology

▶ Psychiatry

▶ Renal

▶ Reproductive

▶ Respiratory

SECTION II

Organ Systems

Cardiovascular

Case 1	138
Case 2	139
Case 3	140
Case 4	141
Case 5	142
Case 6	144
Case 7	145
Case 8	146
Case 9	148
Case 10	140
Case 11	151
Case 12	152
Case 13	154
Case 14	156
Case 15	158
Case 16	159
Case 17	160
Case 18	161
Case 19	162
Case 20	163
Case 21	164
Case 22	166
Case 23	168
Case 24	169
Case 25	170
Case 26	171
Case 27	172
Case 28	174
Case 29	176

▶ **Case 1**

A 75-year-old man visits his physician complaining of lower back pain. He has a history of hyperlipidemia and hypertension. On physical examination, he is obese and has moderately limited range of motion of the back. Magnetic resonance imaging studies demonstrate significant dilation of the abdominal aorta to 4 cm, 200% its expected size.

▪ **What is the most likely diagnosis?**	Abdominal aortic aneurysm.
▪ **What are the major branches of the aorta below the diaphragm?**	Blood flow to the major organs is of special concern with an abdominal aneurysm. The inferior phrenic arteries, celiac trunk, middle suprarenal arteries, renal arteries, superior mesenteric artery, testicular arteries, inferior mesenteric artery, lumbar arteries, and the common iliac arteries are located below the diaphragm (see Figure 5-1).
▪ **What is the three-layer composition of muscular arteries?**	▪ The **tunica intima** is adjacent to the lumen and includes the endothelial layer and the internal elastic lamina. ▪ The **tunica media** includes smooth muscle, collagen, and reticular and elastic fibers. ▪ The **tunica adventitia** contains blood and lymph vessels and nerves supplying the artery.
▪ **Defects in the genes coding for which proteins are associated with an increased risk of this condition?**	**Fibrillin** and **collagen**. Marfan's syndrome is linked to a mutation in the fibrillin-1 gene. Ehlers-Danlos syndrome results from various defects in collagen synthesis or structure. Each of these syndromes is associated with an increased incidence of aortic aneurysms.
▪ **In which space will blood collect if the posterior wall of the aorta ruptures?**	With a rupture, blood will collect in the retroperitoneal space (see Figure 5-2; arrow points to the site of rupture). A confined retroperitoneal bleed from a posterior rupture portends a better prognosis than does bleeding into the peritoneal cavity from a ruptured anterior wall.
▪ **Once the aortic wall is disrupted, how does coagulation proceed?**	Exposure of tissue factor in the vessel wall initiates the extrinsic pathway of coagulation.

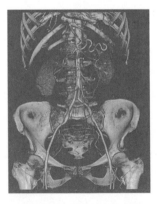

FIGURE 5-1. 3D reconstruction of CT angiogram in a healthy person. (Reproduced, with permission, from Fuster V, Alexander RW, O'Rourke RA, eds; and Roberts R, King SB II, Nash IS, and Prystowsky EN, assoc eds. *Hurst's The Heart*, 11th ed. New York: McGraw-Hill, 2004: 652.)

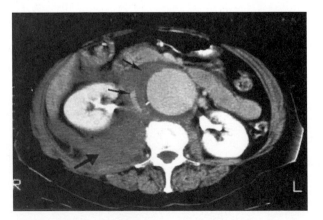

FIGURE 5-2. CT showing abdominal aortic aneurysm rupture. (Reproduced, with permission, from Dean RH, Yao JST, Brewster DC, eds. *Current Diagnosis & Treatment in Vascular Surgery*. Stamford, CT: Appleton & Lange, 1995. Copyright © The McGraw-Hill Companies, Inc.)

A 65-year-old man presents to his cardiologist for evaluation of recurrent episodes of lightheadedness, chest pain, and shortness of breath with exertion. One week earlier, he experienced an episode of syncope while walking up the stairs of his house. Doppler echocardiography demonstrates a heavily calcified aortic valve, with a calculated valve area 40% of normal size.

▪ **What is the most likely diagnosis?**	Aortic stenosis.
▪ **What risk factors increase a person's likelihood of developing this condition?**	Aortic stenosis is commonly associated with older age, male gender, hypercholesterolemia, rheumatic fever, and congenital bicuspid aortic valve.
▪ **What are the qualities of the murmur caused by this condition?**	The murmur of aortic stenosis is a **systolic ejection murmur** at the right upper sternal border, radiating to the neck.
▪ **Which specific qualities of this murmur indicate severe illness?**	Indications of a severely stenosed valve include peaking of the murmur late in systole, a palpable delay of the carotid upstroke, a soft second heart sound (which disappears when the valve is too stiff to open and close properly), and an S_4 gallop.
▪ **How is this condition associated with congestive heart failure?**	Aortic stenosis implies a decreased functional area of the valve, causing a measurable obstruction of outflow. In severe stenosis (<50% of normal size), the obstruction causes a progressive pressure overload on the left ventricle. In response, there is concentric left ventricular hypertrophy, which compromises coronary blood flow during exertion, and can lead to congestive heart failure.
▪ **What symptoms are associated with this condition?**	▪ **Angina:** Without proper intervention, half of patients who present with angina will die within 5 years. ▪ **Syncope with effort:** Half will die within 3 years. ▪ **Dyspnea on exertion:** Half will die within 2 years.
▪ **What is the most appropriate treatment for this condition?**	**Valve replacement** is strongly recommended in patients with symptomatic severe aortic stenosis, as 10-year survival rates after replacement approach rates of the normal population. Mechanical intervention, such as **balloon valvotomy,** provides only temporary symptomatic relief for patients with calcified valves and offers no survival benefit. Sodium restriction along with cautious use of diuretics may be indicated in the setting of congestive heart failure. Excessive volume depletion should be avoided to prevent hypotension.

▶ **Case 3**

A 58-year-old man comes to the physician complaining of occasional chest pain that occurs with strenuous activity. He is obese and has a history of hypertension and diabetes mellitus. During the physical examination, he admits to eating most of his meals at fast-food restaurants. He also reports he has little time for exercise.

▪ What is the most likely diagnosis?	Stable angina, characterized by chest pain with exertion, is often secondary to atherosclerosis.
▪ What risk factors increase a person's likelihood of developing this condition?	Hypertension, diabetes mellitus, age, gender, and hyperlipidemia are major risk factors for atherosclerosis. Family history and smoking are also risk factors. Of note, obesity and lack of exercise have not been firmly linked to increased risk for the development of atherosclerosis.
▪ What is the pathophysiology of this condition?	Endothelial injury resulting from various factors, including hyperlipidemia, smoking, and hypertension, can lead to monocytic and lipid infiltrates into the subendothelium (fatty streaks), release of growth factors leading to smooth muscle cell proliferation into the intima (proliferative plaque), and subsequent development of foam cells and complex atheromas with calcification and ischemia of the intima (see Figure 5-3).
▪ Which arteries are most commonly affected in this condition?	Atherosclerosis preferentially affects the branching points of arteries, or areas of turbulent blood flow, including the proximal coronary arteries, popliteal arteries, renal arteries, carotid arteries, and arteries of the circle of Willis.
▪ What complications are most commonly associated with this condition?	In addition to angina, other complications of atherosclerotic injury include aneurysms, myocardial infarction, stroke, ischemia, and ischemic bowel disease.
▪ How is the patient's symptom classified?	▪ **Stable angina:** Chest pain with exertion; responds to nitroglycerin. ▪ **Unstable angina:** Chest pain at rest secondary to thrombus in a branch. May not completely respond to nitroglycerin; antithrombic agents and heparin may also be required. ▪ **Prinzmetal's angina:** Chest pain at rest, secondary to coronary artery spasm. Treatment includes calcium channel blockers.

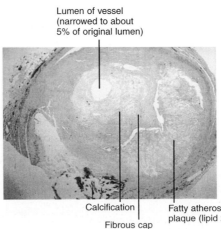

FIGURE 5-3. Cross-section of atherosclerotic coronary artery. (Reproduced, with permission, from Le T, Bhushan V, Rao DA. *First Aid for the USMLE Step 1: 2008.* New York: McGraw-Hill, 2008: Image 132.)

► **Case 4**

A 58-year-old woman comes to the physician's office complaining of feeling lightheaded for the past week. She says she can feel her heart racing in her chest. She mentions she has been staying up late for the past few weeks because of her workload at work. The medical history reveals well-controlled diabetes mellitus. Physical examination reveals an anxious woman with pallor and mild diaphoresis. Cardiac examination reveals an irregularly irregular beat. Vital signs are as follows:

Temperature: 36.1°C (97.0°F)
Respiratory rate: 22/min
Heart rate: 142/min
Blood pressure: 118/55 mm Hg
Glucose: 130 mg/dL

▪ What clinical and ECG abnormalities are most commonly associated with this condition?	The patient has lightheadedness, palpitations, anxiety, pallor, and diaphoresis. Her recent late nights might indicate high caffeine intake, which is a question worth asking the patient. Her heart rate is elevated and she might have borderline hypotension, depending on her baseline blood pressure. The ECG shows an absence of P waves, irregular R-R intervals, and tachycardia (see Figure 5-4).
▪ What is the most appropriate treatment for this condition?	The patient has a high heart rate, which should be slowed down, possibly with β-blockers, calcium channel blockers, or digoxin. Metoprolol is a β_1-blocker that slows conduction through the atrioventricular node, thereby slowing heart rate. One might also consider cardioversion to a normal sinus rhythm. However, care must be taken not to promote thromboembolus formation, which might occur if cardioversion is performed more than 48 hours after the onset of atrial fibrillation. A transesophageal echocardiogram may be done to screen for a left atrial thrombus, or the patient may be given an anticoagulant like warfarin for several weeks before cardioversion is attempted.
▪ How do heparin and warfarin work together to treat this condition?	Given intravenously, heparin activates antithrombin III. Its effectiveness is monitored by measuring the partial thromboplastin time (which reflects activity of the intrinsic pathway). Given orally, warfarin impairs the synthesis of vitamin K–dependent clotting factors (II, VII, IX, and X). It is monitored by measuring the prothrombin time (extrinsic pathway).
▪ Why does paradoxical coagulation sometimes occur after starting warfarin therapy?	Warfarin also inhibits the synthesis of protein C and protein S. Because proteins C and S inhibit factors Va and VIIIa, a deficiency in these proteins promotes coagulation.

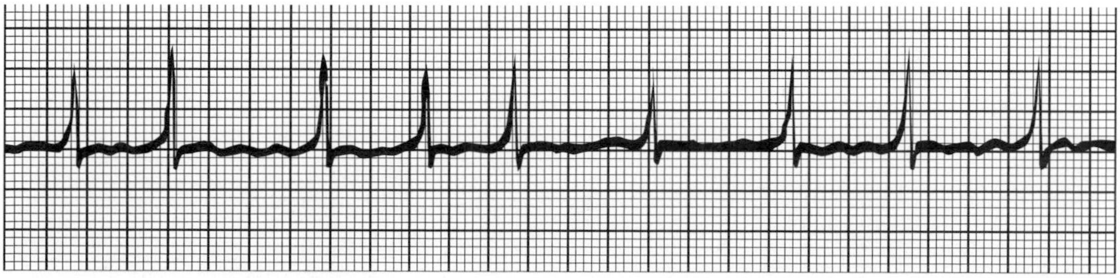

FIGURE 5-4. ECG strip in atrial fibrillation.

▶ **Case 5**

A 50-year-old woman presents to her physician with a several-day history of fever, night sweats, and chills. She also reports increasing dyspnea during her regular walks and transient weakness in her right arm approximately 2 weeks prior, which has spontaneously resolved. She denies any chest pain, arthralgias, myalgias, or rash. Past medical history and family history are unremarkable. Physical examination is notable for a fever of 38°C (100.4°F), heart rate of 90/min, and a respiratory rate of 12/min. On cardiac auscultation, a loud split S_1 is heard, as well as a diastolic third heart sound. Rales and increased tactile fremitus are present in both lung fields.

▪ **What is the most likely diagnosis?**	Cardiac myxoma of the left atrium. Most myxomas arise from the mural endocardium and can measure 1–15 cm.
▪ **What is the epidemiology of this condition?**	Primary tumors of the heart are rare. Myxomas account for approximately 50% of benign tumors in the heart, with the majority located (75%) in the left atrium, although all chambers can be affected. The typical age range is between 30 and 60 years old. Familial occurrences have been reported in about 5% via autosomal dominant transmission. These are associated with a younger age of presentation and higher rates of recurrence.
▪ **What complications may result from this condition?**	Complications from left atrial myxomas can be categorized as: ▪ **Embolization** occurs in 40%–50% with tumor fragments lodging in distal organs (e.g., brain, heart, or extremities). ▪ **Infection** is rare, but may lead to further complications with embolization. ▪ **Obstruction** of the mitral or pulmonary venous orifices may occur, resulting in pulmonary hypertension and right heart failre.
▪ **What conditions should also be included in the differential diagnosis?**	Constitutional symptoms are common with atrial myxomas. However, her transient weakness in her right arm suggests embolization. This combined with her fevers, chills, and sweats raise the possibility of infective endocarditis. A peripheral vasculitis should be considered if the patient has arthralgias, myalgias, or a rash, which are experienced by some people with myxomas. Polyarteritis nodosa can cause multiple arterial aneurysms. Many problems may explain her pulmonary symptoms.

■ **Explain the cardiac examination.**

Splitting of S_1 is accentuated as the tumor is extruded from the mitral orifice. P_2 can also be expected to be louder if the tumor were to obstruct the mitral orifice or pulmonary venous return. The third heart sound is produced by the tumor "plopping" within the atrium during diastole.

▶ **Case 6**

A 55-year-old man comes to his physician for a follow-up visit, after being hospitalized 2 weeks earlier for an inferior wall myocardial infarction. The patient has a history of coronary artery disease. His ECG is shown in Figure 5-5.

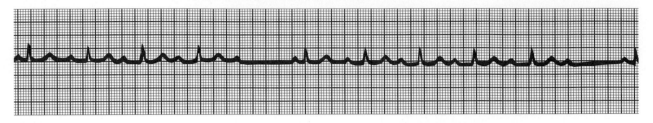

FIGURE 5-5. (Courtesy of Susan Wilansky, MD, Medical Director, Noninvasive imaging, St. Luke's Episcopal Hospital, Houston, TX as published in Fuster V et al (eds). *Hurst's The Heart*, 12th ed. New York: McGraw-Hill, 2008: 2069.)

■ **What pathology does the ECG in Figure 5-5 depict?**	Second-degree atrioventricular (AV) block, also known as **Mobitz type I block** or **Wenckebach block**. As shown in Figure 5-5, note the progressive lengthening of the PR interval from one beat to the next, until finally a beat is dropped (a P wave is not followed by a QRS complex).
■ **What is the pathophysiology of this condition?**	This occurs secondary to impaired conduction at the level of the AV node, such that atrial impulses fail to reach the ventricles. This patient's recent myocardial infarction may have compromised the conductive ability of his AV node.
■ **How is this condition classified?**	■ In **first-degree block,** the PR interval is prolonged but there are no missed beats (a QRS complex follows every P wave). ■ In **second-degree block,** there is intermittent failure of AV conduction. In a **Mobitz type I block,** the PR interval progressively lengthens until a beat is dropped. In a **Mobitz type II block**, there is a sudden loss of impulse conduction without a corresponding change in PR interval. ■ In **third-degree block** (also known as **complete heart block**), there is no conduction via the AV node; atrial impulses do not reach the ventricles, and the ventricles beat at their intrinsic pace. On an ECG, this is reflected as P waves and QRS complexes occurring independently of each other.
■ **What is an escape rhythm?**	Cells in the AV node and His-Purkinje system are capable of generating their own inherent, pacemaking stimuli (**automaticity**), but their rhythm is normally suppressed due to the faster rhythm of the SA node (**overdrive suppression**). In cases where the SA impulse is blocked, the rhythm of the latent pacemakers "escapes" to elicit ventricular contraction. Junctional **escape rhythms** from the AV node or proximal bundle of His have a rate of 40–60/min. Ventricular escape rhythms from more distal pacemakers have rates of 30–40/min and are characterized by wide QRS complexes.
■ **What is the most appropriate treatment for this condition?**	Often, no treatment is necessary in asymptomatic patients with a second-degree Mobitz type I block. In symptomatic patients, atropine or isoproterenol may be used, or a pacemaker may be required.

A 2-week-old baby boy is seen in the pediatrician's office for a well-baby check-up. On physical examination, the baby's femoral pulses are weak and delayed bilaterally

■ **What is the most likely diagnosis?**	Coarctation of the aorta, a condition that occurs two to five times more often in males than in females.
■ **Which part of the aorta is typically affected?**	In the majority of cases, the lesion is in the descending aorta, distal to the origin of the left subclavian artery and in the periductal region. Disease course depends on the degree of obstruction after ductal closure, the presence of collateral circulation, and any associated cardiac anomalies. Less severe forms are characterized by an isolated aortic narrowing and the presence of adequate collateral flow. Less severe forms progress gradually and become symptomatic between the second and third decades of life. Severe, symptomatic disease in early infancy (<10 days old) results if the coarctation is associated with additional cardiac anomalies and/or inadequate collateral flow to compensate for ductal closure. Figure 5-6 shows the anatomic features of aortic coarctation.
■ **What is the characteristic finding on physical examination?**	Auscultation over the chest and/or back may reveal a mid-systolic ejection murmur. A continuous murmur over the chest may also be heard in older individuals who have developed collateral circulation. Weak, delayed pulses in the lower extremities are also characteristic of coarctation.
■ **What chromosomal abnormality is associated with this condition?**	It is associated with Turner's syndrome (45,XO).
■ **What physical examination, ECG, and chest x-ray findings often develop over time in patients with this condition?**	■ Many patients develop hypertension of the upper extremities, with weak, delayed femoral pulses. If the coarctation is proximal to the point of division of the left subclavian artery, the systolic pressure in the patient's right arm may be greater than that in both the lower extremities and the left arm. ■ Left ventricular hypertrophy is a common finding on ECG. ■ Chest radiographs often show an indented aorta and/or notching of the inferior surface of the ribs, usually around age 7. This notching is the result of increased blood flow through the interthoracic and intercostal vessels, which serve as collateral circulation.

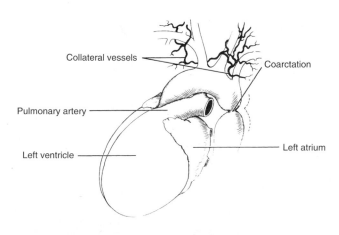

FIGURE 5-6. Anatomic features of aortic coarctation. (Reproduced, with permission, from Cheitlin M, Sokolow M, McIlroy M. *Clinical Cardiology*. New York, NY: Appleton & Lange. Copyright by McGraw-Hill, 1993.)

▶ **Case 8**

A 2-day-old neonate presents with purpuric skin lesions as seen in Figure 5-7. His mother is a recent immigrant from a developing country. Her pregnancy is notable for a flulike illness that was associated with a maculopapular rash involving her face and body several weeks after her last menstrual period. Physical examination reveals a low birth weight, cataracts, and a grade II/VI harsh crescendo-decrescendo systolic murmur most audible at the left upper sternal border with radiation to the axilla and back. Laboratory testing demonstrates thrombocytopenia.

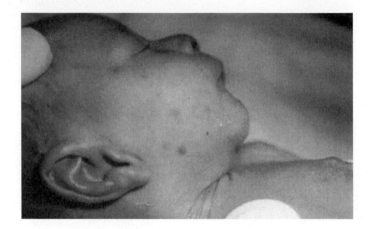

FIGURE 5-7. (Reproduced, with permission, from Lichtman MA, et al. *Lichtman's Atlas of Hematology.* New York: McGraw-Hill, 2007: Figure XI.A.56.)

▪ **What is the most likely diagnosis?**	This constellation of clinical findings, including cardiac manifestations and a "blueberry muffin" rash, along with the maternal history strongly suggest **congenital rubella syndrome** (CRS). Rubella virus (RV) is an RNA virus of the Togaviridiae family, and it is associated with an 85% risk of congenital defects if acquired in the first 12 weeks of pregnancy. The other infections acquired in utero that can present with rash and ocular findings can be recalled with the **TORCH** acronym: Toxoplasmosis, **O**ther infections, **R**ubella, **C**ytomegalovirus infection, and **H**erpes simplex.
▪ **What laboratory test in the newborn is useful for the confirmation of this diagnosis?**	Viral culture of nasal secretions or monthly serology testing for anti-rubella IgM antibody with rising titers can establish a laboratory CRS diagnosis.
▪ **What cardiac anomaly is associated with the murmur seen in this patient?**	The location at the left upper sternal border and radiation of the murmur into the lung fields strongly suggest a valvar (pulmonary valve), supravalvar (immediately distal to the pulmonary valve), or peripheral pulmonary artery stenosis, which is a heart defect commonly seen in CRS. A supravalvar or peripheral pulmonary artery stenosis is more likely in this case given the radiation and the absence of a systolic click, which would otherwise indicate an obstructed or dysplastic valve.

- **What other symptoms are common in patients with this condition?**

Primary rubella infection early in pregnancy results in defective organogenesis. The classic permanent abnormalities include cataracts, retinopathy, heart defects (e.g., patent ductus arteriosus, pulmonary arterial hypoplasia, and pulmonary artery stenosis), and sensorineural deafness. Transient abnormalities include meningoencephalitis, thrombocytopenia with or without purpura, and bony radiolucencies. Since CRS is a persistent infection, more abnormalities, such as developmental difficulties and progressive panencephalitis, can occur.

- **What is the appropriate treatment for this condition?**

No therapy currently exists for CRS. The focus therefore has been on prevention through vaccination. Rubella vaccine contains live, attenuated rubella virus and therefore is contraindicated in pregnant women. Rubella has been eliminated in the United States and Scandinavia, but persists elsewhere due to inadequate vaccination programs.

► **Case 9**

A 56-year-old man suddenly develops chest pressure and pain radiating to his left arm. He has a 50-pack-year history of smoking and a body mass index of 33 kg/m². He calls 911 and is rushed to the hospital, where his ECG shows ST elevation in the precordial leads and his creatine kinase (CK) and CK-MB fraction levels are found to be elevated. He undergoes cardiac catheterization, which reveals his left anterior descending (LAD) artery is occluded.

■ Which area of the heart is affected by this obstruction?

The LAD runs along the anterior interventricular groove and supplies the anterior right and left ventricles, as well as the anterior interventricular (IV) septum. The LAD is the most common coronary artery to become occluded.

■ From what vessel does the LAD originate?

The left coronary artery (LCA) arises as the left main artery, then bifurcates in most people to the LAD and the circumflex artery (see Figure 5-8). In 20% of people, the LCA also gives rise to the **SA nodal artery,** which supplies the sinoatrial (SA) node. Most of the blood flow from the LCA goes to the LAD, which travels along the IV groove to the apex of the heart. The **circumflex artery** is a smaller branch of the LCA. The circumflex artery travels posteriorly to supply the left atrium and left ventricle. The LCA also gives rise to the **left marginal artery,** which runs along the left border of the heart and supplies the left ventricle.

■ What are the branches of the right coronary artery (RCA), and what territories do they supply?

The **RCA** first travels in the atrioventricular groove, then wraps around the inferior border of the heart to the posterior IV groove. In 80% of people, the **SA nodal artery,** which ascends to supply the SA node, is the first branch of the RCA. Other branches of the RCA include the right marginal, posterior descending (in 80% of people), and AV nodal arteries. The **right marginal artery** runs along the inferior margin of the heart to the apex; it supplies the right ventricle and apex. The **posterior descending artery** is the next to branch, and travels in the posterior IV groove to the apex, supplying the posterior right and left ventricles and IV septum. The **AV nodal artery** is a small branch of the RCA that arises near the terminus of the RCA to supply the AV node and bundle of His.

■ What vessel drains the majority of the blood from the cardiac veins back into the chambers of the heart?

The **coronary sinus** receives venous drainage from the great, middle, and small cardiac veins; the left posterior ventricular vein; and the left marginal vein. The coronary sinus lies in the posterior AV groove and opens directly into the right atrium.

■ During which part of the contraction cycle do coronary arteries fill?

The coronary arteries have maximal blood flow during diastole, and minimal flow during systole. This is due to their location above the cusps of the aortic valve, which obstructs flow into the coronary arteries when the valve opens during systole.

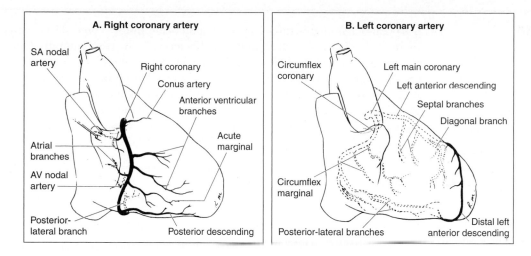

FIGURE 5-8. Arteries of the heart. (Reproduced, with permission, from Doherty GM. *Current Surgical Diagnosis & Treatment*, 12th ed. New York: McGraw-Hill, 2006: 391.)

► **Case 10**

A 65-year-old woman with a 60-pack-year smoking history comes to the physician because she has noticed swelling in both of her feet over the past 3 months. Until recently, she was able to walk four blocks to the grocery store without becoming short of breath; however, now she is only able to walk one block before having to stop and rest. Her sleep has also been poor recently, as she awakens many times each night with difficulty breathing. Sleeping on two pillows relieves her symptoms somewhat. Except for mild edema over her lower extremities, her physical examination is unremarkable. There is no evidence of hepatosplenomegaly or jugular venous distention.

■ **What is the most likely diagnosis?**	Left heart failure (LHF), as evidenced by orthopnea, paroxysmal nocturnal dyspnea, dyspnea on exertion, and mild edema.
■ **What are the common causes of this condition?**	Hypertension, myocardial infarction, valvular heart disease, myocarditis, and cardiomyopathies are associated with the development of LHF.
■ **What symptoms help identify the anatomic source of this condition?**	Right heart failure is characterized by compromised venous return. This can manifest as ascites, significant edema of the lower extremities, jugular venous distention, and hepatosplenomegaly secondary to liver and spleen congestion.
■ **This patient is at risk for which other conditions?**	LHF is the most common cause of right heart failure. In addition, her history of smoking places her at increased risk for chronic lung disease. This can lead to cor pulmonale, characterized by right ventricular hypertrophy and failure due to pulmonary congestion in patients with lung disease or pulmonary hypertension. Emphysema is commonly associated with cor pulmonale.
■ **What are the likely findings on gross pathology?**	Hemosiderin-laden macrophages in the lung are commonly seen in LHF.

A 75-year-old, nonsmoking male status–post recent abdominal surgery suddenly develops calf muscle pain in his left lower extremity (LLE). His hospitalization course since his surgery 3 days ago has been unremarkable. The patient's past medical and family histories reveal no history of cardiovascular disease or malignancy. On physical examination, he is afebrile and is not in acute distress. His LLE is swollen, pale, and mottled with cyanotic discoloration. The skin is warm to the touch and intact throughout. Homans' sign is negative. His right lower extremity is unremarkable. Relevant laboratory test results are as follows:

WBC count: 11,000/mm^3
Hematocrit: 45%
Platelet count: 280,000/mm^3
Prothrombin time: 11 seconds
D-Dimer: 600 ng/mL
   (normal: 0–300 ng/mL)

Blood urea nitrogen: 18 mg/dL
Creatinine: 1.1 mg/dL
Prostate-specific antigen: 2.0 ng/mL
Partial thromboplastin time: 30 seconds

■ **What is the most likely diagnosis?**

Deep venous thrombosis (DVT), which is most common in the lower extremities. Hospitalized patients are at particular risk for DVT and the associated complications of pulmonary embolism. Risk of DVT is higher in surgical patients than medical patients and is particularly high for patients who have had hip or knee surgery.

■ **How is this condition diagnosed?**

The level of D-dimer, a fibrin degradation product, is often elevated in DVT. Assays for D-dimer are highly sensitive and have a low false-negative rate in symptomatic patients. A negative D-dimer test therefore may be sufficient to exclude DVT in low-risk patients. However, in patient populations in which DVTs are especially prevalent (e.g., surgical patients), additional tests are necessary, especially deep venous ultrasonogram with examination for the flow abnormalities (that would be present with a thrombus). Other tests include MRI and venography.

■ **Describe the risk factors of this condition?**

Risk factors of DVT are described by Virchow's triad. **Stasis** may increase secondary to surgery, immobility, paresis, increasing age, heart failure, pregnancy, or obesity. **Vessel injury** may result from smoking, prior DVT, catheterization, or varicose veins. Numerous hereditary conditions result in **hypercoagulability**. Other hypercoagulable states include malignancy, estrogen therapy, acute medical illnesses, inflammatory bowel disease, and nephrotic syndrome.

■ **What conditions should be included in the differential diagnosis?**

Numerous conditions can mimic DVT, including:
■ Muscle strain or tear
■ Drug-induced edema
■ Lymphedema
■ Venous valvular insufficiency
■ Popliteal cysts
■ Cellulitis
■ Derangements of the knee

■ **What is the anatomy of the major deep veins in the lower extremities?**

The deep veins of the lower extremities run parallel to the arteries. Distally, the anterior tibial, posterior tibial, and peroneal veins converge at the lower popliteal fossa to form a single popliteal vein. The latter continues medially and through the adductor hiatus to become the superficial femoral vein. The deep femoral vein runs laterally in the upper leg and joins the superficial femoral and great saphenous vein in the femoral canal to form the common femoral vein.

ORGAN SYSTEMS

CARDIOVASCULAR

▶ **Case 12**

A 50-year-old African-American man presents to his physician complaining of worsening dyspnea on exertion, orthopnea, and paroxysmal nocturnal dyspnea. Past medical history is notable for an anterior myocardial infarction (MI) 15 months prior. Physical examination reveals mild distress and diaphoresis. A holosystolic murmur is audible, particularly at the apex, along with a diastolic rumble. The ECG demonstrates sinus tachycardia at a rate of 110/min; left atrial hypertrophy; left ventricular hypertrophy; and deep (>1 mm), broad Q waves in V_1, V_2, and V_3. Echocardiography shows depressed ejection fraction (EF) and thinning of the left ventricular walls.

▪ **What is the most likely diagnosis?**	Dilated cardiomyopathy (DCM), likely of ischemic etiology. DCM is defined as a left ventricular (LV) ejection fraction (EF) <40% and a ventricular chamber with increased diastolic and systolic volumes. DCM has a prevalence of 36 cases per 100,000. It is a major cause of congestive heart failure in young people. Men and African-Americans are at an increased risk for DCM.
▪ **What are causes of this condition?**	The causes of DCM are too extensive to list here, but can be separated into secondary (i.e., due to known cardiac or systemic processes) and primary (i.e., due to a genetic defect). Common types of secondary DCM include ischemic (e.g., a prior MI as in this patient), hypertensive, and valvular DCM. Primary forms of DCM are typically idiopathic or genetically transmitted via autosomal dominant, autosomal recessive, X-linked, or mitochondrial inheritance. Other causes include drugs (e.g., alcohol, cocaine, and chemotherapeutics, such as doxorubicin), infectious diseases (e.g., Chagas' disease and coxsackievirus), vitamin deficiency (e.g., vitamin B_1 deficiency resulting in wet beriberi), and in women postpartum.
▪ **What typical signs and symptoms are associated with this condition?**	DCM results in depressed systolic pump function and the typical symptoms of myocardial failure seen in this patient. Enlargement of the ventricle dilates the annulus and displaces the papillary muscles. This can result in the holosystolic murmur of mitral regurgitation. The subsequent increase in early diastolic atrium-to-ventricle flow results in the diastolic rumble. Old MIs are characterized by deep, broad Q waves. The presence of Q waves in the precordial leads suggests an old anterior MI.
▪ **What is the pathogenesis of this condition?**	After an MI, it is hypothesized that the reduced peripheral (particularly renal) perfusion leads to fluid retention in an attempt to increase cardiac output. This ultimately results in cardiac remodeling. Figure 5-9 shows the relationship between renin-angiotensin and autonomic nervous systems activation and cardiac myocyte cell death.
▪ **What is the appropriate treatment for this condition?**	Angiotensin-converting enzyme inhibitors and β-blockers are appropriate in symptomatic patients and may slow the remodeling process. Diuretics should be used in volume-overloaded patients. Anticoagulation may be required, as there is a predilection for thrombi to form in a dilated cardiac chamber. Digitalis may also improve the EF, but survival benefits are uncertain.

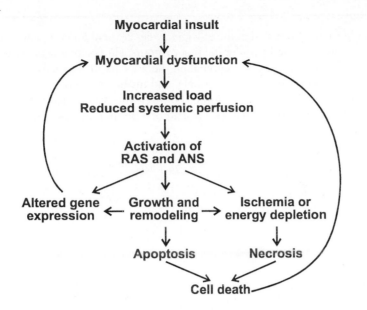

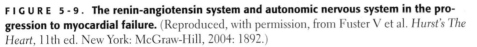

FIGURE 5-9. **The renin-angiotensin system and autonomic nervous system in the progression to myocardial failure.** (Reproduced, with permission, from Fuster V et al. *Hurst's The Heart*, 11th ed. New York: McGraw-Hill, 2004: 1892.)

► **Case 13**

A 30-year-old man is evaluated in the emergency department for complaints of difficulty breathing, chills, and chest pain for the past 24 hours. He denies any previous history of medical problems. On physical examination, he appears ill. His temperature is 40°C (104°F), his blood pressure is 90/50 mm Hg, and his heart rate is 110/min. Cardiac examination reveals a 3/6 diastolic murmur; however, the patient denies any history of a murmur. ECG results are normal. Gram stain of a peripheral blood smear is shown in Figure 5-10.

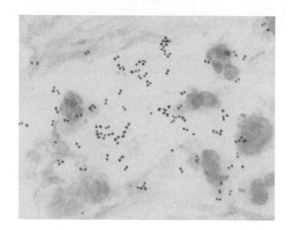

FIGURE 5-10. (Reproduced, with permission, from Le T, Bhushan V, Rao DA. *First Aid for the USMLE Step 1: 2008.* 12th ed. New York: McGraw-Hill, 2004: 1892.)

■ What is the most likely diagnosis?	Acute endocarditis caused by *Staphylococcus aureus*. The man's new heart murmur suggests a possible valvular lesion as the source of infection. In this case, a Gram stain that demonstrates gram-positive organisms in clusters is suggestive of staphylococci.
■ Which valvular structure is most commonly affected in this condition?	In the general population, endocarditis most frequently involves the mitral valve. Common organisms include staphylococcal and streptococcal species. In intravenous drug users, however, the tricuspid valve is most commonly involved. In these cases, venous blood contaminated by nonsterile venipuncture crosses the tricuspid valve first.
■ What other microorganisms are associated with the development of this condition?	**Acute endocarditis** develops in previously normal valves; *S. aureus, Neisseria gonorrhoeae,* and *Streptococcus pneumoniae* are common culprits. **Subacute endocarditis** is diagnosed in previously abnormal or damaged valves, and is often secondary to previous rheumatic fever. *S. viridans, S. epidermidis,* enterococci, and *Candida* are common causes of subacute endocarditis.
■ What is this condition called when it occurs with systemic lupus erythematosus?	**Libman-Sacks endocarditis,** or "sterile endocarditis," occurs with systemic lupus erythematosus. This condition is believed to result from autoimmune damage to cardiac valves.
■ What characteristic of the microbe shown in Figure 5-10 confers resistance to penicillin?	*S. aureus* secretes penicillinase (a β-lactamase), which inactivates penicillin.

- **How does vancomycin resistance develop?**

  S. aureus may acquire a gene that changes the vancomycin binding site from a D-ala D-ala sequence to D-ala D-lac on bacterial cell wall precursors. Loss of the binding site results in resistance to vancomycin.

- **Which of this microbe's virulence factors increases the risk of chordae tendineae rupture?**

  S. aureus secretes hyaluronidase, an enzyme that digests connective tissue.

► **Case 14**

A previously healthy 16-year-old boy presents to the emergency department after experiencing difficulty breathing and substernal chest pain radiating to the neck and shoulder while playing soccer. He currently feels much better. He denies any drug or cigarette use and is not aware of any medical problems in his family beyond two uncles who died suddenly in their youth. Physical examination reveals a heart rate of 70/min, blood pressure of 124/80 mm Hg, and respiratory rate of 12/min. Heart sounds are notable for a normal S_1 and normally split S_2, along with a murmur. The precordial tracings from his ECG are shown in Figure 5-11.

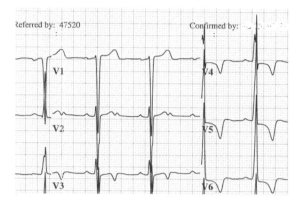

FIGURE 5-11. (Reproduced, with permission, from Fuster V, et al. *Hurst's The Heart*, 12th ed. New York: McGraw-Hill, 2008: 829.)

■ **What is the most likely diagnosis?**	Hypertrophic cardiomyopathy (HCM), as suggested by the patient's age, symptoms, family history of sudden death (a common presentation in young people), murmur, and ECG.
■ **What is the epidemiology of this condition?**	HCM is a disease characterized by the overgrowth of myocardium with myocardial disarray. It is believed to be the most common genetic cardiovascular disorder. Its overall prevalence is estimated to be 1:500 to 1:1000. No gender preference is observed, and clinical manifestation varies by age.
■ **Interpret the ECG in Figure 5-11.**	Normal sinus rhythm. ■ Significant left ventricular hypertrophy, as indicated by the deep S wave in V_1 and tall R wave in V_5 or V_6 (i.e., S wave in V_1 + R wave in V_5 or $V_6 \geq 35$ mm). ■ ST-segment depression with T-wave inversion in V_4 to V_6, which may suggest lateral infarction, given their presence only in these lateral leads.
■ **What is the etiology of this condition?**	Multiple mutations have been associated with HCM, many of which are transmitted in an autosomal dominant pattern. The majority affect the cardiac sarcomere, including β-myosin heavy chain, myosin binding protein C, cardiac troponin T and I, α-tropomyosin, actin, titin, and myosin light chain.

■ **What is the classic murmur associated with this condition?**

The classic murmur is that of left ventricular outflow tract obstruction caused by the hypertrophic septum within a shrunken ventricular cavity. A systolic, crescendo-decrescendo murmur most audible at the left sternal border that ends shortly before S_2 is often heard. This murmur decreases with squatting and increases with subsequent standing. Radiation to the apex and the base of the heart is possible. A mitral valve (MV) regurgitation murmur may also be heard, as the MV leaflets can be pulled into the outflow tract mid-systole.

■ **What major classes of pharmacologic agents may benefit this patient?**

β-Adrenergic antagonists to decrease heart rate, myocardial oxygen consumption, and outflow tract gradient, and to increase diastolic filling time.

Calcium channel blockers to decrease inotropy and chronotropy and improve diastolic relaxation. Verapamil is preferred because it acts primarily on the heart rather than the blood vessels and so has minimal effects on the afterload.

► **Case 15**

A 51-year-old man comes to the physician's office for a routine physical examination. At his last examination 3 years ago, he was advised to make appropriate lifestyle modifications because his blood pressure was 144/87 mm Hg. At the current visit his blood pressure is 150/95 mm Hg. The patient is overweight (body mass index 28 kg/m^2), and he has smoked one pack of cigarettes per day for the past 30 years.

■ What is the most likely diagnosis?	Hypertension.
■ What is the primary treatment for this condition?	Lifestyle modification is attempted before pharmacologic therapy is undertaken. This includes moderate dietary sodium restriction, weight reduction in obese patients, avoidance of excess alcohol intake, and regular aerobic exercise.
■ What is the initial pharmacologic therapy of choice for this condition?	The initial pharmacologic therapy of choice is a **thiazide diuretic**, which inhibits sodium chloride reabsorption in the distal tubule, thereby promoting diuresis. As compared to other classes of diuretics, these drugs (hydrochlorothiazide, chlorothiazide, indapamide, and metolazone) generally cause fewer adverse effects.
■ What are the mechanism of action and major toxicities of angiotensin-converting enzyme (ACE) inhibitors?	**ACE inhibitors,** such as captopril and enalapril, are particularly useful when comorbidities such as diabetes mellitus and cardiovascular disease coexist with hypertension. These drugs work by inhibiting ACE, thereby reducing levels of angiotensin II and preventing inactivation of bradykinin (a vasodilator). Toxicities include cough, angioedema, proteinuria, taste changes, hypotension, fetal renal damage, rash, and hyperkalemia. Angiotensin II receptor blockers such as losartan have a decreased incidence of cough as an adverse effect.
■ What are the mechanism of action and major toxicities of β$_1$-adrenergic blockers?	**β$_1$-Selective blockers** (acebutolol, betaxolol, esmolol, atenolol, and metoprolol) are particularly useful in decreasing mortality after ischemic events. They work by blocking β-adrenergic receptors, slowing the heart rate, and decreasing blood pressure. While β$_1$-specific antagonists have fewer respiratory adverse effects than nonspecific β-blockers (such as propranolol), major adverse effects include bradycardia, congestive heart failure, atrioventricular block, sedation, sleep alteration, and impotence.
■ What are the mechanism of action and major toxicities of calcium channel blockers?	**Calcium channel blockers** such as nifedipine (which is more specific for vasculature than verapamil and diltiazem) block voltage-dependent L-type calcium channels of smooth and cardiac muscle, thus reducing muscle contractility. They are particularly useful when hypertension is not adequately controlled with the above agents. Major toxicities include cardiac depression, peripheral edema, flushing, dizziness, and constipation.

A 3-year-old boy is brought to his pediatrician by his mother because he has had a high fever for the past week. Physical examination reveals bilateral injected conjunctivae, palmar erythema, oral mucositis, cervical lymphadenopathy, and solar erythema.

■ **What is the most likely diagnosis?**	Kawasaki's disease, or mucocutaneous lymph node syndrome.
■ **What symptoms are common at presentation?**	Kawasaki's disease commonly presents with fever lasting >5 days; erythematous rash (usually truncal; see Figure 5-12); edema in the conjunctivae, lips, and mouth ("strawberry tongue"); palmar and solar erythema; cervical lymphadenitis; and mucositis.
■ **Which patients are most commonly affected?**	Kawasaki's disease is most common in children 6 months to 4 years old. Individuals of Asian ancestry are more often affected.
■ **What is the pathophysiology of this disease?**	This acute disorder is characterized by necrotizing vasculitis of small and medium-sized vessels. It is believed to be of autoimmune or infectious origin.
■ **What is the most appropriate treatment for this condition?**	High-dose aspirin and intravenous immunoglobulin G are the preferred treatment. Steroids are used only after a failure in treatment. Patients should be treated as promptly as possible to prevent acute complications, including coronary aneurysm, myocardial infarction, severe heart failure, and hydrops of the gallbladder.
■ **Which other infectious diseases commonly present as palmar and solar erythema?**	Syphilis, Rocky Mountain spotted fever, meningococcemia, and coxsackievirus A infection can also present as palmar and solar erythema.

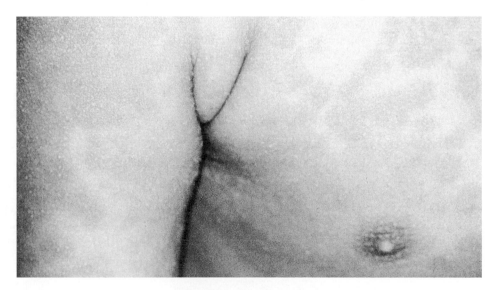

FIGURE 5-12. Erythema in Kawasaki's disease. (Reproduced, with permission, from Wolff K, Johnson RA, Suurmond D. *Fitzpatrick's Color Atlas & Synopsis of Clinical Dermatology*, 5th ed. New York: McGraw-Hill, 2005: 423.)

► **Case 17**

A 45-year-old man presents to his physician for a routine health maintenance visit. He reports that he has experienced intermittent heart palpitations. He denies any chest pain, dyspnea on exertion, or syncope, but he admits to having some anxiety regarding his job security. On physical examination, the patient is well appearing and in no distress. His blood pressure is 110/79 mm Hg. Auscultation of his chest while sitting reveals a late systolic click associated with a high-pitched, late systolic murmur. The systolic click occurs closer to S_1 with standing. His ECG is normal.

■ **What is the most likely diagnosis?**	Mitral valve prolapse (MVP), a condition found in 0.6%–2.4% of the population, is the most common valvular heart disease. Men and women are affected equally. MVP is defined by the echocardiographic measurement of the superior displacement of one or both mitral leaflets into the left atrium (LA).
■ **What symptoms are typically associated with this condition?**	MVP is usually identified by cardiac auscultation in asymptomatic patients or incidentally through echocardiography for other reasons. The most common complaint is palpitation secondary to supraventricular arrhythmias or premature ventricular beats. ECGs, however, are frequently normal. Other manifestations include chest pain that is not associated with myocardial ischemia, exertional dyspnea, syncope, and low blood pressure.
■ **What is the pathogenesis of this condition?**	MVP is multifactorial in origin with an autosomal dominant pattern of inheritance in some families. It can occur as a result of changes within the valvular tissue, geometric disparities between the left ventricle and mitral valve, and connective tissue disorders, such as Marfan's syndrome (prevalence of 91%) and Ehlers-Danlos syndrome (6%).
■ **How does standing and squatting affect the timing of the systolic click?**	In MVP, the systolic click represents the sudden tensing of the mitral valve apparatus as the leaflets prolapse into the LA during systole and occurs when the left ventricle reaches a critical volume (CV) during ventricular contraction. Standing decreases the end-diastolic volume (EDV), thereby allowing the CV to be reached earlier. The click therefore is heard closer to S_1. In contrast, squatting increases the EDV. The click is thus heard closer to S_2.
■ **What are the major complications of this condition?**	MVP typically has a benign prognosis. A poorer prognosis is more likely in male, elderly patients with a systolic murmur, thickened and redundant mitral leaflets, or left atrial or ventricular hypertrophy. Complications include infective endocarditis, sudden cardiac death, severe mitral valve regurgitation, and cerebrovascular ischemic events. Risk stratification by clinical examination and echocardiography is necessary.

► **Case 18**

A 35-year-old man presents to the emergency department complaining of a sudden on-set of substernal chest pain that radiates to his shoulder and began shortly after he awoke for work. He also reports a several-day history of headaches and dizziness 1 month prior, and a recurrence of these symptoms over the weekend. The patient exercises regularly and denies any history of smoking or any cardiovascular disease in his family. Physical examination reveals a mildly diaphoretic, slender man with a heart rate of 120/min and blood pressure of 140/80 mm Hg. His heart and lung sounds are normal. At the conclusion of the examination, he expresses concern about missing a day of work at the local munitions plant because he is a new employee there.

▪ **Exposure to what chemical is of concern in this patient?**	Nitroglycerin. In its pure form, it is highly explosive and therefore utilized in the manufacture of munitions. Exposure in work environments can result in dependence, such that temporary removal from the workplace for periods of 24–72 hours (e.g., the weekend) leads to the withdrawal symptoms seen in this patient that is also known as "Monday disease." Had this patient returned to work, he likely would have seen his symptoms be relieved.
▪ **What is the mechanism of action of this compound?**	Nitrates such as nitroglycerin undergo denitration that results in the liberation of nitric oxide (NO) in vivo. NO activates guanylyl cyclase, thereby increasing cyclic guanosine monophosphate (cGMP) concentrations and stimulating cGMP-dependent protein kinases. In smooth muscles this results in the dephosphorylation of myosin light chains, inhibition of calcium entry, and increases potassium channel activity. This ultimately leads to vasorelaxation. At low levels, nitroglycerin has been shown to affect veins preferentially rather than arterioles.
▪ **What are the major determinants of myocardial oxygen consumption?**	▪ Left ventricular wall tension (determined by preload and after load) ▪ Heart rate ▪ Contractility
▪ **How do therapeutic levels of this compound relieve angina?**	Nitroglycerin is useful in the treatment of angina because it is readily administered (e.g., sublingually) and reaches therapeutic levels rapidly. Angina is relieved primarily through the reduction of myocardial oxygen consumption by a decrease in ventricular wall tension. Nitroglycerin also reduces preload by increasing venous capacitance, which results in lower end-diastolic volumes. Afterload is attenuated, as arteriolar resistance is also decreased to a certain extent. Another, albeit modest, way in which nitroglycerin may also benefit is through both the dilation of coronary arteries and the increase in flow to ischemic subendocardial areas.
▪ **Explain the clinical presentation seen in this scenario.**	Initial exposure to nitrates in healthy persons results in headaches, due to the dilation of meningeal arteries, and reflex tachycardia, secondary to the postural hypotension induced by the dilation of blood vessels. Tolerance develops within 2 weeks of repeated exposure. Dependence results in withdrawal symptoms when exposure ends suddenly, including headaches (possibly from meningeal venous constriction or spasm), decreased exercise tolerance, and worse yet, coronary vasospasms. Acute coronary artery syndrome or sudden death may result. Long-term nitrate therapy therefore should not be discontinued abruptly in patients for fear of dependence.

▶ **Case 19**

A 56-year-old woman presents to the emergency department complaining of severe pain in her lower jaw and neck that has developed over the past hour. The pain is not sharp, and it is not relieved by rest or by changes in position. She took ibuprofen at home without relief. She also complains of nausea that began shortly before the onset of jaw and neck pain. On further questioning, she admits to a "heavy" feeling in her chest, which she describes as a squeezing or crushing sensation. She is profusely diaphoretic.

■ What is the most likely diagnosis?	Acute myocardial infarction (AMI).
■ How does this condition typically present?	Pain is the most common presenting symptom in patients with AMI. The pain is typically felt substernally or in the epigastrium and is described by patients as "crushing" or "squeezing," and less commonly as "stabbing" or "burning" pain. An AMI may also present as pain in the left arm and/or jaw, sudden onset of shortness of breath, fatigue, or adrenergic symptoms.
■ What serum markers are useful in making this diagnosis?	Serum cardiac markers such as creatinine kinase-MB fraction (CK-MB), cardiac-specific troponin I (cTnI), aspartate aminotransferase, and lactate dehydrogenase are released into the blood at varying times in response to cardiac tissue necrosis after AMI. **cTnI**, which is more specific than the other markers for AMI, is used within the first 4 hours, and cTnI levels may remain elevated for 7–10 days. **CK-MB** levels peak about 20 hours after the onset of coronary artery occlusion.
■ What test is the gold standard for diagnosing this condition in the first 6 hours after symptom onset?	Electrocardiogram is used to diagnose AMI soon after onset. Figure 5-13 gives an example of ST-segment elevation on a ECG. Total occlusion of an artery causing an AMI results in ST-segment elevation. If there is subtotal occlusion, if the occlusion is transient, or if there is adequate collateral circulation, then ST-segment elevation does not occur. Most patients who present with ST-segment elevation eventually develop Q waves on ECG, unless they are treated rapidly.
■ What complications are associated with this condition?	Complications of AMI include cardiac arrhythmia, left ventricular failure, thromboembolus as a result of a mural thrombus, cardiogenic shock (if the infarct involves a large area), and death. In addition, cardiac structures, including the ventricular wall, interventricular septum, or papillary muscles, may rupture. Fibrinous pericarditis and cardiac tamponade are additional possible complications.

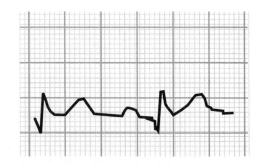

FIGURE 5-13. ECG in acute myocardial infarction showing ST-segment elevation.

► **Case 20**

A 47-year-old man presents to the emergency department after experiencing substernal chest pain. The pain is worsened with inspiration and is relieved only when he leans forward. He says he recently recovered from an upper respiratory infection. Cardiac examination reveals a friction rub and distant heart sounds.

▪ What is the most likely diagnosis?	Pericarditis.
▪ What is an ECG likely to show?	Diffuse ST-segment elevations are consistent with pericarditis (see Figure 5-14). This is in contrast to ST-segment elevations in some myocardial infarctions, in which the elevations are limited to ischemic regions. Another classic finding with pericardial effusion is PR-segment depression.
▪ How is this patient's condition classified?	Preceding viral infection is a possible cause of serous pericarditis in this patient. Other causes of **serous pericarditis** include systemic lupus erythematosus, rheumatoid arthritis, and uremia. Causes of **fibrinous pericarditis** include uremia, myocardial infarction, and rheumatic fever. Causes of **hemorrhagic pericarditis** include tuberculosis and malignancy.
▪ Which physical examination and ECG findings would be suspicious for cardiac tamponade in this patient?	**Tamponade** is compression of the heart by fluid in the pericardium. This compression causes an equilibration of pressure in all four chambers of the heart and a reduction in blood pressure. **Pulsus paradoxus,** a decrease in arterial blood pressure by >10 mm Hg during inspiration, is a sign of tamponade. Electrical **alternans,** or beat-to-beat variations in the amplitude of the QRS complex, may also be noted (see Figure 5-15).
▪ Why would an increase in jugular venous pressure on inspiration be of concern with this patient?	This sign, known as the **Kussmaul's sign,** indicates constrictive pericarditis, which can lead to compromise of cardiac output.
▪ What diagnosis would be considered if the patient had had a myocardial infarction 2 weeks earlier?	**Dressler's syndrome,** or post-infarction pericarditis, describes the development of fibrinous pericarditis several weeks after myocardial infarction or cardiac surgery. It is likely an autoimmune response to myocardial antigens.

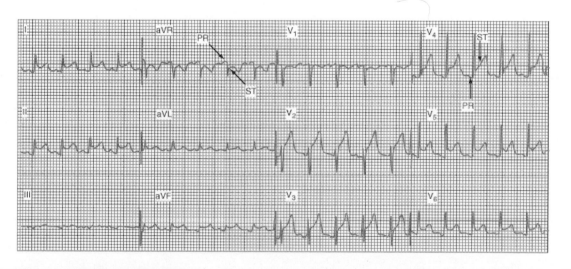

FIGURE 5-14. ECG strip in pericarditis. (Reproduced, with permission, from Kasper DL, et al. *Harrison's Principles of Internal Medicine,* 16th ed. New York: McGraw-Hill, 2005: 1318.)

▶ **Case 21**

A 62-year-old woman comes to the emergency department with "excruciating" abdominal pain that began suddenly, waking her up from sleep early the same morning. She has no history of colitis or irritable bowel, and had an appendectomy as a teenager, but has had no surgeries since. On physical examination, she appears very uncomfortable, and her abdomen is slightly distended with hypoactive bowel sounds. She has only minimal pain on palpation, in the mid-epigastric area. She has no rebound or guarding. She denies changes in bowel habits, but her stool is heme positive.

■ What is the most likely diagnosis?	This is a case of mesenteric ischemia, as suggested by the patient's severe gastrointestinal symptoms being out of proportion to the physical signs elicited. Given the sudden onset, this is most likely an embolic event. Ischemia affecting the small bowel will initially present with severe pain, with peritoneal signs developing later. Ischemia of the large bowel is less painful, and typically presents with hematochezia.
■ What organs are most likely affected by this condition?	This case most likely represents ischemia of the midgut, which is supplied by the superior mesenteric artery (SMA) (see Figure 5-15). The SMA supplies part of the duodenum and part of the head of the pancreas (the territory of inferior pancreaticoduodenal artery), jejunum, ileum, ascending colon, and proximal two-thirds of the transverse colon.
■ What is the vascular supply of the hindgut?	The inferior mesenteric artery (IMA) supplies the hindgut, which includes the distal third of the transverse colon, the descending colon, the sigmoid colon, and the rectum. The IMA gives off the left colic (LCA) and sigmoid arteries (SA) before becoming the superior rectal artery. The LCA supplies the descending colon, and the SA supplies the sigmoid colon. The superior rectal artery supplies the proximal part of the rectum. The middle and inferior rectum are supplied by branches of the internal iliac and pudendal arteries, respectively. The anal canal below the pectinate line is supplied by the inferior rectal artery.
■ What is the venous drainage of the midgut?	The midgut is drained by the superior mesenteric vein, which lies anterior and to the right of the superior mesenteric artery. The superior mesenteric vein unites with the splenic vein behind the neck of the pancreas to form the portal vein.
■ After evaluating the patient, the surgeon decides to operate. Through what layers will the surgeon incise if he makes an incision 4 cm below the umbilicus?	A midline incision through the anterior abdominal wall inferior to the umbilicus will cut through skin, superficial fascia and fat, the anterior layer of the rectus sheath (which is formed by the aponeuroses of the external oblique, internal oblique, and the transversus abdominis), then transversalis fascia, and finally peritoneum. Note that at the umbilicus and above, there is also a posterior layer of the rectus sheath.

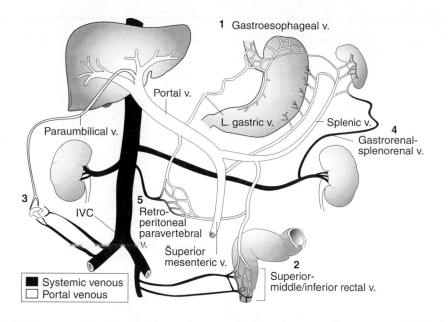

1 Gastroesophageal v.

Portal v.

Paraumbilical v.

L. gastric v.

Splenic v.

4 Gastrorenal-splenorenal v.

3

IVC

5 Retro-peritoneal paravertebral v.

Superior mesenteric v.

2 Superior-middle/inferior rectal v.

■ Systemic venous
□ Portal venous

FIGURE 5-15. **Portal-systemic anastomoses.** Left gastric-azygos (1), superior-middle/inferior rectal (2), paraumbilical-inferior epigastric (3), retroperitoneal renal (4), and retroperitoneal-paravertebral (5). (Reproduced, with permission, from Le T, Bhushan V, Rao DA. *First Aid for the USMLE Step 1: 2008*. New York: McGraw-Hill, 2008: 293.)

▶ **Case 22**

A 2-month-old boy is brought to his physician's office because of poor feeding since discharge from the hospital on his second day of life. The mother reports that he seems to tire easily. His medical history is notable for an uncomplicated 38-week gestation, and a normal, spontaneous vaginal delivery. On physical examination, the patient is small for his age, but is otherwise well appearing and breathing comfortably without cyanosis. Palpation reveals a hyperdynamic precordium and wide, bounding peripheral pulses. A grade III/VI continuous, machine-like murmur that peaks at the second heart sound is audible over the left sternal border and below the left clavicle.

■ **What is the most likely diagnosis?**

Patent ductus arteriosus (PDA). This is indicated by the characteristic continuous murmur and by the physical examination. The incidence of PDA is increasing due to the improved survival of premature infants. PDA is also associated with exposure to rubella virus in the first trimester in an unimmunized mother or birth at high altitudes.

■ **What is the purpose of the ductus arteriosus?**

The ductus arteriosus (DA) typically originates from the origin of the left pulmonary artery to connect to the lower aspect of the aortic arch at the origin of the left subclavian artery. Prior to birth, it serves to shunt blood away from the pulmonary vasculature, as the lungs are fluid filled and do not provide oxygenation. Patency is maintained during fetal life by the low arterial oxygen content and circulating prostaglandins produced largely by the placenta.

■ **What typical signs and symptoms are associated with this condition?**

Clinical manifestation of PDA depends on the size (diameter and length) of the PDA and the gestational age. A small PDA may be asymptomatic in infancy or childhood because of the restriction of excessive flow into the lungs. In such cases, the only symptom may be a murmur. A large PDA that is nonrestrictive to blood flow could cause respiratory distress or failure to thrive in a full-term infant, in addition to the manifestations seen in this case. PDAs tend to affect premature infants earlier and more severely, with apnea, tachypnea, poor perfusion, and complications, such as necrotizing enterocolitis. Heart failure can also occur earlier with prematurity.

■ **What is the pathogenesis of this condition?**

The DA typically closes within 2–3 days after birth and becomes the ligamentum arteriosum. This spontaneous closure occurs from a combination of factors, including the increased partial pressure of oxygen secondary to lung-mediated oxygenation, the removal of the vasodilatory effects of prostaglandin E_2 (PGE_2) derived from the placenta, and a decreased number of PGE_2 receptors. Inadequate closure of the DA results in a PDA and permits a left-to-right blood shunt that places an increased volume load on the left ventricle and the pulmonary arteries.

■ **What is the prognosis of this condition?**

The additional stress upon the heart and lungs derived from the left-to-right shunt eventually results in left ventricular hypertrophy and ultimately heart failure, vascular damage, and pulmonary hypertension. A PDA, regardless of size, also increases the risk for infective endocarditis. Pharmaceutical closure can often be achieved with a prostaglandin inhibitor, such as indomethacin. Otherwise, a surgical or catheter-based closure may be required.

■ **What is the nerve that is associated with the ligamentum arteriosum?**

The recurrent laryngeal nerve, a branch of the left vagus nerve, wraps around the ligamentum arteriosum (embryonically derived from the sixth aortic arch). On the right, the recurrent laryngeal nerve loops around the right subclavian artery (derived from the fourth aortic arch).

▶ **Case 23**

A 35-year-old woman presents to her physician complaining of fatigue and fever. She also reports occasional abdominal pain, headaches, and muscle pain, and has lost 7 kg (15 lb) over the past 2 months. On physical examination, her blood pressure is 154/92 mm Hg. Retinal examination reveals cotton-wool spots, and skin examination is notable for palpable purpura. Her laboratory values are as follows:

Erythrocyte sedimentation rate: 121 mm/h
Alanine aminotransferase (ALT): 1700 IU/L
Aspartate aminotransferase (AST): 1200 IU/L

▪ What is the most likely diagnosis?	Polyarteritis nodosa.
▪ What is the pathophysiology of this disease?	Polyarteritis nodosa is an autoimmune disorder characterized by segmental, transmural inflammation of small and medium-sized arteries due to necrotizing immune complexes. Vessels supplying the kidneys, heart, liver, and gastrointestinal tract are most often involved.
▪ What laboratory test would be helpful in establishing a diagnosis?	The presence of **P-ANCA** (perinuclear pattern of antineutrophil cytoplasmic antibodies) correlates with disease activity. P-ANCAs are more commonly seen in small-artery disease.
▪ What syndrome should be suspected if eosinophilia were also present?	**Churg-Strauss syndrome;** this is a variant of polyarteritis nodosa characterized by eosinophilia and asthma.
▪ What is the relevance of the ALT and AST levels?	About 30% of cases of polyarteritis nodosa are associated with hepatitis B virus infection.

► **Case 24**

A 33-year-old woman who recently emigrated from India presents to her physician complaining of profound shortness of breath. Over the past few weeks, she has been progressively unable to walk up a flight of stairs without stopping to catch her breath. For the past few nights, she has been waking up suddenly, gasping for air. She also notes that she has recently been unable to fit into her dress shoes. The patient says she is generally healthy, leads an active lifestyle, and takes no medication except for vitamin supplements. Her past medical history is significant only for a 2-week hospitalization when she was a teenager for fever, sore throat, and joint pain. On physical examination her blood pressure is 110/80 mm Hg, heart rate is 100/min, and respiratory rate is 24/min. Jugular venous distention is noted, as are diffuse wheezes and rales at both lung bases. There is trace edema of her ankles bilaterally. Heart auscultation reveals a low-pitched, diastolic murmur with an opening snap, heard best at the apex.

▪ What is the most likely diagnosis?	Mitral stenosis (fish-mouth buttonhole deformity), resulting from a previous rheumatic fever infection. **Rheumatic heart disease** primarily affects the mitral and aortic valves; involvement of tricuspid and pulmonary valves is rare.
▪ What histologic changes are likely present in the myocardium in this condition?	The histologic hallmark of rheumatic heart disease is **Aschoff bodies,** which are areas of fibrinoid and collagen necrosis surrounded by multinucleated giant cells and other large mononuclear cells (**Anitschkow myocytes**) (see Figure 5-16).
▪ What hemodynamic changes occur in the heart in this condition?	Left atrial diastolic pressure increases in cases of mitral stenosis because the left atrium must pump against a small, stiff valve. This can result in increased pulmonary hydrostatic pressure and, eventually, right heart failure.
▪ What pathogen is responsible for the underlying infection in this condition?	Rheumatic heart disease is a result of group A β-hemolytic streptococci infection. Valvular heart disease, as in this patient, often occurs many years after the acute infection. Antistreptolysin O antibodies are often seen in patients long after the acute infection resolves.
▪ What is the most appropriate treatment for this condition?	Cautious use of diuretics and sodium restriction to relieve pulmonary congestion is recommended. Surgery for valve replacement may be indicated for patients with severe symptoms. Prophylactic antibiotics for endocarditis may also be indicated.

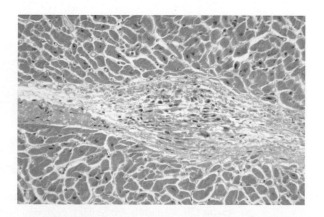

FIGURE 5-16. Aschoff bodies. (Reproduced, with permission, of the Pathology Education Instructional Resource Digital Library [http://peir.net] at the University of Alabama, Birmingham.)

► **Case 25**   A 59-year-old woman consults her physician because she has recently begun experiencing brief episodes of blurred vision in her right eye when reading the newspaper. On further questioning, she reports she has recently started to have headaches, which worsen at night.

▪ What is the most likely diagnosis?	Temporal arteritis.
▪ How is this condition diagnosed?	An elevated erythrocyte sedimentation rate and elevated C-reactive protein levels are nonspecific markers associated with temporal arteritis. Definitive diagnosis, however, requires biopsy of the temporal artery.
▪ Which histopathologic features are associated with this condition?	Temporal arteritis is a systemic vasculitis of large and medium-sized vessels. One would expect to find mononuclear infiltrates in vessel walls and frequent giant cell formation (see Figure 5-17).
▪ What is the most appropriate treatment for this condition?	Corticosteroids should be started as soon as possible. Nonsteroidal anti-inflammatory drugs can be given for pain.
▪ What complications are associated with this condition?	Blindness in one or both eyes is the most common complication of untreated temporal arteritis, due to involvement of the ophthalmic artery or posterior ciliary arteries. Patients may also have fever, fatigue, new-onset headache, and jaw or arm claudication. More serious complications, such as thoracic aneurysm, occur less frequently. Additionally, temporal arteritis is often associated with **polymyalgia rheumatica**.

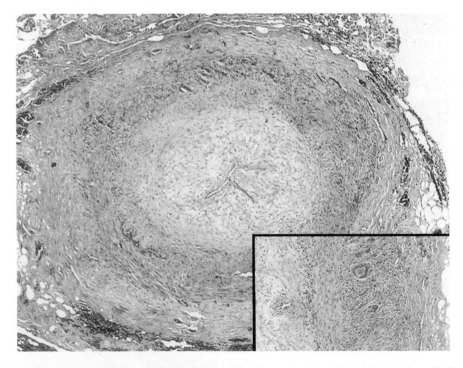

FIGURE 5-17. Histology of temporal arteritis. (Reproduced, with permission, from Hellmann DB. Vasculitis. In: Stobo J, et al, eds. *Principles and Practice of Medicine*. Norwalk, CT: Appleton & Lange. Copyright by McGraw-Hill, 1996.)

► **Case 26**   A 13-month-old boy is brought to the pediatrician by his mother, who reports that he hyperventilates and becomes blue around his lips and in his fingertips after crying, eating, or any exertion. She has also noticed he tends to squat when he gets these symptoms.

■ **What is the most likely diagnosis?**	Tetralogy of Fallot (cyanotic congenital heart disease) presents as dyspnea on exertion, such as feeding or crying. Exertion results in systemic vasodilation, which lowers left-sided resistance, therefore increasing the right-to-left shunting of blood. Bypass of oxygen exchange in the lungs causes hypoxia and cyanosis.
■ **What anatomic findings are characteristic of this condition?**	**PROVe** is the mnemonic to recall anatomic findings in tetralogy of Fallot (refer to Figure 5-18): **P**ulmonary stenosis (1), **R**ight ventricular hypertrophy (2), **O**verriding aorta (deviation of the origin of the aorta to the right) (3), and **V**entricular septal defect (VSD; 4).
■ **Which congenital defect is responsible for this condition?**	VSD is responsible. Specifically, the infundibular septum (portion of the septum adjacent to the outflow tracts) is anteriorly and superiorly displaced, leaving a hole in the ventricular septum. This displacement also causes pulmonary stenosis by blocking flow to the pulmonary artery. This results in increased pressure on the right side of the heart and right ventricular hypertrophy. Right-to-left shunting is increased when pressures on the left are decreased.
■ **What is the characteristic radiologic finding in this condition?**	Chest radiographs typically show a boot-shaped heart, due to right ventricular hypertrophy and the absence of a pulmonary artery shadow above the left side of the heart.
■ **What additional physical finding is commonly associated with this condition?**	Clubbing of the fingers in an adult (see Figure 5-19) also suggests chronic hypoxemia.

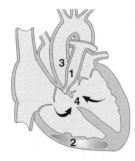

FIGURE 5-18. Drawing of heart in tetralogy of Fallot. (Adapted, with permission, from Chandrasoma P, TaylorCR. Concise Pathology, 3rd ed. Stamford, CT: Appleton &Lange, 1997: 345. Copyright © The McGraw-Hill Companies, Inc.)

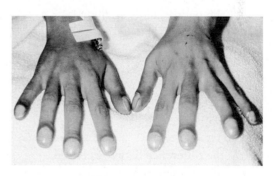

FIGURE 5-19. Clubbing of the fingers. (Courtesy of Alan B. Storrow, MD, as published in Knoop KJ. Stack LB, Storrow AB. *Atlas of Emergency Medicine*, 2nd ed. New York: McGraw-Hill, 2002: 369.)

► **Case 27**   A full-term baby girl presents from the well-baby nursery with bluish discoloration of her lips. Her caretakers report that she becomes sweaty with feeding. Her prenatal history is notable for the lack of prenatal care. Her physical examination reveals tachycardia and tachypnea. Her S_2 heart sound is single and loud. An early systolic ejection click is audible at the left sternal border. Her hips are maintained in flexion, and her extremities are warm and well perfused.

■ What is the most likely diagnosis for this condition?	Truncus arteriosus (TA), a condition that accounts for 1% of congenital cardiac malformations. It is also associated with DiGeorge syndrome.
■ What is the characteristic anatomy in this condition?	The TA is the embryologic precursor to the aorta and pulmonary artery. Therefore, both ventricles eject blood into a common vessel in patients with a persistent TA, which can be seen in Figure 5-20A. A ventricular septal defect (VSD) is always present, and in lieu of separate aortic and pulmonary valves, there is one truncal valve with two to six leaflets. Surgical repair of these defects is required for survival (see Figure 5-20B); the prognosis is good with repair.
■ What are the reasons for the symptoms seen in this patient?	The clinical presentation depends on the amount of pulmonary flow. High pulmonary flow ultimately increases the arterial oxygen saturation, and therefore patients are less likely to be cyanotic. However, this patient likely has low pulmonary flow, which results in central cyanosis and earlier presentation with congestive heart failure, which is indicated by the tachycardia and respiratory distress. The single S_2 heart sound with ejection click is produced by the truncal valve. The cyanosis is central because there is a systemic arterial oxygen desaturation from the mixing of right and left ventricular outflow.
■ What is the pathogenesis of this condition?	TA is caused by failure of development of the spiral septum. In the early embryonic heart, both ventricles eject blood into the TA. Neural crest cells that are present in the TA grow in a spiral formation, separating the two outflow tracts and forming the intertwined aorta and pulmonary artery. If this septum fails to form, a single outflow tract persists. If this septum forms, but does not develop in a spiral fashion, the result is transposition of the great arteries.
■ What is the difference between central and peripheral cyanosis?	Cyanosis requires the presence of 5 g/dL or more of deoxyhemoglobin and is usually not seen above an arterial oxygen saturation of 85%. **Central cyanosis** involves highly vascularized tissue such as the lips and mucous membranes. It results from systemic arterial oxygen desaturation. Cardiac output can be normal. **Peripheral cyanosis** occurs in the setting of normal systemic arterial oxygen saturation, but increased levels of oxygen extraction peripherally due to slowed movement of blood through the capillary bed (e.g., vasoconstriction).
■ What changes may be expected on the ECG?	Waveforms associated with combined ventricular hypertrophy or isolated right ventricular hypertrophy can be expected, as both ventricles simultaneously encounter systemic and pulmonary resistance.

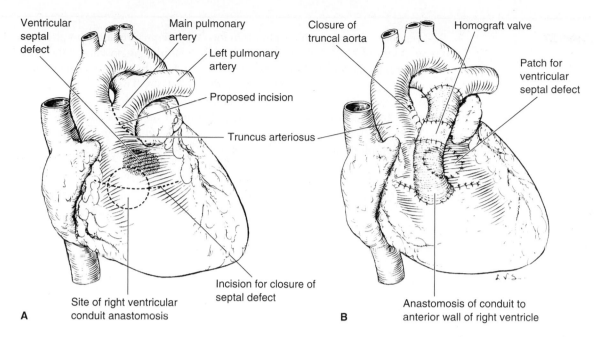

Ventricular septal defect

Main pulmonary artery

Left pulmonary artery

Proposed incision

Truncus arteriosus

Site of right ventricular conduit anastomosis

Incision for closure of septal defect

A

Closure of truncal aorta

Homograft valve

Patch for ventricular septal defect

Anastomosis of conduit to anterior wall of right ventricle

B

FIGURE 5-20. Truncus arteriosus. (**A**) The main pulmonary artery derives from the truncus arteriosus. A ventricular septal defect (VSD) is present. (**B**) In this method of repair, an artificial conduit connects the right ventricle to the main pulmonary artery that has been separated from the truncus arteriosus. The VSD is closed with a patch and serves to direct blood from the left ventricle to the truncus arteriosus. (Reproduced, with permission, from Doherty GM, et al. *Current Surgical Diagnosis & Treatment*, 12th ed. New York: McGraw-Hill, 2007: 438.)

► **Case 28**

A 22-year-old man comes to his physician for a routine pre-employment physical examination. Medical history reveals he is generally healthy, has no known medical conditions, and takes no medications. However, he admits he has recently experienced a few episodes of shortness of breath, dizziness, and palpitations. These episodes have no clear triggers. Results of physical examination are unremarkable. However, the patient's ECG is notable for the following: normal sinus rhythm at 65/min; a shortened PR interval (<0.12 sec); a prolonged QRS complex (>0.12 sec); and a slurred, slow-rising onset of the QRS complex (known as a **delta wave**; see Figure 5-21).

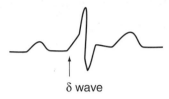

δ wave

FIGURE 5-21. (Reproduced, with permission, from Le T, Bhushan V, Rao DA. *First Aid for the USMLE Step 1: 2008*. New York: McGraw-Hill, 2008: 251.)

■ **What is the most likely diagnosis?**	Wolff-Parkinson-White (WPW) syndrome, or pre-excitation syndrome.
■ **What is the pathophysiology of this condition?**	The presence of an abnormal band of myocytes creates an accessory conduction pathway, distinct from the atrioventricular (AV) node, between the atrial and ventricular systems. Because this accessory pathway is often faster than the AV node, the ventricles are excited more quickly than usual, causing the "pre-excitation" syndrome. The presence of an accessory pathway, and the fact that accessory pathways have shorter refractory periods, predispose patients to reentrant tachycardias, atrial fibrillation, and atrial flutter.
■ **Why is the PR interval on ECG shortened in this condition?**	The PR interval is the interval between atrial contraction (the P wave) and ventricular contraction (the QRS complex). Thus, it is analogous to the conduction time through the AV node. It is shortened in WPW syndrome because AV conduction occurs via a faster, accessory pathway (frequently, the bundle of Kent), which bypasses the AV node.
■ **What ion channels are predominantly responsible for the upstroke in an action potential of a pacemaker cell in the AV node?**	Pacemaker cells depolarize due to the opening of voltage-gated calcium channels. These slow channels produce a slow conductance through the AV node, allowing for an interval between atrial and ventricular contraction. Without this interval, ventricles would not have time to fill. Atrial and ventricular myocytes (non-pacemaker cells), in contrast, depolarize via fast voltage-gated sodium channels; this produces the characteristic rapid upstroke of myocyte action potentials.

- Why are class II and class IV antiarrhythmic drugs potentially not useful in this condition?

Class II and IV antiarrhythmics, the β-blockers and calcium channel blockers, may not be useful in patients with WPW syndrome because they act by increasing AV node refractoriness and decreasing AV node conduction velocity. They do **not** slow conduction over accessory pathways, and may even shorten the refractory period for accessory pathways. This may exacerbate atrial fibrillation or flutter, causing hemodynamic collapse. Rather, quinidine, disopyramide, and procainamide may be used to control arrhythmias in this syndrome.

- What is the most appropriate treatment for this condition?

For most patients with WPW syndrome, electrophysiologic ablation is performed to ablate the accessory pathway. Cure is achieved in 90% of cases with no need for medication.

▶ **Case 29**

A 61-year-old man with chronic sinusitis presents to his physician with cough and hemoptysis of 3 weeks' duration. He also complains of frequently becoming short of breath. Laboratory tests reveal his level of circulating antineutrophil cytoplasmic antibodies (C-ANCA) is elevated, and urinalysis reveals hematuria with RBC casts.

▪ What is the most likely diagnosis?	Wegener's granulomatosis.
▪ What is the pathophysiology of this disease?	Necrotizing granulomatous vasculitis of small and medium-sized vessels leads to manifestations in the kidney and lungs (see Figure 5-22).
▪ What laboratory test would be helpful in establishing the diagnosis?	The presence of C-ANCA is associated with Wegener's granulomatosis. In particular, Wegener's granulomatosis must be differentiated from **Goodpasture's syndrome,** an autoimmune disorder that also presents with hemoptysis and renal disease secondary to anti–glomerular basement membrane antibodies.
▪ What are the likely findings on gross pathology?	Renal involvement in Wegener's granulomatosis commonly manifests as a pauci-immune or type III rapidly progressive glomerulonephritis. Immunofluorescence would reveal no antibodies or immune complex deposition.
▪ If this patient also had severe renal dysfunction, which treatment should be avoided?	Methotrexate can be nephrotoxic in patients with Wegener's granulomatosis. Preferred treatments include cyclophosphamide and corticosteroids.
▪ What other findings are common in patients with this condition?	Perforation of the nasal septum (the so-called "saddle-nose" deformity; see Figure 5-23), chronic sinusitis, mastoiditis, cough, hemoptysis, hematuria, and RBC casts are common findings in patients with Wegener's granulomatosis.

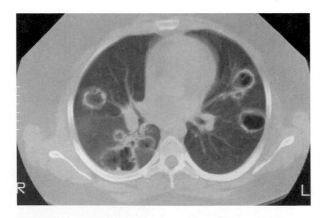

FIGURE 5-22. Lung findings in Wegener's granulomatosis. (Reproduced, with permission, from Kasper DL, et al. *Harrison's Principles of Internal Medicine*, 16th ed. New York: McGraw-Hill, 2005: 2004.)

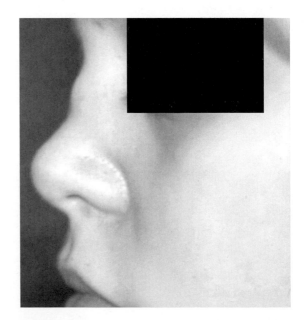

FIGURE 5-23. Nasal septum perforation in Wegener's granulomatosis. (Reproduced, with permission, from Imboden J, Hellmann DB, Stone JH. *Current Rheumatology Diagnosis & Treatment.* New York: McGraw-Hill, 2004: 249.)

Endocrine

Case 1   178

Case 2   180

Case 3   181

Case 4   183

Case 5   184

Case 6   185

Case 7   186

Case 8   188

Case 9   189

Case 10   190

Case 11   191

Case 12   192

Case 13   194

Case 14   196

Case 15   198

Case 16   199

Case 17   200

Case 18   201

Case 19   202

Case 20   203

Case 21   204

► **Case 1**

A 4-year-old girl is brought to her pediatrician for a routine check-up. The child is found to have high blood pressure. Upon chart review, the physician finds that the patient was born with ambiguous genitalia, namely clitoral enlargement and labial fusion. Laboratory tests reveal the following:

Sodium: 142 mEq/L
Potassium: 3.1 mEq/L
Chloride: 102 mEq/L
Bicarbonate: 25 mEq/L

▪ What enzyme deficiency is responsible for this condition?	11β-Hydroxylase deficiency, as suggested by the constellation of **hyper**tension, masculinization, and **hypo**kalemia.
▪ How might this condition be differentiated from a more common, but similar, enzyme deficiency?	**21β-Hydroxylase deficiency** presents with **hypo**tension and **hyper**kalemia. Both deficiencies present with masculinization of the external genitalia. A review of adrenal steroid synthesis is shown in Figure 6-1.
▪ How does this enzyme deficiency result in hypertension?	11β-Hydroxylase converts 11-deoxycorticosterone into corticosterone, and 11-deoxycortisol into cortisol. 11β-Hydroxylase deficiency results in a lack of cortisol and aldosterone. However, the precursor 11-deoxycortisone is a weak mineralocorticoid and causes hypertension.
▪ What is the most appropriate treatment for this condition?	Administration of dexamethasone or hydrocortisone to replace the missing corticosteroid. The patient should be treated with the lowest effective dose to avoid the Cushingoid adverse effects of glucocorticoids, including bone demineralization and growth retardation.
▪ What is the mode of inheritance of this condition?	11β-Hydroxylase deficiency is inherited in an autosomal recessive manner, with mutations in the *CYP11B1* gene. All of the congenital adrenal hyperplasias are inherited in an autosomal recessive manner.

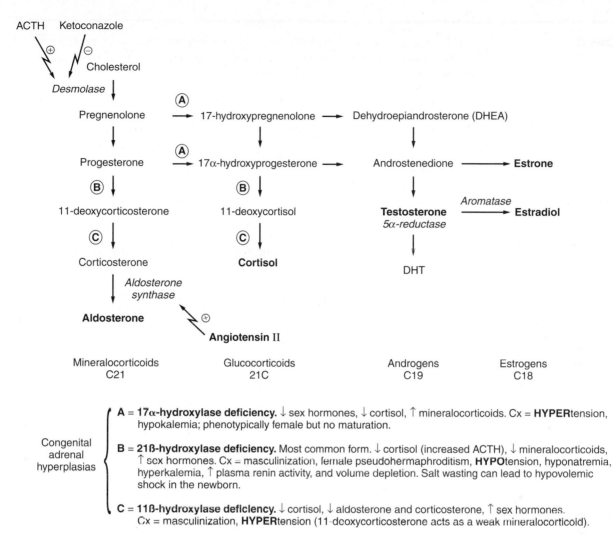

ACTH   Ketoconazole

⊕   ⊖
Cholesterol

Desmolase ↓

Pregnenolone ⟶ (A) 17-hydroxypregnenolone ⟶ Dehydroepiandrosterone (DHEA)

↓   ↓   ↓

Progesterone ⟶ (A) 17α-hydroxyprogesterone ⟶ Androstenedione ⟶ **Estrone**

(B) ↓   (B) ↓   ↓

11-deoxycorticosterone   11-deoxycortisol   **Testosterone** ⟶ **Estradiol**
                                Aromatase
                                5α-reductase

(C) ↓   (C) ↓   ↓

Corticosterone   **Cortisol**   DHT

Aldosterone synthase ↓

Aldosterone ⟵ ⊕

Angiotensin II

Mineralocorticoids   Glucocorticoids   Androgens   Estrogens
C21   21C   C19   C18

Congenital adrenal hyperplasias

A = **17α-hydroxylase deficiency.** ↓ sex hormones, ↓ cortisol, ↑ mineralocorticoids. Cx = **HYPER**tension, hypokalemia; phenotypically female but no maturation.

B = **21ß-hydroxylase deficiency.** Most common form. ↓ cortisol (increased ACTH), ↓ mineralocorticoids, ↑ sex hormones. Cx = masculinization, female pseudohermaphroditism, **HYPO**tension, hyponatremia, hyperkalemia, ↑ plasma renin activity, and volume depletion. Salt wasting can lead to hypovolemic shock in the newborn.

C = **11ß-hydroxylase deficiency.** ↓ cortisol, ↓ aldosterone and corticosterone, ↑ sex hormones. Cx = masculinization, **HYPER**tension (11-deoxycorticosterone acts as a weak mineralocorticoid).

FIGURE 6-1. Adrenal steroid synthesis. (Reproduced, with permission, from Le T, Bhushan V, Rao DA. *First Aid for the USMLE Step 1: 2008.* New York: McGraw-Hill, 2008: 277.)

► **Case 2**

A baby is born without complications to a healthy mother. Physical examination reveals a dangerously hypotensive neonate with ambiguous genitalia, fused labia, and an enlarged and masculinized clitoris. Intravenous fluids are started.

▪ What is the most likely diagnosis?	Congenital adrenal hyperplasia, as suggested by the ambiguous external genitalia (masculinization) and **hypo**tension. These signs are caused by lack of cortisol and aldosterone.
▪ What enzyme deficiency is responsible for this condition?	The defective enzyme is 21β-hydroxylase, an enzyme in the pathway that converts cholesterol into aldosterone and cortisol (see Figure 6-1). This leads to excess substrates, which are shunted towards synthesis of sex hormones. Decreased cortisol leads to loss of feedback inhibition, increased adrenocorticotropic hormone, and further stimulation of the conversion of cholesterol into sex hormone precursors.
▪ What are the likely findings on laboratory testing?	**Hyponatremia** and **hyperkalemia,** because mineralocorticoids (which are low in these patients) are responsible for the retention of sodium and the excretion of potassium. Salt wasting causes hypotension, which leads to activation of the renin-angiotensin system, resulting in elevated serum renin levels.
▪ Is this an example of hermaphroditism or pseudohermaphroditism?	**Pseudohermaphroditism,** which is defined as having the gonads of one sex and the external genitalia of the opposite sex. The baby will have normal female gonads, but ambiguous, male-like external genitalia. **True hermaphroditism** (rare) occurs when the child has both male and female gonadal tissue.
▪ What is the most appropriate treatment for this condition?	Treatment consists of replacement of the deficient hormones.

► **Case 3**

A 40-year-old woman visits her physician because of fatigue, weakness, nausea, and constipation of several weeks' duration. She says she often feels lightheaded when she first gets out of bed in the morning. Review of symptoms is otherwise negative. Physical examination reveals several patches of hyperpigmentation on the skin (see Figure 6-2). Relevant laboratory findings are as follows:

Sodium: 126 mEq/L   Cortisol: 4.3 mg/dL
Bicarbonate: 19 mEq/L   Chloride: 97 mEq/L
Potassium: 5.2 mEq/L

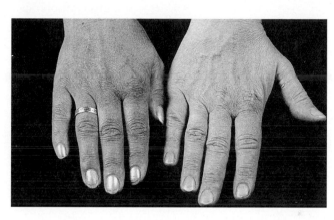

FIGURE 6-2. (Reproduced, with permission, from Wolff K, Johnson RA, Suurmond D. *Fitzpatrick's Color Atlas & Synopsis of Clinical Dermatology*, 5th ed. New York: McGraw-Hill, 2005: 445.)

▪ **What is the most likely diagnosis?**	Addison's disease, or primary adrenal insufficiency. This diagnosis is suggested by the clinical history of weakness and orthostatic hypotension, as well as hyperpigmentation, hyponatremia, hyperkalemia, and low serum cortisol level.
▪ **What are common etiologies of this disease?**	Most cases of Addison's disease are idiopathic/autoimmune-related. Other causes include: ▪ Disseminated intravascular coagulation ▪ **Waterhouse-Friederichsen syndrome** (hemorrhagic necrosis of the adrenal gland, classically due to meningococcemia) ▪ Granulomatous diseases such as tuberculosis ▪ Human immunodeficiency virus infection ▪ Neoplasm ▪ Trauma ▪ Iatrogenic vascular causes
▪ **What is the cause of this patient's metabolic abnormalities?**	Adrenal insufficiency causes a deficiency of cortisol. Hyponatremia, hyperkalemia, and a low bicarbonate level can result from low aldosterone levels associated with primary adrenal insufficiency.

■ How would this patient's cortisol level change if she were administered adrenocorticotropic hormone (ACTH)?

The cortisol level should not change appreciably, as the levels are low due to a **primary** adrenal insufficiency (i.e., the problem is within the adrenal gland itself). This is suggested by the **hyperpigmentation**, which is due to the pituitary gland's attempt to overcome the cortisol deficiency by increasing ACTH production. ACTH, in turn, stimulates the release of melanocyte-stimulating hormone, causing hyperpigmentation.

■ What are the secondary and tertiary forms of this condition?

Secondary adrenal insufficiency is caused by decreased ACTH secretion by the pituitary gland. Administration of ACTH *will* result in a cortisol response. This syndrome does *not* cause hyperpigmentation. **Tertiary adrenal insufficiency** is caused by a decrease in corticotropin-releasing hormone production by the hypothalamus.

▶ **Case 4**

A 35-year-old woman presents to her internist complaining of recent episodes of weakness and tingling in her extremities. She also complains of polyuria, nocturia, and polydipsia. Although her blood pressure was normal in the past, her blood pressure on the day of her visit is 160/100 mm Hg. Laboratory studies reveal a serum sodium level of 147 mEq/L, a potassium level of 2.8 mEq/L, and very low serum renin activity.

■ **What is the most likely diagnosis?**

Primary hyperaldosteronism, also known as Conn's syndrome, as suggested by the patient's history and her hypertension, hypernatremia, and hypokalemia. About 30%–60% of these cases are due to solitary adrenal adenomas in the zona glomerulosa, the aldosterone-secreting layer of the adrenal cortex. Bilateral hyperplasia of the zona glomerulosa can also cause Conn's syndrome.

■ **How is aldosterone regulated?**

Renin, produced by the **juxtaglomerular cells** of the kidney, cleaves **angiotensinogen** (produced by the liver) to form **angiotensin I.** Angiotensin I, in turn, is cleaved by angiotensin-converting enzyme (**ACE**) to form **angiotensin II.** In response to volume contraction, **angiotensin II** is a potent stimulator of aldosterone synthase, a key enzyme in aldosterone synthesis.

Two other key stimuli for aldosterone secretion are decreased plasma sodium and increased plasma potassium.

■ **Another patient presents with similar symptoms, but his laboratory tests show increased serum renin activity. What is his most likely diagnosis?**

Secondary hyperaldosteronism, due to extra-adrenal hyperstimulation of aldosterone secretion. Causes include: a renin-secreting tumor, renovascular disease (renal artery stenosis, malignant hypertension), and a decreased effective circulating volume (as in congestive heart failure, cirrhosis, nephrotic syndrome, hypovolemia, or the use of diuretics).

In primary hyperaldosteronism, renin is decreased, and in secondary hyperaldosteronism it is increased.

■ **Given the patient's serum potassium level, what are the most likely findings on ECG?**

The typical ECG findings (see Figure 6-3) include:
■ Prominent U waves
■ Flattened T waves
■ ST-segment depression

■ **What is the most appropriate treatment for this condition, and what are the side effects?**

If the patient is found to have a solitary, aldosterone-secreting adrenal adenoma, surgical resection (adrenalectomy) is indicated. Bilateral adrenal hyperplasia is treated medically with spironolactone. Spironolactone is an aldosterone antagonist of the principal cells of the collecting tubule. Major adverse effects are due to its antiandrogen effects, including gynecomastia, loss of libido, menstrual irregularities, and impotence.

Hypokalemia

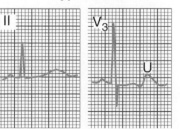

FIGURE 6-3. ECG in hypokalemia. (Reproduced, with permission, from Kasper DL, et al. *Harrison's Principles of Internal Medicine,* 16th ed. New York: McGraw-Hill, 2005: 1319.)

► **Case 5**

A 36-year-old woman with a history of hypertension, easy bruising, hirsutism, amenorrhea, and acne presents to her physician for a check-up. Physical examination reveals central obesity, proximal weakness, edema, and abdominal striae. Relevant laboratory findings are as follows:

Sodium: 140 mEq/L
Bicarbonate: 25 mEq/L
Potassium: 3.4 mEq/L
Glucose: 225 mg/dL
Chloride: 92 mEq/L

■ **What is the most likely diagnosis?**

Cushing's syndrome, caused by excess glucocorticoids, either from increased cortisol production or exogenous glucocorticoid therapy. Common causes include:
  ■ Iatrogenic (e.g., steroid ingestion, most common).
  ■ Pituitary adenoma (**Cushing's disease).**
  ■ Adrenal tumor/hyperplasia.
  ■ Adrenocorticotropic hormone (ACTH)-producing tumor (most commonly secondary to small cell lung cancer).

■ **What laboratory tests can help confirm the diagnosis?**

  ■ 24-hour urine test: Demonstrates hypercortisolism.
  ■ Dexamethasone suppression test: Oral administration of low-dose dexamethasone will not result in cortisol suppression.

■ **What diagnostic tests can elucidate the source of this patient's hormonal abnormalities?**

Serum ACTH levels:
  ■ High ACTH: Pituitary adenoma or an ectopic ACTH-producing neoplasm
  ■ Low ACTH: Adrenal tumor/hyperplasia, or exogenous glucocorticoid administration

A pituitary adenoma may be differentiated from an ectopic ACTH-producing tumor by administering a high-dose **dexamethasone suppression test.** Pituitary adenomas are suppressed by high-dose ACTH, whereas ectopic ACTH-producing tumors usually are not.

■ **What are the most appropriate treatments for this condition?**

The most appropriate treatment for adrenal tumors is surgery. For nonresectable tumors or hyperplasia:
  ■ Ketoconazole: Inhibits glucocorticoid production.
  ■ Metyrapone: Inhibits cortisol formation in adrenal pathway.
  ■ Aminoglutethimide: Inhibits the synthesis of steroids.

► **Case 6**

A mother brings her 7-year-old child in to see the pediatrician. She says the boy has been less active, taking more naps, and wetting his bed, which he had stopped doing 2 years prior. Chart review reveals that within the past year the patient's weight dropped from the 75th percentile curve to the 50th percentile; however, the mother reports that he has been eating and drinking even more than usual. Relevant laboratory findings include:

WBC count: 11,400/mm³,
  normal differential
Chloride: 100 mEq/L
Sodium: 132 mEq/L

Blood urea nitrogen: 14 mg/dL
Creatinine: 1.2 mg/dL
Potassium: 5.0 mEq/L
Glucose: 350 mg/dL

■ **What is the most likely diagnosis?**

Type 1 diabetes mellitus. Autoimmune destruction of pancreatic islet cells results in insulin deficiency (see Figure 6-4). Common presenting symptoms include: polydipsia, polyphagia, weight loss, and polyuria (osmotic diuresis secondary to glucosuria).

■ **What are the two types of this condition, and how do they differ?**

While **Type 1 diabetes** is characterized by absolute insulin deficiency, **Type 2 diabetes** is characterized by insulin resistance and increased insulin levels. Type 1 diabetes typically presents in thin individuals <30 years old, and is HLA linked. Type 2 diabetes typically affects obese individuals >30 years old (although increasingly this disease is seen among obese individuals <30 years old). Both types of diabetes can result in retinopathy, nephropathy, and neuropathy.

■ **What are the major risks of rapid insulin therapy in this patient?**

■ Cerebral edema from rapidly decreasing extracellular osmolality and subsequent influx of water into neurons
■ Hypokalemia from insulin driving potassium into cells
■ Hypoglycemia from too much insulin

■ **What is DKA?**

DKA (**diabetic ketoacidosis**) is a life-threatening complication of uncontrolled diabetes mellitus. In the absence of insulin, increased levels of fatty acids are delivered to the liver, where ketogenesis occurs. This lowers the pH of the blood. Presenting symptoms include **Kussmaul's hyperpnea** (deep respirations), abdominal pain, dehydration, and nausea/vomiting. Patients may have a sweet/fruity/alcoholic odor to their breath.

■ **What is the most appropriate treatment for this condition?**

Lifelong insulin replacement is the treatment for Type 1 diabetes. Oral hypoglycemic agents, which are effective for treating Type 2 diabetes, will not work in patients with Type 1 diabetes. Pancreatic transplantation (rare) may also be considered in some patients.

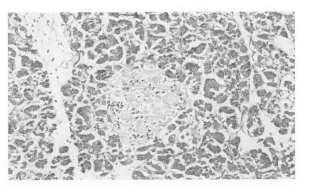

FIGURE 6-4. **Pancreatic islet cells in Type 1 diabetes mellitus.** (Reproduced, with permission, from Le T, Bhushan V, Rao DA. *First Aid for the USMLE Step 1: 2008.* New York: McGraw-Hill, 2008: Color Image 67B.)

▶ **Case 7**

A worried mother brings her 12-year-old son to the pediatrician with concerns that he is "too tall." Both she and the patient's father are relatively short, as are other members of the family. The patient, an avid Little League player, complains only that his baseball cap, mitt, and shoes do not fit any more. On physical examination, the patient is above the growth curve for his age, has large hands and feet, frontal bossing of the cranium, prominent jaw, and coarse facial features with very oily skin.

■ What is the most likely diagnosis?	Gigantism. The disease is called **acromegaly** in patients with fused epiphyses (i.e., growth plates). In older patients, physical changes may go unnoticed, until hats, gloves, and shoes do not fit anymore.
■ What is the pathophysiology of this condition?	Excess growth hormone (GH) can arise from pituitary excess, hypothalamic growth hormone–releasing hormone (GHRH) excess, or an ectopic source. A genetic component of the disease is suggested by the high levels of GH seen in **McCune-Albright syndrome** and multiple endocrine neoplasia type I.
■ Why is this patient extremely tall?	GH stimulates chondrocytes, heavily concentrated in the epiphyseal growth plates, to divide. By virtue of endochondral ossification, excess secretion of GH will cause rapid, excessive linear growth.
■ How is growth hormone produced?	GH is produced and stored in the acidophilic cells of the anterior pituitary. To remember which cells in the anterior pituitary are acidophilic and basophilic, remember **B-FLAT**, **B**asophils: **F**SH (folllicle-stimulating hormone), **L**H (luteinizing hormone), **A**CTH (adrenocorticotropic hormone), **T**SH (thyroid-stimulating hormone). Acidophils: GH and prolactin.
■ How is secretion of growth hormone controlled?	GH is released in a **pulsatile** fashion. Secretion is controlled by the hypothalamus (see Figure 6-5). GHRH stimulates GH production. Somatostatin interferes with its effect on the pituitary. Insulin-like growth factor-1 (IGF-1) exerts negative feedback to inhibit GH secretion. At puberty, the frequency and amplitude of GH secretory pulses increase due to gonadal hormones. The combination drives the "growth spurt."
■ How is this condition diagnosed?	It is diagnosed with an **oral glucose tolerance test**. In normal patients, GH levels will be suppressed. In patients with gigantism or acromegaly, GH values may rise, remain unchanged, or suppress only partially. However, the best screening test is for **IGF-1**. Patients will have elevated IGF-1 levels, as IGF synthesis is dependent on GH. Unlike GH, serum IGF-1 levels remain constant throughout the day.

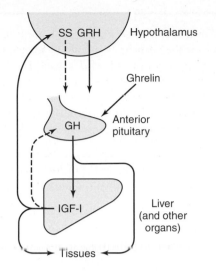

FIGURE 6-5. Feedback control of growth hormone secretion. Stimulatory effects (solid line) and inhibitory effects (dashed line). IGF-1 stimulates the secretion of somatostatin (SS) from the hypothalamus, which in turn acts directly on the pituitary to inhibit GH secretion. (Reproduced, with permission, from Ganong WF. *Review of Medical Physiology*, 22nd ed. New York: McGraw-Hill, 2005; 405.)

▶ **Case 8**

A 40-year-old man presents to the clinic complaining of pain in his left big toe. He claims the pain is so severe that he is unable to walk normally. The pain began suddenly that same morning and woke him from sleep. He denies trauma or insect bites to the area; however, the night before, he and his fiancée had a dinner of liver paté, cheese, and wine. Physical examination reveals a warm, erythematous, and exquisitely tender left metatarsophalangeal joint. Arthrocentesis of the affected toe is performed. Laboratory studies are significant for a serum uric acid level of 9 mg/dL.

■ **What is the most likely diagnosis?**	Gout, secondary to hyperuricemia. Gout characteristically causes monarticular arthritis, often of the first metatarsophalangeal joint (**podagra**).
■ **What is the pathophysiology of this condition?**	Hyperuricemia, secondary to overproduction (breakdown product of purine metabolism), or underexcretion of uric acid. Urate crystal deposition in the joints leads to acute and chronic inflammation.
■ **What are some common causes of this condition?**	**Uric acid overproduction**: ■ Excessive cell turnover (such as myelo- or lymphoproliferative disease, chronic hemolytic anemia, cytotoxic drugs, or severe muscle exertion). ■ Excessive alcohol intake. ■ Excessive dietary purine intake. ■ Inherited enzyme defects. ■ Lesch-Nyhan syndrome (hypoxanthine guanine phosphoribosyltransferase [HGPRT] deficiency). ■ Phosphoribosylpyrophosphate (**PRPP**) synthetase overactivity. **Uric acid underexcretion**: ■ Dehydration. ■ Impaired renal function. ■ Lactic acidosis. ■ Use of certain drugs (diuretics, salicylates, cyclosporine A).
■ **What are the most likely findings on arthrocentesis of the big toe in this case?**	Needle-shaped **negatively birefringent crystals** are diagnostic for gout. In contrast, findings of pseudogout include basophilic rhomboid crystals of calcium pyrophosphate composition. Pseudogout typically occurs in larger joints, such as the knees.
■ **What are the most appropriate treatments for this condition?**	■ Nonsteroidal anti-inflammatory drugs (naproxen, sulindac, indomethacin) to reduce inflammation. ■ Colchicine to treat acute gout attacks. This depolymerizes microtubules, thus impairing leukocyte chemotaxis. ■ **Note:** In patients with impaired renal clearance, acute attacks may need to be treated with steroids, due to the negative renal effects of NSAIDs and colchicine. ■ Probenecid is for chronic gout. This inhibits renal reabsorption of uric acid. ■ Allopurinol is also used in chronic gout. It inhibits conversion of xanthine to uric acid by xanthine oxidase. (Allopurinol is contraindicated in patients taking mercaptopurine and thiazide diuretics and should not be initated during an acute attack.) ■ Diet control, including reduced intake of purine-rich foods (e.g., meat, beans, and spinach) and alcohol, and avoidance of dehydration.

► **Case 9**   A 30-year-old woman visits her physicians complaining of a "racing heart." She also reports sweating much more than usual, to the point of soaking her clothes. Physical examination reveals marked proptosis, and sparse, fine hair. She appears anxious, and on further questioning reports that her anxiety and feelings of restlessness have begun to cause problems at her workplace.

■ What is the most likely diagnosis?	Graves' disease.
■ What demographic group does this condition typically affect?	Graves' disease occurs eight times more frequently in women than men. The prevalence is higher in populations with a high iodine intake. The disease rarely occurs before adolescence and typically affects those in the fourth to sixth decades of life.
■ What is the pathophysiology of this condition?	It is caused by autoimmune-induced hyperthyroidism. Immunoglobulins mimic thyroid-stimulating hormone (TSH) and activate the TSH receptor.
■ What are other common causes of hyperthyroidism?	■ Iatrogenic ■ Silent thyroiditis ■ Struma ovarii ■ Subacute thyroiditis ■ Thyroid adenoma ■ Toxic multinodular goiter (**Plummer's disease**) **Note:** Infiltrative ophthalmopathy and pretibial myxedema are seen only in hyperthyroidism caused by Graves' disease.
■ What are the most appropriate treatments for this condition?	Graves' disease can remit and recur. Definitive treatment includes radioactive iodine ablation or thyroidectomy. Propylthiouracil (PTU) and methimazole inhibit iodine organification and coupling in the thyroid. PTU and steroids also inhibit the peripheral conversion of thyroxine to triiodothyronine.
■ What is thyroid storm?	**Thyroid storm** is an acute, life-threatening surge of thyroid hormone in the blood, usually precipitated by surgery, trauma, infection, acute iodine load, or long-standing hyperthyroidism. Manifestations include tachycardia (>140/min), heart failure, fever, agitation, delirium, psychosis, stupor, and/or coma. Gastrointestinal symptoms can also be present. This condition is treated with the methimazole and agents to reduce peripheral conversion of T_4 to triiodothyronine.

▶ **Case 10**

A 62-year-old woman presents with a month-long history of vague abdominal pain, constipation, and nausea and vomiting. She also has experienced diffuse bone pain over the past month, but attributed this symptom to "just getting old." Physical examination reveals diffuse abdominal tenderness. Relevant laboratory findings are as follows:

Sodium: 140 mEq/L
Calcium: 12.3 mg/dL
Chloride: 110 mEq/L
Bicarbonate: 26 mEq/L
Potassium: 4.0 mEq/L
Phosphate: 2.0 mg/dL
Blood urea nitrogen/creatinine: 20/1.2 mg/dL

■ What is the most striking laboratory finding?	Hypercalcemia. Common causes may be remembered with the mnemonic **MISHAP**: **M**alignancy, **I**ntoxication with vitamin D, **S**arcoidosis, **H**yperparathyroidism, **A**lkali syndrome, and **P**aget's disease of bone.
■ How is calcium regulated in the body?	■ **Parathyroid hormone (PTH)** stimulates osteoclasts to resorb calcium from bone; increased calcium reabsorption in the distal convoluted tubules of the kidney; increased production of 1,25-$(OH)_2$ vitamin D by the kidney; and decreased renal reabsorption of phosphate. ■ **Vitamin D** promotes calcium reabsorption from bone and the small intestine. ■ **Calcitonin**, though probably not important in normal calcium homeostasis, inhibits osteoclast activity, thereby decreasing reabsorption of calcium from bone.
■ The patient is found to have an elevated PTH level and normal creatinine. How does this help explain the patient's overall clinical presentation?	The patient has primary **hyperparathyroidism**, as evidenced by high PTH, high calcium, and normal renal function. A useful mnemonic for the symptoms of hyperparathyroidism (and hypercalcemia in general) is: "Painful **bones**, renal **stones** (nephrolithiasis), abdominal **groans** (abdominal pain, nausea, vomiting, and anorexia), psychic **moans** (changes in mental status, concentration, and mood), and fatigue **overtones**."
■ What are the most appropriate treatments for acute, severe hypercalcemia?	Hydration. If the electrolyte abnormality persists, a loop diuretic can be used (to increase calcium excretion). If needed, calcitonin and bisphosphonates can also be prescribed.
■ What are the three forms of this condition?	■ **Primary hyperparathyroidism** is often (80%) due to a PTH-producing parathyroid adenoma. The tumors are not responsive to normal feedback regulation via an increased calcium concentration. ■ **Secondary hyperparathyroidism** is the term given to a high production of PTH as a response to decreased calcium levels, as in renal failure, and is most commonly due to parathyroid gland hyperplasia. ■ **Tertiary hyperparathyroidism** is autonomous hyperparathyroidism in the setting of long-standing secondary hyperparathyroidism, as seen in end-stage renal failure.
■ What is the best long-term treatment for this patient?	Parathyroidectomy. Surgery for primary hyperparathyroidism has cure rates of 96%–98%.

A 52-year-old woman presents to the clinic complaining of several months of generalized weakness, cold intolerance, and weight gain. Physical examination reveals alopecia, a thick and beefy tongue, myxedema, and delayed deep tendon reflexes. Her heart rate is 55/min and her blood pressure is 100/70 mm Hg. She is not taking any medications. Relevant laboratory findings are as follows:

Free thyroxine (T_4): 4.5 pmol/L (normal is 10.3–35 pmol/L)
Thyroid-stimulating hormone (TSH): 31 µU/mL (normal is 0.8–2 µU/mL)
Cholesterol: 230 mg/dL

■ **What is the most likely diagnosis?**	Primary hypothyroidism, as suggested by her cold intolerance, weight gain, myxedema, fatigue, and the prolonged relaxation phase of deep tendon reflexes.
■ **What is the most common cause of this condition?**	**Hashimoto's thyroiditis** (autoimmune destruction of the thyroid gland). Patients are typically positive for **antithyroid peroxidase (antimicrosomal) antibodies.** Additional causes of hypothyroidism include Riedel's thyroiditis, subacute thyroiditis, and silent thyroiditis.
■ **What endocrine disorder is associated with low free T_4 and low serum TSH levels?**	Low T_4 levels in the setting of low or normal TSH levels implies **secondary hypothyroidism,** the most common cause of which is **hypopituitarism.** Other manifestations of hypopituitarism include sexual dysfunction and diabetes insipidus.
■ **What is the most appropriate treatment for this condition?**	Levothyroxine (synthetic T_4 hormone). Levels of T_4 typically take 4–6 weeks to reach steady state after initiating therapy.

▶ **Case 12**

A 14-year-old Hispanic-American boy presents to the pediatrician for a mandatory school physical examination. He has no medical complaints, but has been told that he needs a tetanus shot. He does not participate in sports, receives B's in school, and otherwise reports being "fine." Physical examination reveals an obese male with a large pannus and abdominal striae. His body mass index (BMI) is 36 kg/m², pulse is 100/min, and blood pressure is 140/95 mm Hg. In addition he has a fine, velvety-appearing, and darkly pigmented skin pattern in the skin folds at the nape of his neck and axilla (see Figure 6-6). In addition to updating the patient's vaccinations for school, the physician decides to run additional tests.

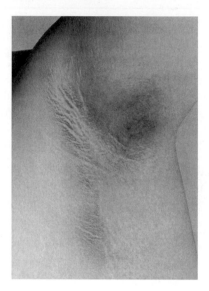

FIGURE 6-6. (Reproduced, with permission, from Wolff K, Johnson RA, Suurmond D. *Fitzpatrick's Color Atlas & Synopsis of Clinical Dermatology*, 5th ed. New York: McGraw-Hill, 2005: 87.)

■ **What is the most likely diagnosis?**	Metabolic syndrome (MS), aka dysmetabolic syndrome, syndrome X, and insulin resistance syndrome.
■ **What are the criteria for diagnosing this condition?**	According to the National Cholesterol Education Program Adult Treatment Panel (ATP) III, the definition for MS includes any three of the following five traits: ■ Abdominal obesity (male >40 inches, female >35 inches). ■ Hypertriglyceridemia (≥150 mg/dL) or prescription medication for elevated triglycerides. ■ Low HDL cholesterol (Male <40 mg/dL, female <50 mg/dL) or prescription for low HDL. ■ Blood pressure ≥130/85 mm Hg, or prescription for high blood pressure. ■ Fasting glucose ≥110 mg/dL or prescription for high plasma glucose.
■ **What do the skin findings represent?**	**Acanthosis nigricans**, a common physical sign of insulin resistance, particularly in Hispanics and African-Americans. It may be due to high levels of circulating insulin on insulin-like growth factor receptors in the skin. Other conditions with acanthosis nigricans include **polycystic ovarian syndrome** (PCOS) and some visceral **malignancies**.

■ **What is insulin resistance?**	Insulin resistance is the state in which endogenous or exogenous insulin produces a less-than-expected biological effect. Thus, patients have elevated blood glucose with normal to elevated insulin levels. Insulin resistance (IR) is nearly universal in obese individuals and is correlated with amount of intra-abdominal fat. There are several proposed mechanisms for IR in obesity: ■ Insulin receptor downregulation. ■ Intracellular lipid accumulation. ■ Increased free fatty acids that impair insulin action. ■ Cytokines and "adipokines," which modify insulin's effect.
■ **What other tests are appropriate to order for this patient?**	Given the acanthosis nigricans, central obesity, and hypertension, it is reasonable to order a fasting plasma glucose level and a serum lipid panel as this patient likely has metabolic syndrome. Hypercortisolemia is also in the differential diagnosis.
■ **Is there a certain class of drugs that should be avoided in patients with this condition?**	Atypical antipsychotics, such as **clozapine**, have been associated with the metabolic syndrome, particularly causing weight gain and hypertriglyceridemia. Even for patients without weight gain, the effect on serum triglycerides is significant enough to cause increased risk for adverse cardiovascular events.

► **Case 13**

A 40-year-old woman presents to her physician with a 2-month history of hoarseness and occasional palpitations and headaches. Her blood pressure is 170/90 mm Hg. Physical examination reveals a lump at the base of her neck. Results of biopsy of the mass are shown in Figure 6-7. Laboratory values are significant for hypercalcemia. Family history is not contributory, as the patient is adopted.

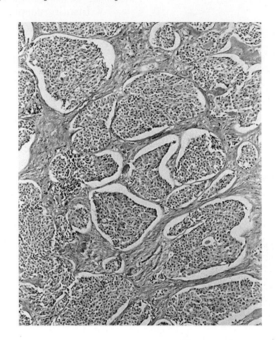

FIGURE 6-7. (Reproduced with permission of the Pathology Education Instructional Resource Digital Library [http://peir.net] at the University of Alabama, Birmingham.)

■ **What is the most likely diagnosis?**	Multiple endocrine neoplasia (MEN) type IIA, or **Sipple's** syndrome. This syndrome is characterized by medullary carcinoma of the thyroid, pheochromocytoma, and hyperparathyroidism (due to either hyperplasia or tumor). Figure 6-7 shows the lobular pattern of growth of this tumor, which is accentuated to some degree by shrinkage artifact.
■ **What are the likely findings on gross pathologic examination of the neck mass?**	Medullary carcinoma of the thyroid is characterized by nests of cells in amyloid stroma.
■ **What genetic screening tests would be useful in confirming the diagnosis?**	The presence of the *RET* oncogene mutation in the setting of medullary carcinoma would be diagnostic for MEN IIA. A variant of the *RET* mutation is also seen in MEN IIB, characterized by pheochromocytoma, medullary carcinoma, and mucocutaneous neuromas. These patients have early childhood development of medullary thyroid cancer, and often have a Marfanoid body habitus. However, parathyroid hyperplasia (hyperparathyroidism) is not a feature of MEN IIB.

■ **What additional laboratory tests would be useful in confirming the diagnosis?**	■ Elevated calcitonin and carcinoembryonic antigen (CEA) levels due to medullary carcinoma. ■ Elevated parathyroid hormone and calcium levels from parathyroid hyperplasia or adenoma. ■ Elevated urinary levels of catecholamines and catecholamine metabolites (vanillylmandelic acid, metanephrine, and normetanephrines) in pheochromocytoma. ■ Elevated plasma levels of metanephrines and normetanephrines in pheochromocytoma.
■ **If this patient and her father have the *RET* mutation what is the probability of her children's developing this condition?**	MEN IIA is an autosomal dominant disease. Thus, the probability of her children's having the mutation is 50%.

► **Case 14**

A 30-year-old African-American woman presents for a physical examination. She is a new patient, having just moved to the area. She claims to be in good health, but has noticed she is urinating more frequently and has had several urinary tract infections in the past year. She has a past medical history of hypertension, for which she takes metoprolol. Her family history is significant for heart attacks in her father and grandmother, and diabetes in her mother, aunt, and sister. Morbid obesity is noted on examination (body mass index ~48 kg/m²) and a urine dipstick reveals 2+ glucosuria.

▪ What is the most likely diagnosis?	Non-insulin-dependent (Type 2) diabetes (NIDDM).
▪ What are the criteria for diagnosing someone with this condition?	Random plasma glucose >200 mg/dL with symptoms or Fasting plasma glucose >126 mg/dL on two separate occasions or Plasma glucose >200 mg/dL 2 hours after a glucose tolerance test
▪ Describe the production and structure of insulin.	Insulin is originally produced as **pre-proinsulin** in the pancreas. During post-translational processing, a signal peptide is removed, producing **proinsulin**. Proinsulin contains two polypeptide chains connected by two sulfhydryl bonds (cysteine to cysteine) and a **C-peptide**. In the conversion from proinsulin (the zymogen) to active insulin, the C-peptide is cleaved off (see Figure 6-8). Synthetic insulin lacks the C-peptide. Therefore, measuring C-peptide is useful in patients in whom surreptitious insulin injection is suspected (factitious hypoglycemia).
▪ How does insulin exert its effects on organs?	The insulin receptor is a heterodimer of α and β subunits. The β subunit is a **tyrosine kinase**. When insulin binds, this subunit autophosphorylates itself, leading to activation of downstream signaling cascades. Insulin stimulates glucose storage as glycogen in the liver, triglyceride storage in adipose tissue, and amino acid storage as protein in muscle. It also promotes utilization of glucose in muscle for energy (see Figure 6-9).
▪ What is the first-line treatment for this condition?	The number one reason this patient has NIDDM is her obesity. Nonpharmacologic treatments such as diet, weight reduction, and exercise must be employed. However, these have limited long-term success. Pharmacologic treatment for type 2 diabetics includes **oral hypoglycemic agents**. Only in refractory cases is insulin added to the regimen (Table 6-1 lists common drugs for both Type 1 and Type 2 diabetes). Tight glucose control markedly reduces microvascular and neurologic complications of diabetes. The goal is a hemoglobin A_{1c} level <7%.

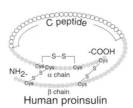

FIGURE 6-8. Structure of human insulin. (Reproduced, with permission, from Le T, Bhushan V, Rao DA. *First Aid for the USMLE Step 1: 2008*. New York: McGraw-Hill, 2008: 105.)

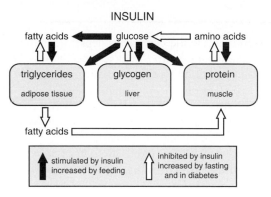

FIGURE 6-9. Actions of insulin on human tissues. (Reproduced, with permission, from Brunton, LL, Lazo, JS, Parker KL. *Goodman & Gilman's The Pharmacological Basis of Therapeutics*, 11th ed. New York: McGraw-Hill, 2006: 1621.)

TABLE 6-1. Common Pharmacologic Agents for the Treatment of Type 1 and 2 Diabetes Mellitus.

DRUG CLASSES	ACTION	CLINICAL USE	TOXICITIES
Insulin: Lispro (short-acting) Insulin (short-acting) NPH (intermediate) Lente (long-acting) Ultralente (long-acting)	**Bind insulin receptor** (tyrosine kinase activity). Liver: ↑ glucose stored as glycogen. Muscle: ↑ glycogen and protein synthesis, K⁺ uptake. Fat: aids TG storage.	Type 1 DM. Also life-threatening hyperkalemia and stress-induced hyperglycemia.	Hypoglycemia, hypersensitivity reaction (very rare).
Sulfonylureas: First generation: Tolbutamide Chlorpropamide Second generation: Glyburide Glimepiride Glipizide	Close K⁺ channel in β-cell membrane, so cell depolarizes → **triggering of insulin release** via ↑ Ca²⁺ influx.	Stimulate release of endogenous insulin in type 2 DM. Require some islet function, so useless in type 1 DM.	First generation: disulfiram-like effects. Second generation: hypoglycemia.
Biguanides: Metformin	Exact mechanism is unknown. Possibly ↓ **gluconeogenesis,** ↑ glycolysis, ↓ serum glucose levels.	Used as oral hypoglycemic. Can be used in patients without islet function.	Most grave adverse effect is lactic acidosis.
Glitazones: Pioglitazone Rosiglitazone	↑ target cell response to insulin.	Used as monotherapy in type 2 DM or combined with above agents.	Weight gain, edema. Hepatotoxicity (troglitazone—no longer used).
α-glucosidase inhibitors: Acarbose Miglitol	**Inhibit intestinal brush border α-glucosidases.** Delayed sugar hydrolysis and glucose absorption lead to ↓ postprandial hyperglycemia.	Used as monotherapy in type 2 DM or in combination with above agents.	GI disturbances.

(Reproduced, with permission, from Le T, Bhushan V, Rao DA. *First Aid for the USMLE Step 1: 2008.* New York: McGraw-Hill, 2008: 287.)

▶ **Case 15**

A 50-year-old woman presents to the emergency department complaining of two hours of vertigo, headache, palpitations, blurry vision, and diaphoresis. She has a history of occasional tension headaches, but no significant cardiac history. She does not smoke and has no history of hypertension. At presentation her blood pressure is 200/140 mm Hg, heart rate is 120/min, and she is afebrile. Her skin is sweaty and flushed. Non-contrast imaging of the brain is negative for blood or other mass lesions. Her blood pressure is stabilized pharmacologically. Laboratory testing reveals increased plasma metanephrine and normetanephrine levels. Results of a serum thyroid-stimulating hormone test are within normal limits. 24-hour urine catecholamines and meta/normetanephrines are elevated.

▪ What is the most likely diagnosis?	Pheochromocytoma, a catecholamine-secreting tumor of chromaffin cells of the adrenal medulla.
▪ What are the key steps in epinephrine catabolism?	Catecholamines are substrates for monoamine oxidase (MAO) and catechol-O-methyltransferase (COMT) (see Figure 6-10). Epinephrine can undergo two paths of catabolism. In the first, COMT converts epinephrine into metanephrine, which MAO then converts into 3-methoxy-4-hydroxymandelic acid. In the second, MAO converts epinephrine into dihydroxymandelic acid, which COMT then converts into 3-methoxy-4-hydroxymandelic acid (the same product as the first pathway).
▪ What receptors do catecholamines act on to produce hypertension?	Catecholamines act on α_1 and β_1 receptors. Activation of α_1 receptors leads to vascular smooth muscle contraction, and activation of β_1 receptors in the heart increases heart rate, conduction velocity, and contractility.
▪ During removal of an adrenal gland, the surgeon must secure the adrenal vasculature, especially the adrenal vein. Describe the blood supply to the adrenal gland.	The arterial blood supply to the adrenal gland can be variable, with blood supply from the superior suprarenal artery originating from the inferior phrenic artery; the middle suprarenal artery originating from the aorta; and the inferior suprarenal artery originating from the renal artery. The adrenal gland typically has a dominant vein, which empties into the left renal vein (left adrenal gland) and the IVC (right adrenal gland).
▪ What is the probability that this patient's condition is malignant?	Approximately 10%. Remember the **"rule of 10's"** for pheochromocytomas: 10% are malignant, 10% bilateral, 10% extra-adrenal, 10% calcify, 10% are pediatric, 10% are familial, and they are 10 times more likely to appear on the boards than in real life!

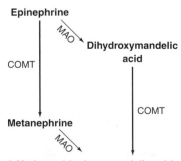

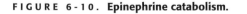

FIGURE 6-10. Epinephrine catabolism.

A 10-year-old girl is brought to her pediatrician for a work-up of new-onset seizure. The patient had been in her usual state of health until 3 months previously, when she developed numbness and tingling in her fingertips and frequent muscle cramps. Last week, she had a grand mal seizure. CT of the head at that time revealed no intracranial lesions. Family history is negative for seizure. Physical examination is notable for short stature, shortened fourth and fifth metacarpals, and positive Chvostek's and Trousseau's signs. Relevant laboratory findings include:

Calcium: 7 mg/dL
Phosphate: 6 mg/dL
Parathyroid hormone (PTH): 100 pg/dL (normal is 10–60 pg/dL)

▪ **What is the most likely diagnosis?**	Pseudohypoparathyroidism (type 1a), characterized by renal unresponsiveness to PTH. A genetic cause of this disorder results from a mutation in the G_s-α_1 protein of adenylyl cyclase. **McCune-Albright's hereditary osteodystrophy** is also present in type 1a pseudohypoparathyroidism, and some patients have growth hormone–releasing hormone resistance.
▪ **What would hypocalcemia with a low serum PTH level suggest?**	**Primary hypoparathyroidism,** usually caused by accidental removal or injury of the parathyroid glands during thyroid surgery, causes decreased PTH levels, which results in decreased serum calcium levels.
▪ **What are Chvostek's and Trousseau's signs?**	**Chvostek's sign** (twitching of ipsilateral facial muscles upon tapping of the facial nerve just anterior to the ear) and **Trousseau's sign** (carpal contractions provoked by inflating a blood pressure cuff above systolic blood pressure for over 3 minutes) are signs of hypocalcemia.
▪ **How is the serum calcium level regulated?**	It is regulated by PTH and vitamin D. **PTH** has two major sites of action: bone and kidney. In bone, PTH increases bone turnover, liberating calcium. In the kidney, PTH increases enzymatic formation of 1,25-$(OH)_2$-cholecalciferol from vitamin D, phosphate excretion, and calcium reabsorption. The active form of **vitamin D** stimulates calcium and phosphate absorption in the gut as well as bone resorption.
▪ **Where is PTH synthesized?**	It is synthesized in the **chief cells** of the parathyroid glands.

► **Case 17**

A 32-year-old woman is postpartum day 4 after delivery of her fourth child. The delivery was complicated by massive hemorrhage. She desires to breast-feed, but her breast milk has not come in (normally it begins by ~24–48 hours postpartum). She breast-fed all of her other children without delay. In addition, she complains of intense fatigue, mental sluggishness, lightheadedness, and a racing heartbeat. On physical examination she is pale, diaphoretic, and weak. Vital signs are: temperature 36.2°C (97.1°F); pulse 100/min supine, 115/min sitting, and 130/min standing; and blood pressure 90/70 mm Hg supine, 80/60 mm Hg sitting, and 70/50 mm Hg standing.

▪ **What is the most likely diagnosis?**	Sheehan's syndrome.
▪ **What is the likely cause?**	Massive hemorrhage during pregnancy leads to ischemia and necrosis of the pituitary gland.
▪ **What hormones are secreted by the pituitary gland?**	The pituitary gland can be separated into anterior and posterior components. The anterior pituitary (adenohypophysis) is derived from ectoderm and produces follicle-stimulating hormone (FSH), luteinizing hormone (LH), adrenocorticotropic hormone (ACTH), growth hormone (GH), thyroid-stimulating hormone (TSH), melanotropin, and prolactin. Know the role of each of these hormones. The posterior component (neurohypophysis) is derived from neuroectoderm and produces antidiuretic hormone (ADH) and oxytocin. **Oxytocin** is required for **lactation** and **contraction** of the uterus.
▪ **What are the clinical manifestations of this condition?**	The presentation can be broken down into deficiencies of each of the pituitary hormones. Severe presentations can present within the first days to weeks after delivery with profound lethargy, anorexia, weight loss, cardiovascular instability, and inability to lactate. Less severe cases may present months to years after the event with hypothyroidism, menstrual irregularities, and other hormonal disturbances.
▪ **What is the significance of the patient's vital signs?**	The patient is displaying **orthostatic hypotension**, defined as a systolic blood pressure decrease of at least 20 mm Hg systolic (or a diastolic blood pressure decrease of 10 mm Hg) within 3 minutes of standing. There is a compensatory increase in heart rate to maintain peripheral perfusion. The cause for hypotension in this patient is **loss of cortisol**, which is required for maintenance of peripheral vascular tone. This is a medical emergency, as the patient is at risk for vascular collapse.
▪ **What other laboratory abnormalities can be expected in this patient?**	Hyponatremia and hyperkalemia, due to loss of ACTH (secondary hypoaldosteronemia), hypocortisolism, hypothyroidism, and FSH and LH deficiency are all seen. Lifelong hormone replacement is required.

► **Case 18**   A 13-year-old girl presents 2 weeks after an upper respiratory infection with a complaint of a "lump in her neck." Physical examination demonstrates a round, freely mobile, slightly tender midline mass that elevates with swallowing. The remainder of the examination is within normal limits. Her birth and developmental history are unremarkable.

▪ **What is the most likely diagnosis?**	Thyroglossal duct cyst.
▪ **What is the differential diagnosis?**	The differential for benign midline neck masses is vast, including thyroglossal duct cysts, dermoid cysts, sebaceous cysts, ectopic thyroid tissue, midline branchial cleft cysts (usually are lateral), lipomas, and lymphadenopathy.
	Hint for the USMLE: If a scenario describes a **lateral** neck mass in a patient with a webbed neck, shield chest, short stature, and coarctation of the aorta, think Turner's syndrome. The neck mass is likely to be a **cystic hygroma**.
▪ **How does the thyroid gland form during development?**	The thyroid is derived from **endoderm** at the **foramen cecum**, the junction between the developing anterior and posterior tongue. The thyroid descends to its final position over the trachea by the seventh week of gestation, and its pharyngeal connection forms a stalk called the thyroglossal duct (see Figure 6-11).
▪ **What is the pathophysiology of this condition?**	The thyroglossal duct should degenerate by the tenth week of gestation. However, in some individuals cystic remnants of the tract remain. Most never become clinically relevant. However, many cysts are detected in patients with recent upper respiratory tract infections, either because infection leads to cyst inflammation, or simply because the cysts are found incidentally on examination of the neck.
▪ **Where is the most common location for this neck mass?**	Thyroglossal duct cysts are in close relation with the hyoid bone and the thyrohyoid membrane. More than 50% are at the level of the hyoid bone within 2 cm of the midline.
▪ **Where is the most common site for ectopic thyroid tissue?**	It is commonly found in the tongue (**lingual thyroid**). If ectopic foci of thyroid tissue will be surgically removed, one must first ensure that the ectopic tissue is not the only thyroid tissue the patient has, as thyroid hormone is necessary for survival.

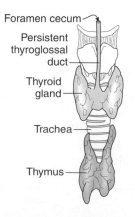

Foramen cecum

Persistent thyroglossal duct

Thyroid gland

Trachea

Thymus

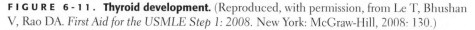

FIGURE 6-11. Thyroid development. (Reproduced, with permission, from Le T, Bhushan V, Rao DA. *First Aid for the USMLE Step 1: 2008.* New York: McGraw-Hill, 2008: 130.)

▶ **Case 19**

As part of Federal Aviation Administration requirements, a 55-year-old pilot presents for a complete check-up. Upon examination of his neck the physician notes a firm nodule in the right upper lobe that remains fixed with swallowing. Ultrasound-guided fine-needle aspiration (FNA) reveals papillary thyroid cancer.

■ What is the prevalence of thyroid nodules?	Thyroid nodules are very common. Clinically, the prevalence is ~5%, but on autopsy studies it can be as high as 50%. Thyroid nodules are more common in women than men.
■ What is the prevalence of thyroid cancer?	Thyroid cancer represents ~1% of all human cancers. **Papillary** thyroid cancer is the most common type (~85%). Other types include **follicular** (~10%), **medullary** (5%), and **anaplastic** (1%). Papillary and follicular types make up the well-differentiated thyroid cancers, whereas the medullary and anaplastic types are considered poorly differentiated.
■ How is the diagnosis of thyroid cancer made?	Careful physical examination, serum thyroid function tests, ultrasound, and FNA of the thyroid are required. **Note:** Thyroid-stimulating hormone (TSH) levels do not make the diagnosis of cancer, but are necessary in the work-up of any thyroid nodule.
■ What characteristic features of papillary thyroid cancer would a pathologist likely see on excisional biopsy?	There is no single pathognomonic feature of papillary carcinoma. However, the combination of "**ground-glass**" cytoplasm, "**Orphan Annie**" inclusion bodies, prominent nuclei with clefts and grooves, and calcified **psammoma bodies** point to the diagnosis.
■ What are the risk factors for this condition?	■ Male gender (while women are more likely to have thyroid nodules, a thyroid nodule in a man is more likely to be cancerous). ■ Age <20 years or >60 years. ■ Prior **radiation exposure** (i.e., for acne treatment as a child, victims of Hiroshima, and frequent flyers). ■ Past medical or family history of thyroid cancer (especially medullary thyroid cancer).
■ How should the patient be treated?	Treat with total thyroidectomy (with/without lymph node dissection) and postoperative radioactive iodine ablation. The radioactive iodine is necessary to destroy microsatellites of disease that may have been left behind at surgery. Lumpectomy and lobectomy are no longer recommended in the surgical management of thyroid cancer.
■ The patient's pathology slides were mistaken for another patient's. The new report says "large polygonal Hurthle cells, abundant microfollicles with little to no colloid, possibly concerning for follicular cancer." How should the patient be counseled?	It is impossible to diagnose follicular thyroid cancer on FNA alone, as follicular adenoma (benign) and follicular carcinoma appear similar. Frozen section/surgical pathology is necessary. The diagnosis of follicular cancer is made if the tumor shows **capsule or vascular invasion**. Therefore, the patient needs surgery to be certain.

A 55-year-old woman with a history of external neck radiation therapy as a child presents to her physician for her yearly check-up. Physical examination reveals a nodule in the neck. Ultrasound reveals several bilateral thyroid nodules, the largest one measuring in 1.5-cm in the left lobe. Biopsy of the 1.5-cm nodule confirms the presence of papillary carcinoma. Two weeks later, the patient undergoes total thyroidectomy.

■ How many parathyroid glands are there?	Most people (85%) have four parathyroid glands. However, 13%–15% have more than four glands, and <2% have fewer than four glands.
■ What is the embryologic origin of the parathyroid glands?	The superior parathyroid glands are derived from the fourth pharyngeal pouch. The inferior parathyroids are derived from the third pharyngeal pouch. Most ectopic sites are derived along the embryologic descent path (e.g., carotid sheath and mediastinum).

■ What layers of muscle are encountered during a thyroidectomy?	■ Platysma (facial nerve innervation).
	■ Cervical fascia.
	■ The muscles listed below are flat and are referred to as "strap" muscles:
	  ■ Sternohyoid
	  ■ Sternothyroid
	  ■ The other two strap muscles (thyrohyoid and omohyoid) are not commonly encountered during routine thyroidectomy.

■ What nerves in this region are particularly at risk during thyroidectomy?	Damage to the **recurrent laryngeal nerve** in the tracheoesophageal groove results in a hoarse voice. The external laryngeal artery branch of the superior laryngeal nerve accompanies the superior thyroid artery and therefore can be ligated with the artery in thyroid surgery (see Figure 6-12). It is spared by ligating the artery close to the gland. Damage results in changes in pitch and reduction in voice volume.
■ After total thyroidectomy, this patient will require lifelong thyroid hormone replacement. What are some other causes of hypothyroidism?	■ Autoimmune (Hashimoto's thyroiditis) ■ Alcohol ■ Drugs (amiodarone and lithium) ■ Infection

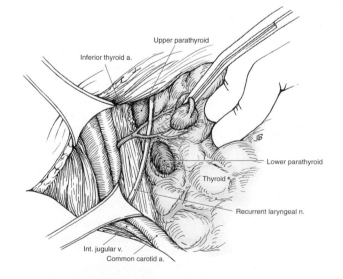

FIGURE 6-12. Relationship of the parathyroids to the recurrent laryngeal nerve. (Reproduced, with permission, from Brunicardi FC, et al. *Schwartz's Principles of Surgery*, 8th ed. New York: McGraw-Hill, 2005: 1402.)

► **Case 21**

A 77-year-old man is brought in by a concerned neighbor to evaluate a large neck mass. According to the neighbor, the patient lives alone and keeps to himself. The neighbor has noticed the neck mass to be enlarging over several months. Meanwhile, the patient has lost approximately 12 lb (5.4 kg) and has developed noticeable tremor when he reaches for his morning paper or walks his dog. On physical examination, the man is thin with a large goiter containing many palpable nodules. ECG reveals atrial fibrillation. Exophthalmos and pretibial myxedema are absent. Thyroid function tests reveal elevated free thyroxine (T_4) and barely detectable thyroid-stimulating hormone (TSH) levels.

■ What is the most likely diagnosis?	Plummer's disease (aka toxic multinodular goiter [TNG]), which is the second most common cause of hyperthyroidism in the Western world after Graves' disease, and the number one cause among the elderly or in endemic areas of iodine deficiency. This is not to be confused with the uncommon **Plummer-Vinson syndrome** (esophageal web + iron deficiency anemia).
■ How does the physical examination help in the formulation of a differential diagnosis?	Patients with Graves' disease typically have a diffusely enlarged, painless goiter, rather than a multinodular goiter. Exophthalmos, pretibial myxedema, and acropachy (thickening of peripheral tissues), characteristic of Graves' disease, are absent in TNG. Subacute thyroiditis (aka de Quervain's thyroiditis) presents with an enlarged **painful** goiter (see Figure 6-13), neck pain, and fever, frequently after a viral illness such as mumps or coxsackievirus. The erythrocyte sedimentation rate is typically elevated, and the condition resolves with time and nonsteroidal anti-inflammatory drug use.
■ What are the signs and symptoms of local compression by a neck mass?	**Symptoms**: Dysphagia (difficulty swallowing), dysphonia (hoarseness), and dyspnea (difficulty breathing).
	Signs: Stridor, tracheal deviation, superior vena cava syndrome. (Pemberton's sign is engorgement of the facial and neck veins upon simultaneous raising of the arms overhead, secondary to superior vena cava compression at the thoracic inlet.)
■ What would a radioactive iodine scan likely show?	A thyroid scan with radioactive iodine or Tc^{99m} will likely show **patchy uptake**, with multiple "**hot**" **nodule**s interspersed among areas with decreased uptake. A "hot" nodule means that the activity of the thyroid tissue in that area is elevated. Patients with Graves' disease will have homogenously high uptake on thyroid scan, whereas patients with thyroiditis (de Quervain's or silent lymphocytic thyroiditis) will have low uptake on thyroid scan. In general, nodules containing thyroid cancer tend to be "cold" nodules and should be biopsied via fine-needle aspiration.
■ What is the most appropriate treatment for this condition?	Given the size of his goiter, signs of local compression, and symptoms of hyperthyroidism, **thyroidectomy** should be performed. This will alleviate the symptoms of hyperthyroidism in ~90% of cases and will rapidly relieve the compression. Preoperatively the patient should be treated with **antithyroid medication** (such as methimazole) and **β-blockers** in order to render him euthyroid and to alleviate the atrial fibrillation.

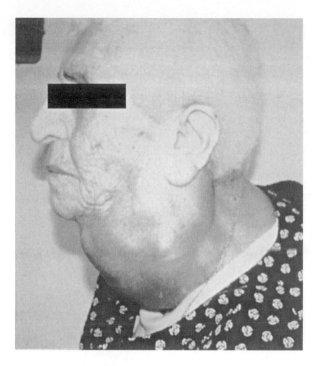

FIGURE 6-13. A large multinodular goiter. (Reproduced, with permission, from Bruni-cardi FC, et al. *Schwartz's Principles of Surgery*, 8th ed. New York: McGraw-Hill, 2005: 1413.)

Gastrointestinal

Case 1	208
Case 2	209
Case 3	210
Case 4	212
Case 5	213
Case 6	214
Case 7	216
Case 8	218
Case 9	220
Case 10	221
Case 11	222
Case 12	223
Case 13	224
Case 14	225
Case 15	226
Case 16	227
Case 17	228
Case 18	229
Case 19	230
Case 20	232
Case 21	233
Case 22	234
Case 23	236
Case 24	237
Case 25	238
Case 26	239
Case 27	240
Case 28	241
Case 29	242
Case 30	244

► **Case 1**

A 50-year-old man presents to his physician complaining of problems swallowing for the past several months. Solid foods are the most difficult for him to swallow and recently liquids have also become problematic. He often has chest discomfort after eating and occasionally will regurgitate bits of undigested food. His physical examination is unremarkable.

■ **What is the most likely diagnosis?**	Achalasia.
■ **What type of imaging or testing could help confirm this diagnosis?**	A barium esophagogram in a patient with achalasia will demonstrate a "**bird's beak**" appearance of the esophagus (as shown in Figure 7-1 below). Esophageal manometry confirms the diagnosis and reveals complete absence of peristalsis and failure of the lower esophageal sphincter (LES) to relax after swallowing.
■ **What other conditions should be considered in the differential diagnosis?**	**Chagas' disease** is indistinguishable from idiopathic forms of achalasia and should be considered in a patient from endemic areas (e.g., Central and South America). Certain malignancies affect the gastroesophageal junction and produce "**pseudoachalasia.**" Diffuse **esophageal spasm** and esophageal scleroderma should also be ruled out.
■ **What is the pathophysiology of this condition?**	Achalasia is an idiopathic motility disorder caused by impaired relaxation of the LES and loss of smooth muscle peristalsis in the lower two-thirds of the esophagus. It is thought that nitric oxide–producing inhibitory neurons are lost in the myenteric plexus, resulting in the clinical picture described above.
■ **What is the most appropriate treatment for this condition?**	Pneumatic dilation of the LES provides effective relief in most patients. Surgical myotomy and an antireflux procedure are also effective. In patients who are not surgical candidates, treatment includes multiple injections of botulinum toxin in the LES.

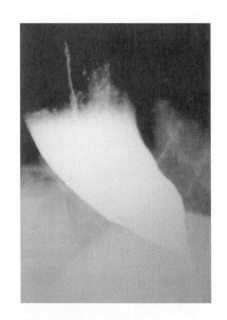

FIGURE 7-1. "Bird's beak" appearance of the esophagus in achalasia. (Reproduced, with permission, from Lalwani AK. *Current Diagnosis & Treatment in Otolaryngology—Head & Neck Surgery*, 2nd ed. New York: McGraw-Hill, 2008: 489.)

► **Case 2**   A 48-year-old man with human immunodeficiency virus (HIV) presents to his primary care physician with a 1-day history of nausea and vomiting. He also has severe epigastric pain radiating to the back, which is worse when lying down. Review of the patient's medical history reveals that he is taking the reverse transcriptase inhibitor didanosine. Laboratory testing reveals an amylase level five times higher than normal and a lipase level six times higher than normal.

■ **What is the most likely diagnosis?**	Acute pancreatitis.
■ **What are the most common causes of this condition?**	Acute pancreatitis occurs when pancreatic enzymes (trypsinogen, chymotrypsinogen, and phospholipase A) are activated in pancreatic tissue rather than in the lumen of the intestine, resulting in the autodigestion of pancreatic tissue. The most common causes are **G**allstones, **E**tOH, **T**rauma, **S**teroids, **M**umps, **A**utoimmune diseases, **S**corpion stings, **H**yperlipidemia, and certain **D**rugs, including antiretrovirals (mnemonic: **GET SMASHeD**).
■ **What other conditions should be considered in the differential diagnosis?**	■ Cholelithiasis ■ Diabetic ketoacidosis ■ Dissecting aortic aneurysm ■ Intestinal obstruction ■ Mesenteric ischemia ■ Myocardial infarction ■ Nephrolithiasis ■ Perforated ulcer In this patient, the elevated amylase and lipase levels are sensitive and specific for acute pancreatitis.
■ **Why is there an increased incidence of this condition in patients with HIV infection?**	Patients with HIV or acquired immunodeficiency syndrome (AIDS) are often infected with organisms such as cytomegalovirus, *Mycobacterium avium* complex, and *Cryptosporidium*, all of which can cause pancreatitis. Antiretroviral agents such as didanosine, pentamidine, and trimethoprim-sulfamethoxazole can also cause acute pancreatitis.
■ **What is the most appropriate treatment for this condition?**	Most cases (85%–90%) are self limited and spontaneously resolve within 4–7 days of the start of treatment. Typical treatment for acute pancreatitis includes avoiding oral intake, aggressive intravenous fluid resuscitation, pain control, and possibly nasogastric tube placement to decrease the amount of gastric secretions in the stomach. Antibiotics are not recommended in uncomplicated pancreatitis, but may be used prophylactically in cases of severe acute pancreatitis.

► **Case 3**

A 42-year-old man presents to his doctor for a regular check-up after several years without medical care. His past medical history is significant for extensive smoking, alcohol, and intravenous drug abuse. On review of systems, the patient reports bleeding from his gums and increased bruising. Physical examination reveals an overweight white male who appears older than his stated age, mild gynecomastia, palmar erythema, and pitting edema of his lower extremities. Abdominal examination reveals shifting dullness. Relevant laboratory findings are as follows:

WBC count: 3200/mm^3
Chloride: 98 mEq/L
Platelets: 90,000/mm^3
Bicarbonate: 24 mEq/L
Hemoglobin: 9 g/dL
Blood urea nitrogen (BUN):
  36 mg/dL
Hematocrit: 28%
Creatinine (Cr): 1.5 mg/dL
Prothrombin time (PT):
  14 seconds

Albumin: 3.3 g/dL
Partial thromboplastin time (PTT):
  40 seconds
Aspartate aminotransferase (AST):
  100 U/L
Sodium: 138 mEq/L
Alanine aminotransferase (ALT):
  60 U/L
Potassium: 4.0 mEq/L

■ **What is the most likely diagnosis?**	Alcoholic cirrhosis of the liver. The ascites, palmar erythema, and gynecomastia all suggest liver failure. The moderately elevated transaminase levels suggest a chronic process (too many hepatocytes have already died to cause the dramatic rise that would be seen in an acute process). Further indicators of chronicity include: a decreased albumin level, elevated PT and PTT, thrombocytopenia, and decreased hematocrit. An AST level > ALT level suggests an alcoholic, rather than viral, etiology (mnemonic: To**AST**ed).
■ **What are the causes of this patient's gynecomastia and bleeding gums?**	The liver normally degrades estrogen. In liver failure, circulating serum levels of estrogen are higher, thus explaining the gynecomastia. Bleeding gums are likely due to thrombocytopenia secondary to splenic sequestration.
■ **How does ascites form?**	**Ascites** (an abnormal accumulation of serous fluid in the abdominal cavity) forms as a result of increased intrahepatic sinusoidal pressure secondary to intrahepatic obstruction within the cirrhotic liver; decreased degradation of aldosterone by the liver leading to sodium and water retention; and decreased plasma osmotic pressure due to decreased hepatic production of albumin. Signs of ascites include: shifting dullness, bulging flanks, and a fluid wave.
■ **What do the laboratory findings show regarding renal function?**	Elevated BUN and Cr levels (BUN:Cr ratio >20) suggest prerenal failure. The kidneys are not perfused appropriately because of decreased intravascular volume (as a result of the patient's ascites).
■ **Describe the findings in Figure 7-2 below.**	Micronodular architecture and broad fibrous bands are typical findings of alcoholic liver damage and represent areas of liver regeneration (nodules) separated by scar (bands).

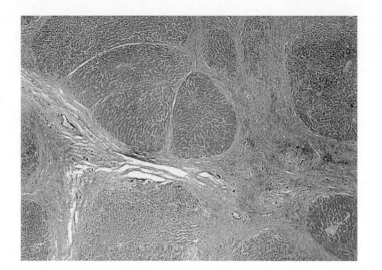

FIGURE 7-2. Cirrhosis on microscopy. Regenerative lesions are surrounded by fibrotic bands of collagen ("bridging fibrosis"), forming the characteristic nodularity. (Reproduced, with permission, of the Pathology Education Instructional Resource Digital Library [http://peir.net] at the University of Alabama, Birmingham.)

► **Case 4**

A 25-year-old woman presents to her physician complaining with a 3-day history of crampy abdominal pain that started in the epigastrum. She also reports nausea, low-grade fever, and loss of appetite. She denies changes in frequency of urination, dysuria, or recent contact with a sick person. Her last menstrual period was 2 weeks ago. Relevant laboratory findings are as follows:

WBC count: 13,000/mm³
β-Human chorionic gonadotropin: negative
Urinalysis: negative for blood, WBCs, leukocyte esterase, and protein

▪ What is the most likely diagnosis?	Appendicitis.
▪ Which conditions should be considered in the differential diagnosis?	▪ Genitourinary: Ruptured Graafian follicle, ectopic pregnancy, pelvic inflammatory disease, ovarian torsion. ▪ Gastrointestinal: Crohn's disease, Meckel's diverticulitis, perforated bowel, *Yersinia enterocolitica* infection, intussusception. ▪ Renal: Urinary tract infection, renal colic. ▪ Lymphatics: Mesenteric lymphadenitis.
▪ What is the pathophysiology of this condition?	Appendicitis results from **obstruction** or **infection.** The appendiceal lumen may become obstructed by mucosal secretions or a fecolith, resulting in a distended appendix. Alternatively, bacteria may attack the wall of the appendix, blocking the venous system, creating increased intraluminal pressure and subsequent arterial insufficiency.
▪ What is McBurney's point?	**McBurney's point** is one-third the distance from the right anterior superior iliac spine to the umbilicus, and is where the pain from acute appendicitis classically localizes.
▪ Which antibiotics are used to cover against enteric organisms?	Ampicillin and sulbactam are empirically used to treat *Escherichia coli* and *Bacteroides fragilis* infections. Gentamicin, clindamycin, imipenem, second-generation cephalosporins, and piperacillin/tazobactam are also effective.
▪ What is the most appropriate treatment for this condition?	The most likely cause of the appendicitis in this patient is obstruction, as her presentation is typical and her laboratory results are not indicative of infection. Surgery is the preferred treatment, along with supportive intravenous fluids and empiric antibiotics (in case of rupture). The gold standard for diagnosis is CT of the abdomen with contrast; Figure 7-3 below shows calcified appendolith.

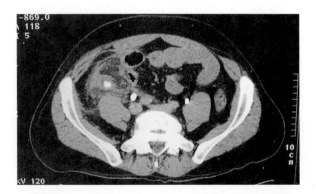

FIGURE 7-3. Contrast-enhanced CT showing a calcified appendolith. (Reproduced, with permission, from Stone CK, Humphries RL. *Current Emergency Diagnosis & Treatment*, 5th ed. New York: McGraw-Hill, 2004: 269.)

A 55-year-old man presents to his physician with a complaint of burning chest pain that typically occurs after eating and radiates to the neck. Occasionally, the pain awakens him from sleep. He also complains of difficulty swallowing, particularly solid foods. The patient has had these symptoms for several years, but they seem to be worsening. Endoscopy reveals gastric columnar epithelium in the distal esophagus.

▪ What is the most likely diagnosis?	Gastroesophageal reflux disease (GERD), complicated by Barrett's esophagus.
▪ In the absence of positive findings on endoscopy, what other conditions should be considered in the differential diagnosis?	▪ Angina pectoris ▪ Erosive esophagitis ▪ Esophageal stricture ▪ Peptic ulcer disease ▪ Pill esophagitis ▪ Malignancy ▪ Schatzki's ring
▪ What type of epithelium is normally found in the distal esophagus?	Nonkeratinized squamous epithelium. In Barrett's esophagus (intestinal metaplasia), the squamous epithelium is replaced by gastric (columnar) epithelium, due to chronic injury from refluxed stomach acid (see Figure 7-4 below). Intestinal metaplasia typically begins at the squamocolumnar junction, or "Z line," which is the border between the squamous epithelium of the esophagus and the columnar epithelium of the stomach.
▪ Patients with this condition are at greatly increased risk for what other condition?	Esophageal adenocarcinoma. Compared to the general population, patients with Barrett's esophagus are 30 times more likely to develop this condition (approximately 1%).
▪ What factors increase the risk of developing esophageal cancer?	Barrett's esophagus is the major risk factor for esophageal adenocarcinoma, whereas alcohol and cigarette smoking are major risk factors for esophageal squamous cell carcinoma. The risk factors for esophageal cancer may be remembered with the mnemonic **ABCDEF**: **A**chalasia/**A**frican-American male, **B**arrett's esophagus, **C**orrosive esophagitis/**C**igarettes, **D**iverticuli (i.e., Zenker's diverticulum), **E**sophageal web/**E**tOH, and **F**amilial.

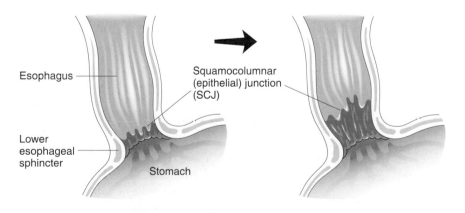

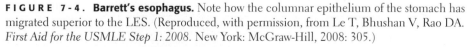

FIGURE 7-4. Barrett's esophagus. Note how the columnar epithelium of the stomach has migrated superior to the LES. (Reproduced, with permission, from Le T, Bhushan V, Rao DA. *First Aid for the USMLE Step 1: 2008*. New York: McGraw-Hill, 2008: 305.)

ORGAN SYSTEMS

GASTROINTESTINAL

► **Case 6**

A 42-year-old obese woman presents to the urgent care facility with a sudden onset of right upper quadrant and epigastric pain that began 8 hours earlier. The pain is steady in nature, worsened by eating, and radiates to the right shoulder. Physical examination reveals inspiratory arrest with deep palpation of the right upper quadrant (**Murphy's sign**). Relevant laboratory findings are as follows:

Total bilirubin: 2 mg/dL
Blood urea nitrogen: 16 mg/dL
Aspartate aminotransferase [AST]: 44 U/L
Creatinine: 1.05 mg/dL
Alanine aminotransferase [ALT]: 49 U/L

■ What is the most likely diagnosis?	Choledocholithiasis (a gallstone lodged in the common bile duct). **Note:** The presence of gallstones is termed *cholelithiasis*. Gallbladder disease is very common in the United States and manifests as a spectrum of disorders from asymptomatic cholelithiasis to biliary colic, cholecystitis, choledocholithiasis, and cholangitis (infection of the biliary tree). Biliary colic usually resolves within a few hours. The fact that the patient has had unremitting pain for 8 hours suggests obstruction.
■ Infection with which bacteria may result from this condition?	*Escherichia coli*, *Enterobacter cloacae*, *Enterococcus*, and *Klebsiella* are commonly implicated in infection of the gallbladder secondary to obstruction (cholecystitis).
■ What are the risk factors for this condition?	**Cholesterol gallstones** are most common in the United States and occur when bile is supersaturated with cholesterol, allowing crystals to form.
	Risk factors for gallstones include the **Four F's: F**at, **F**ertile, **F**emale, and **F**orty. Other risk factors include oral contraceptive use, spinal cord injury, or diabetes mellitus, all of which cause decreased gallbladder emptying. Intestinal and liver diseases are also risk factors. Worldwide, **pigmented gallstones** are the most common form. These form secondary to bile duct/gallbladder infection, hemolysis, or impaired hepatic synthesis of bilirubin.
■ What is the pathophysiology of the patient's pain?	Gallstones produce visceral pain by obstructing the ampulla of Vater or the cystic duct, causing distention of the gallbladder, and irritation of surrounding structures.
■ Which structures are adjacent to the gallbladder?	The **gallbladder** lies immediately below the liver and above the **right kidney.** The **cystic duct** from the gallbladder joins the common hepatic duct to form the common bile duct. The common bile duct joins with the pancreatic duct and terminates in the **ampulla of Vater**—the site where bile is excreted into the duodenum.
■ What is the most appropriate treatment for managing this patient's pain?	Gallstone pain is relieved when the gallstone moves back into the gallbladder, moves into the common bile duct, or passes through the ampulla of Vater. Pain of biliary colic accompanies spasms of the sphincter of Oddi. Therefore, **meperidine** should be given for pain, as morphine causes spasms of the sphincter of Oddi.

■ **The hepatoduodenal ligament includes which three structures?**

Three structures run through the hepatoduodenal ligament (see Figure 7-5 below):

■ **Portal vein:** Brings blood from the digestive tract to the liver.
■ **Hepatic artery:** Brings oxygen and nutrients to the liver.
■ **Common bile duct:** Connects the liver and gallbladder to the small intestine.

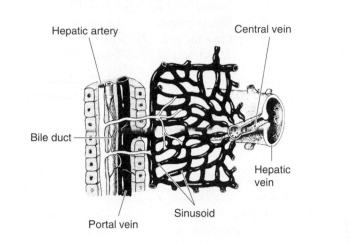

FIGURE 7-5. Vascular anatomy of the liver lobule. (Reproduced, with permission, from Doherty GM. *Current Surgical Diagnosis & Treatment*, 12th ed. New York: McGraw Hill, 2006: 542.)

► **Case 7**

A 6-day-old girl born to a Jewish couple is brought to her pediatrician because she "looks yellow," seems weak and floppy, and sleeps all the time. Physical examination reveals a jaundiced infant with scleral icterus, without other obvious abnormalities. Relevant laboratory findings are as follows:

Total bilirubin: 34 mg/dL
Alanine aminotransferase (ALT): 12 U/L
Direct bilirubin: Undetectable
Coombs' test: Negative
Aspartate aminotransferase (AST): 10 U/L

▪ What is the most likely diagnosis?	Crigler-Najjar syndrome.
▪ What is the pathophysiology of this condition?	This disease is an inherited disorder of bilirubin metabolism. It is the result of a mutation in **glucuronyl transferase**, the enzyme responsible for conjugating bilirubin with glucuronic acid. Unconjugated bilirubin is less water soluble than conjugated bilirubin and is less easily excreted in urine and bile.
▪ What are the two subtypes of this condition, and how do they differ in severity?	▪ **Crigler-Najjar type I:** Glucuronyl transferase activity is completely absent, which results in a high likelihood of death in the first year of life. ▪ **Crigler-Najjar type II:** Glucuronyl transferase activity is present but low. Patients with this form of the disease have a better prognosis than those with type 1 (see Table 7-1).

TABLE 7-1. Principal Differential Characteristics of Crigler-Najjar Syndromes

FEATURE	CRIGLER-NAJJAR SYNDROME	
	TYPE I	TYPE II
Total serum bilirubin, mg/dL	18–45 (usually >20)	6–25 (usually ≤20)
Routine liver tests	Normal	Normal
Response to phenobarbital	None	Decreases bilirubin by >25%
Kernicterus	Usual	Rare
Hepatic histology	Normal	Normal
Bile characteristics		
Color	Pale or colorless	Pigmented
Bilirubin fractions	>90% unconjugated	Largest fraction (mean: 57%) monoconjugates
Bilirubin UDP-glucuronosyl transferase activity	Typically absent; traces in some patients	Markedly reduced: 0%–10% of normal
Inheritance (both autosomal)	Recessive	Predominantly recessive

Modified, with permission, from Kasper DL, et al. *Harrison's Principles of Internal Medicine,* 16th ed. New York: McGraw-Hill, 2005: 1819.

- This patient is at risk for what life-threatening complication?

Kernicterus, or an abnormal accumulation of bile pigment in the central nervous system leading to irreversible brain damage and even death. Unconjugated bilirubin penetrates the blood-brain barrier to cause neuronal death.

- What is the most appropriate treatment for this condition?

In Crigler-Najjar type I, liver transplantation is the only cure. Phototherapy may be employed to prevent kernicterus. In type II, the hyperbilirubinemia often responds to **phenobarbital.**

► **Case 8**

A 64-year-old woman presents to her physician complaining of gas, constipation, and left lower abdominal discomfort. The pain increases after meals but persists throughout the day. She also complains of lightheadedness and fatigue for the past week. The patient has a history of chronic constipation, but the current symptoms are worse than normal. She denies bloody stools currently, but did have a massive gastrointestinal (GI) bleed last year. During that hospitalization she received a barium enema; her roentgenogram is shown in Figure 7-6. Her only medication is one baby aspirin per day. On physical examination, she is febrile to 38.6°C (101.5°F), with a blood pressure of 110/70 mm Hg, heart rate of 105/min, and respiratory rate of 18/min. Relevant laboratory findings are as follows:

WBC count: 13,400/mm^3 Bicarbonate: 24 mEq/L
Potassium: 4.3 mEq/L   Hematocrit: 38%
Platelets: 250,000/mm^3 Creatinine: 1.2 mg/dL
Chloride: 100 mEq/L   Sodium: 136 mEq/L
Hemoglobin: 13 g/dL   Stool guaiac test: Negative

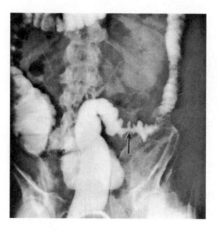

FIGURE 7-6. (Reproduced, with permission, from Doherty GM, Way LW. *Current Surgical Diagnosis & Treatment*, 12th ed. New York: McGraw-Hill, 2006: 715.)

■ **What is the most likely diagnosis?**	Diverticulitis. The patient has known diverticulae in her distal colon, as per her roentgenogram. The previous GI bleed was likely secondary to a diverticular bleed.
■ **Which of the clinical signs and symptoms help confirm the diagnosis?**	Constipation, flatus, left-sided abdominal pain, tenderness, fever, tachycardia, and elevated WBC count are characteristic of diverticulitis.
■ **What tests could help confirm the diagnosis?**	Abdominal x-ray should be ordered to rule out free air (which indicates diverticular rupture and is a surgical emergency). In the absence of a "surgical abdomen," a CT of the abdomen may be ordered. Radiographic findings would include: bowel wall thickening, fistulas, and/or abscesses. Colonoscopy is contraindicated in the acute setting, as it may cause perforation; however, colonoscopy should be completed on follow-up.

■ **What factors increase the risk of this condition, and what steps can prevent recurrence?**

Advanced age, chronic constipation, previous diverticulosis, and aspirin use all heighten her risk for diverticular disease. A high-fiber diet and good hydration reduce the risk of developing diverticulae and subsequent diverticulitis.

■ **What is the most appropriate treatment for this condition?**

Broad-spectrum antibiotics, such as metronidazole and ciprofloxacin, a clear liquid diet for 1 week, and adequate analgesia. A follow-up colonoscopy should be performed after the acute symptoms resolve.

► **Case 9**

The emergency department (ED) triage nurse calls the on-call intern to ask how she should triage a 42-year-old woman with a history of hereditary spherocytosis, fever, and mental status changes. She was brought to the ED by her husband, after he found her disoriented and sick appearing in bed. The patient is unable to provide a good history. Vital signs are notable for a temperature of 102°F (38.9°C), heart rate of 125/min, blood pressure of 80/50 mm Hg, and respiratory rate of 24/min. She is overweight, diaphoretic, slightly yellow appearing, and oriented only to person. Physical examination is notable for tenderness and guarding in the right upper quadrant (RUQ).

■ Where should this patient be placed on the triage list?	This patient is sick and requires **immediate attention**. Even without laboratory data, her vital signs (fever, tachycardia, hypotension, and tachypnea) and toxic appearance should raise suspicion of sepsis.
■ What is the most likely diagnosis?	**Cholangitis,** or infection of the bile ducts secondary to ductal obstruction (see Figure 7-7). Most commonly, the common bile duct is obstructed by a gallstone. Other causes include stricture, biliary cancer, and infection (e.g., *Clonorchis*).
■ How does the physical examination help confirm the diagnosis?	The patient displays **Charcot's triad** and **Reynolds' pentad**, which are classic for cholangitis. Charcot's triad: RUQ pain, jaundice, and fever. Reynold's pentad: Charcot's triad, hypotension, and mental status changes.
■ What risk factors in this patient's history predisposed her to this condition?	The patient likely has underlying cholelithiasis (gallstones). In addition to the **4F's** (Fat, Fertile, Forty, and Female), the patient has an additional risk factor; hereditary spherocytosis (HS). Due to chronic hemolysis, patients with HS are predisposed to develop **pigment gallstones**. Pigment gallstones are radiopaque due to their composition of calcium bilirubinate. The high iron content from the hemolyzed red blood cells may also help these stones to be visualized on x-ray.
■ What laboratory values are expected?	■ Elevated WBC ■ Hyperbilirubinemia (total and direct) ■ Elevated alkaline phosphatase ■ Positive blood cultures
■ What is the appropriate treatment for this condition?	As this patient is displaying severe symptoms, every effort should be made to relieve the obstruction and decompress the biliary tree. Endoscopic retrograde cholangiopancreatography (**ERCP**) is the tool of choice, as it is both diagnostic and therapeutic.

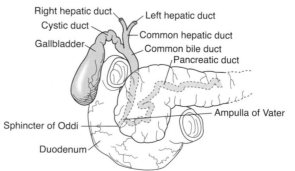

FIGURE 7-7. Anatomy of the biliary tree. (Reproduced, with permission, from Le T, Bhushan V, Rao DA. *First Aid for the USMLE Step 1: 2008.* New York: McGraw-Hill, 2008: 294.)

▶ **Case 10**

The mother of a newborn girl complains to the pediatrician that the infant is coughing, drooling excessively, and vomiting immediately after every feeding. The woman's pregnancy was complicated by gestational polyhydramnios. The physician attempts to place a nasogastric tube in the infant, but chest x-ray reveals that it cannot pass to the stomach, which is distended with air.

▪ What is the most likely diagnosis?	Esophageal atresia with tracheoesophageal fistula. As depicted in Figure 7-8 below, this variant accounts for 85% of these malformations.
▪ How did the patient's polyhydramnios develop?	Normally, fetuses swallow amniotic fluid in utero. The fluid is absorbed by the infant's gastrointestinal (GI) tract and is returned to the mother via the placenta, or eliminated through the urinary system. When a fetus is unable to swallow, amniotic fluid builds up, resulting in **polyhydramnios**. Polyhydramnios can also result from disorders of the urinary tract, as in neonatal Bartter's syndrome.
▪ Lung buds are derived from which embryonic structure?	The lung buds, which will become the bronchial tree, begin as evaginations from the primitive foregut, which also gives rise to the esophagus. Thus, abnormalities anywhere along this developmental pathway can result in a variety of tracheoesophageal fistulae.
▪ Which pathogens are most likely to cause pneumonia in this patient?	**Anaerobes,** given the increased risk of aspiration of GI contents from frequent vomiting and pooling of fluids in the esophageal pouch.
▪ What other congenital condition is associated with polyhydramnios and bilious vomiting?	**Duodenal atresia,** which has an increased incidence in infants with trisomy 21 (Down syndrome). Bilious vomiting is indicative of gastrointestinal obstruction distal to the opening of the bile duct.

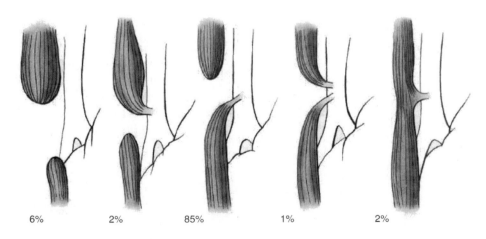

6% 2% 85% 1% 2%

FIGURE 7-8. Variants of esophageal atresia and their prevalence. (Reproduced, with permission, from Brunicardi FC, et al. *Schwartz's Principles of Surgery*, 8th ed. New York: McGraw-Hill, 2005: 1481.)

► **Case 11**

A 65-year-old woman presents to her physician with left lower quadrant pain, a 3-week history of nausea and vomiting, diarrhea, and an unintentional 15.9-kg (35-lb) weight loss over the past month. Her medical history is complicated by Type 2 diabetes, hypertension, breast cancer, erosive esophagitis, and chronic peptic ulcer disease. She takes several medications, including a β-blocker. CT of the abdomen reveals a 5 × 5-cm mass in the head of the pancreas. Relevant laboratory findings are as follows:

Gastric pH: <2.0
Gastrin: 97 pg/mL (normal: <90 pg/mL)
Hematocrit: 26%
Basal gastric acid output: >15 mEq/h (normal: <15 mEq/h)

▪ **What is the most likely diagnosis?**	Gastrinoma, a gastrin-secreting, non–β islet cell tumor of the pancreas or duodenum. These tumors cause gastric hypersecretion of hydrochloric acid, which results in disseminated gastrointestinal ulcers.
▪ **What are the two most common neuroendocrine tumors?**	Gastrinoma (two-thirds are malignant) and insulinoma (usually benign).
▪ **What signs and symptoms are diagnostic of these tumors?**	▪ Diarrhea ▪ Epigastric pain ▪ Gastroesophageal reflux disease ▪ Hematemesis ▪ Hematochezia ▪ Increased resting gastrin level ▪ Melena ▪ Nausea/vomiting ▪ Peptic ulcer disease ▪ Ulcers in unusual locations such as the proximal jejunum ▪ Weight loss
▪ **With what syndrome are these tumors commonly associated?**	**Zollinger-Ellison syndrome**, of which the classical triad includes: increased gastric acid secretion, peptic ulcer disease, and diarrhea.
▪ **What is the most appropriate treatment for this tumor?**	▪ Surgical: Whipple's procedure, duodenotomy. ▪ Medical: Proton pump inhibitors, somatostatin. Octreotide is a somatostatin analogue with a longer half-life. Both somatostatin and octreotide act by inhibiting release of somatotropin, insulin, gastrin, glucagons, and vasoactive intestinal peptide.

► **Case 12**

A 36-year-old male presents with erectile dysfunction, decreased libido, achy joints, increased thirst, and frequency of urination. His wife also notes that despite it's being January, he looks like he has a tan. On physical examination, his skin appears bronze in color. Relevant laboratory studies are as follows:

Blood glucose: 242 mg/dL
Serum iron: 1200 mg/dL
Transferrin saturation: 99%

■ **What is the most likely diagnosis?**	Hemochromatosis. The classic triad is: ■ Micronodular pigment cirrhosis ■ Diabetes mellitus ■ Skin pigmentation The last two symptoms give this disease the nickname "**bronze diabetes.**"
■ **How is this condition inherited?**	Hereditary (primary) hemochromatosis is an **autosomal recessive** disease caused by a defect in the *Hfe* gene of chromosome 6. There is also an acquired (secondary) form, in which iron overload results from chronic transfusion therapy, such as for hemolytic anemias.
■ **Do the presentations differ between men and women?**	Yes. Women tend to present later and/or with milder forms, as iron is lost with monthly menstruation.
■ **What is the pathophysiology of this condition?**	In the primary disorder, excess iron is stored in parenchymal cells of the visceral organs, particularly the: ■ Liver, leading to **cirrhosis.** ■ Pancreas, leading to **diabetes mellitus.** ■ Heart, leading to restrictive **cardiomyopathy** and congestive heart failure. ■ Joints, leading to arthritis and **arthralgias.** ■ Gonads, leading to **testicular atrophy.**
■ **What would liver biopsy likely show?**	Extensive hemosiderin deposits within the hepatocytes and Kupffer cells. Hemosiderin and other iron-containing compounds stain with **Prussian blue.**
■ **What is the most appropriate treatment for this condition?**	Repeated phlebotomy and an iron chelator such as deferoxamine.
■ **How is this condition differentiated from Wilson's disease?**	In Wilson's disease, a decrease in circulating **ceruloplasmin** causes copper to accumulate in the liver, brain, and cornea (e.g., hepatolenticular degeneration). Like hemochromatosis, patients are at risk of developing hepatocellular carcinoma. Wilson's disease is characterized by **ABCD**: ■ **A**sterixis. ■ **B**asal ganglia degeneration (parkinsonian features, choreiform movements, and hemiballismus). ■ **C**orneal deposits in Descemet's membrane and cirrhosis. ■ **D**ementia and other mental status disturbances. Wilson's disease is treated with penicillamine.

► **Case 13**

A 34-year-old man with a history of alcohol and drug abuse comes to the emergency department complaining of nausea and vomiting. He notes no recent change in diet or lifestyle and has been in a monogamous relationship for the past year. Physical examination reveals a fever of 38.3°C (101°F), a heart rate of 80/min, and a respiratory rate of 18/min. Icterus is present and there is tenderness in the right upper quadrant and mid-epigastric region. Work-up is negative for gonorrhea and chlamydia. Relevant laboratory findings are as follows:

Alanine aminotransferase (ALT): 1310 U/L
Aspartate aminotransferase (AST): 1200 U/L
Alkaline phosphatase: 98 U/L

- HBsAg: Negative
- HBeAg: Negative
- Anti-HBeAg antibody: Positive
- Anti-HBcAg antibody: Positive
- Anti-HBsAg antibody: Negative

▪ What is the most likely diagnosis?	Hepatitis.
▪ What is the etiology of this condition?	Hepatitis can be caused by alcohol, viral infection, ischemia, congestive heart failure, or toxins such as acetaminophen or aflatoxin. The history and the roughly equivalent increases of serum transaminases (by >1000 U/L), suggest a viral etiology. In contrast, in alcoholic hepatitis. AST is typically elevated more than ALT, but does not often rise above 1000 U/L.
▪ Does the patient have HBV infection?	The patient is in the "window phase" of HBV infection, which occurs after HBsAg has disappeared but before anti-HBsAg antibody is detectable. This is indicated by the presence of anti-HBeAg and anti-HBcAg antibodies. The patient is not a carrier because he is negative for HBsAg. The patient is not highly infective because he is negative for HBeAg. Finally, the patient is not immune because he does not yet have anti-HBsAg.
▪ What percentage of patients with this acute condition progress to chronic infection?	Ten percent of adults with acute HBV infection develop chronic hepatitis, while 90% of affected neonates develop the chronic disease.
▪ What are the most appropriate treatments for this condition?	▪ Adefovir ▪ α-Interferon ▪ Lamivudine

T A B L E 7 - 2 . Serologic Responses to Hepatitis B Virus Infection

TEST	ACUTE DISEASE	WINDOW PHASE	COMPLETE RECOVERY	CHRONIC CARRIER
HBsAg	+	−	−	+
HBsAb	−	−	+	−b
HBcAb	+a	+	+	+

a IgM in acute stage; IgG in chronic or recovered stage.

b Patient has surface antibody but available antibody is bound to HBsAg.

Reprinted, with permission, from Bhushan V, Le T, Rao DA. *First Aid for the USMLE Step 1: 2008.* New York: McGraw-Hill, 2008: 168.

► **Case 14**

A nursing student gives a patient an intramuscular injection, and while attempting to re-cap the needle accidentally sticks himself. The patient is known to have chronic, active hepatitis C virus (HCV) infection. At Occupational Health, the student has blood drawn for antibody testing, which is found to be negative for anti-HCV antibody. Four weeks later, the nursing student is still negative for anti-HCV antibody, but at 12 weeks, results of antibody testing are positive.

■ Was the third antibody test falsely positive? Why or why not?	No, this patient has acute HCV infection. It takes weeks to months for the body to develop an antibody response to HCV (see Figure 7-9). The two prior negative tests simply indicated that he did not have a pre-existing HCV infection or prior exposure.
■ What other laboratory findings are typically found in patients with this condition?	Transaminitis (elevated aspartate aminotransferase [AST] and alanine aminotransferase [ALT]), secondary to damaged liver cells releasing intracellular enzymes. HCV RNA may also be de-tectable in the serum by reverse transcriptase-polymerase chain reaction.
■ What is the course of acute HCV infection?	The majority of patients with acute HCV infection are asymptomatic. About 25% of patients will become jaundiced. The patient may have flulike symptoms lasting between 2 and 12 weeks. While only a small percentage of those exposed to HCV by needlestick will develop acute hepatitis, 60%–80% of those who develop acute hepatitis will develop chronic infection. **Chronic infection** has a variable but slowly progressive course, with ~20% of patients developing cirrhosis. Excessive alcohol consumption further increases the risk of cirrhosis in this patient population.
■ What are the most appropriate treatments for this condition?	A combination of ribavirin and pegylated α-interferon (IFN) is ~40% effective for inducing remission of chronic, active HCV in-fection. Ribavirin is a guanosine analog that inhibits viral mRNA synthesis. Pegylated α-IFN is an endogenous cytokine that induces antiviral host enzymes and causes significant flulike symptoms.

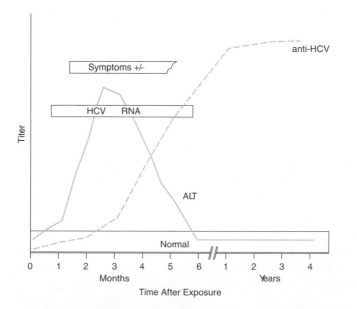

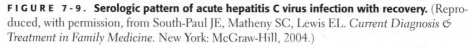

FIGURE 7-9. Serologic pattern of acute hepatitis C virus infection with recovery. (Repro-duced, with permission, from South-Paul JE, Matheny SC, Lewis EL. *Current Diagnosis & Treatment in Family Medicine.* New York: McGraw-Hill, 2004.)

▶ **Case 15**

A 50-year-old alcoholic male with known chronic liver disease presents with increasing weight loss and ascites. Physical examination reveals spider angiomas, palmar erythema, shrunken scrotum, and hemorrhoids. The liver edge is nonpalpable. A CT of the abdomen shows a nodular liver and a 3×4-cm single mass in the left lobe.

■ **What is the likely diagnosis?**	Hepatocellular carcinoma (HCC), also known as hepatoma. (Don't let the "oma" fool you into thinking that this tumor is benign.)
■ **What risk factors are associated with this condition?**	■ Hepatitis B and C infection ■ Aflatoxin (produced by *Aspergillus flavus*) ■ Cirrhosis ■ Wilson's disease ■ Hemochromatosis ■ α_1-Antitrypsin deficiency
■ **What serum marker may be of assistance in the diagnosis?**	**α-Fetoprotein (AFP)**. This is not specific for HCC, as elevated serum AFP also occurs in pregnancy, germ cell tumors, and other liver diseases. However, for Step 1, hepatic tumor + AFP = hepatoma.

■ **How can the physical examination findings be explained?**	Functional hyperestrogenemia and portal hypertension. The liver is responsible for the degradation of estrogen. Alcoholics have higher circulating estrogens, leading to:
	■ Spider angiomata
	■ Palmar erythema
	■ Testicular atrophy
	■ Gynecomastia
	■ Portal hypertension, which leads to the opening of collaterals to bypass the obstructed liver, and results in:
	  ■ Esophageal varices
	  ■ Caput medusae
	  ■ Hemorrhoids

■ **What nutritional deficiencies are likely to be present in this patient?**	While alcoholics may be deficient in several vital nutrients, it is very common to see the following deficiencies: ■ Thiamine (Vitamin B_1) ■ Vitamin B_{12} ■ Folate ■ Calcium ■ Magnesium In addition to the substitution of alcohol for nutrient-containing foods, abusers' gastrointestinal tracts are altered by alcohol, thereby further reducing absorption.
■ **What role does thiamine play in the metabolism of carbohydrates and amino acids?**	Thiamine is present in cells as thiaminpyrophosphate (TPP), which is necessary for the metabolism of pyruvate to acetyl-CoA, and α-Ketoglutarate to succinyl-CoA. It is also used for the oxidative decarboxylation of branched-chain amino acids (leucine, isoleucine, and valine), and the pentose-phosphate shunt.
■ **Why must alcoholics receive thiamine whenever glucose-containing intravenous fluids are given?**	To prevent **Wernicke's encephalopathy**. Thiamine is necessary for the metabolism of glucose. There is a high level of TPP in the mammillary bodies. If glucose is administered, the remaining thiamine in the mammillary bodies is consumed, leading to irreversible damage. The triad of Wernicke's encephalopathy is **confusion, ataxia,** and **ophthalmoplegia (nystagmus)**.

► Case 16

An otherwise healthy 36-hour-old boy born at 37 weeks' gestation to a G3P2 mother is noted to have yellowed skin over his entire body. A complete blood count (CBC) reveals a slightly low hematocrit, but normal WBC and platelet counts. Other relevant laboratory findings are as follows:

Direct bilirubin: 0 mg/dL
Serum total bilirubin (STB): 19 mg/dL (95th percentile of normal at this age is 11 mg/dL)
Direct Coombs' test: Weakly positive
Mother's blood type: O+
Infant's blood type: B+

▪ What is the most likely diagnosis?	Hyperbilirubinemia.
▪ Is this patient's condition likely due to cholestatis?	No, because the infant's direct bilirubin level is 0 mg/dL, indicating that conjugated bilirubin is being excreted properly.
▪ The patient is given phototherapy. Why is this effective?	Phototherapy irreversibly converts unconjugated bilirubin into **lumirubin**, which is similar to conjugated bilirubin in that it is soluble and able to be excreted in bile and urine.
▪ The patient is given a blood transfusion for his anemia. What ABO blood types of the packed RBC donor and of the plasma donor should be chosen in order to minimize hemolysis upon transfusion?	The RBC donor should be type O to avoid hemolysis of donor cells by maternal anti-B antibodies in the infant's blood. The plasma donor should be type B or AB, so that the plasma will not contain anti-B antibodies, which would be incompatible with the infant's blood.
▪ Which drugs, when ingested by the mother, increase the baby's risk of kernicterus?	Drugs that are highly bound to albumin—such as aspirin, ceftriaxone, and sulfa-based drugs—may displace bilirubin from albumin, thus increasing the level of neurotoxic free bilirubin in the blood.
▪ Despite phototherapy, the infant's total serum bilirubin climbs to 26 mg/dL, An infusion of albumin followed by an exchange transfusion is ordered. Why is this treatment effective?	Infused albumin binds free bilirubin, helping to draw extravascular bilirubin from tissues into the blood, which will then be removed by the exchange transfusion.

ORGAN SYSTEMS

GASTROINTESTINAL

▶ **Case 17**

An 18-year-old man presents with a 2-year history of abdominal pain and increasingly frequent bloody diarrhea. He has unintentionally lost 5.4 kg (12 lb) over 6 months and now complains of joint and lower back pain. He reports that several relatives have had similar complaints, and recently his 40-year-old uncle was diagnosed with colon cancer. Physical examination reveals diffuse voluntary guarding, no rebound tenderness, no masses, and no rectal fistulas. Colonoscopy reveals inflamed mucosa with friable pseudopolyps from the rectum to the splenic flexure.

■ **What is the most likely diagnosis?**

Inflammatory bowel disease. In this case, ulcerative colitis (UC) is more likely than Crohn's disease (CD).

■ **How can these two conditions be differentiated from one another?**

UC:
- Bimodal age distribution.
- Possibly autoimmune in origin.
- Males > females.
- Involvement of the rectum.
- **Continuous lesions** confined to the **mucosa.**
- Friable mucosal **pseudopolyps**, on gross morphology and crypt abscesses and ulcers on microscopic morphology.
- No strictures or fistulas, but may cause a "**lead pipe**" colon without haustra and colon shortening.
- Colectomy is curative.

CD:
- Involvement of the entire gastrointestinal (GI) tract, including the mouth (oral ulcers) and anus (bloody diarrhea or constipation).
- Distal ileum is often affected.
- **Transmural** inflammation and thickening ("string sign" on x-ray), **cobblestone** mucosa, **skip lesions**, and creeping fat.
- Frequently causes strictures, fistulas, and perianal disease.
- **Noncaseating granulomas** on histology.
- Surgery not curative, as disease may develop anywhere along the GI tract.

■ **How should this patient be counseled about his risk of developing colon cancer?**

There is a significantly increased risk of developing colorectal cancer (CRC) among patients with UC. The risk depends on duration and extent of disease, especially ~8–10 years after onset of symptoms. Incidence of CRC is 5%–10% after 20 years, and up to 30% at 35 years after onset. People with CD are also thought to be at risk of developing CRC; however, the magnitude of this risk is not yet clear.

■ **What extraintestinal manifestations are possible in this patient?**

Extraintestinal manifestations in UC relate to its association with **HLA-B27**: arthritis, ankylosing spondylitis, uveitis, Reiter's syndrome, primary sclerosing cholangitis (PSC), and pyoderma gangrenosum. Patients with PSC have an even greater risk of developing CRC.

■ **What further screening is recommended for the future?**

Patients should undergo colonoscopy and biopsy ~8 years after first diagnosis, and if negative, undergo a repeat examination every 1–3 years thereafter.

A 75-year-old woman presents to the emergency department (ED) after passing two bright red, plum-sized clots of blood. There was no stool passed with the clots. The patient denies any abdominal discomfort or cramping, but states she becomes lightheaded upon standing. She also reports she has been very constipated over the past few months. She takes one 81-mg aspirin per day. In the ED, her hematocrit is 28% and her blood pressure is 110/70 mm Hg supine, 80/50 mm Hg standing.

▪ **Where is the likely origin of the blood?**	The blood is most likely from the lower gastrointestinal (GI) tract. **Hematochezia** (maroon or bright red blood/clots per rectum) is a hallmark of a lower GI bleed. **Hematemesis** (vomiting of blood or coffee grounds–like material) and/or **melena** (black, tarry stools) are characteristic of an upper GI bleed. While this distinction is not absolute, it is a good rule of thumb.
▪ **What conditions should be considered in the differential diagnosis?**	▪ Anatomic (diverticulosis, hemorrhoids). ▪ Inflammatory (infectious, ischemic, idiopathic inflammatory bowel disease, and radiation). ▪ Neoplastic (polyp, carcinoma). ▪ Ulcers. ▪ Vascular (angiodysplasia, radiation-induced telangiectasia).
▪ **What is the most likely cause of this patient's bleeding?**	Diverticulosis. The most common causes of acute lower GI bleeding are: diverticulosis (33%), cancers/polyps (19%), colitis/ulcers (18%), angiodysplasia (8%), and anorectal/hemorrhoids (4%). By age 85, about 65% of the population has diverticulae. Additionally, 30%–50% of massive rectal bleeding is caused by diverticulosis. Suspect hemorrhoids in a younger patient.
▪ **What is the pathophysiology of this condition?**	Diverticulosis occurs when **diverticulae** (sac-like protrusions of the colonic wall) form, exposing the surrounding arterial vasculature to injury and causing thinning of the media. This predisposes to rupture, arterial bleeding, and rapid loss of blood per rectum. This is in contrast to **angiodysplasia**, which can cause venous intestinal bleeding. Although most diverticula form in the left colon, right-sided diverticula are more likely to bleed. Risk factors for diverticular formation include: nonsteroidal anti-inflammatory drugs, lack of dietary fiber, older age, and constipation.
▪ **What is the initial diagnostic test for this condition?**	Colonoscopy can be both diagnostic and therapeutic. Additional tests include radionuclide imaging and mesenteric angiography.

▶ **Case 19**

A worried mother rushes her 2-year-old son to the clinic after finding a large amount of bright red blood in his diaper. She notes that over the past week the child has been intermittently extremely irritable, curling into a ball with his legs pulled to his chest. His irritability resolves after vomiting (bilious) or passing a small stool. On examination, the child's vital signs are within normal limits, and he is in no apparent distress. Dried blood is noted at the anus. He is slightly uncomfortable with abdominal palpation, although no masses are appreciated.

▪ What is the most likely diagnosis?	Meckel's diverticulum acting as a nidus for intussusception.
▪ What is the embryonic origin of this structure?	A Meckel's diverticulum is the most common congenital abnormality of the small intestine, resulting from failure of the **vitelline duct** to close. The role of the vitelline duct is to connect the developing midgut to the yolk sac. Normally, the duct should close and obliterate by ~7 weeks' gestation.
▪ Where is this structure most likely located?	Meckel's diverticulum classically follows the **"rule of 2's"**: ▪ Occurs in 2% of the population, the majority of whom are <2 years of age. ▪ 2% will develop a complication. ▪ Male:female ratio is 2:1. ▪ Found within 2 feet of the ileocecal valve. ▪ Are ~2 inches long.
▪ Why is the patient intermittently irritable, and why does he "ball up?"	**Intussusception**, or telescoping of one portion of the bowel into another, makes the child irritable. The classic presentation on the boards will be an inconsolable child with a sausage-like palpable abdominal mass and "currant-jelly" stools. Children may appear completely well between episodes of obstruction. A barium enema can be both diagnostic and therapeutic. There is an association between intussusception and adenovirus infection, as well as the rotavirus vaccine.
▪ What is the cause of the bright red rectal bleeding?	The two most common tissue types found in a Meckel's diverticulum are gastric (80%) or pancreatic (~20%). The heterotopic gastric tissue releases gastric enzymes into the surrounding sensitive intestinal mucosa, which can lead to ulceration, pain, and bleeding. The most common presentation of symptomatic Meckel's diverticulum in children is painless, massive rectal bleeding, which is often maroon (40%) or bright red (35%). If the bleed is brisk, the stool may resemble currant jelly, while a slow bleed will be black and tarry (melena).
▪ Is this a true or false diverticulum?	This is a true diverticulum, in that it involves all layers of the intestinal wall (see Figure 7-10).

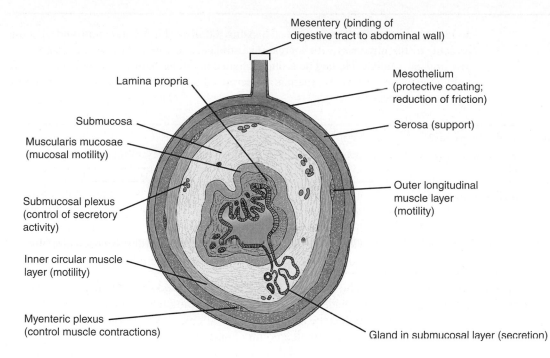

Mesentery (binding of digestive tract to abdominal wall)

Lamina propria

Submucosa

Muscularis mucosae (mucosal motility)

Submucosal plexus (control of secretory activity)

Inner circular muscle layer (motility)

Myenteric plexus (control muscle contractions)

Mesothelium (protective coating; reduction of friction)

Serosa (support)

Outer longitudinal muscle layer (motility)

Gland in submucosal layer (secretion)

F I G U R E 7 - 1 0 . Layers of the bowel wall.

▶ **Case 20**

A 53-year-old man with a history of hepatitis C virus (HCV) infection and cirrhosis presents to his physician with increasing jaundice, increased abdominal girth, weight loss, and early satiety. He says he is often fatigued and feels lightheaded when he stands. Laboratory testing reveals anemia, hyperbilirubinemia, and an increased serum α-fetoprotein level.

▪ What is the most likely diagnosis?	Primary hepatocellular carcinoma (HCC). HCC is increased in patients HCV who develop cirrhosis. In contrast, patients who are infected with hepatitis B virus may develop HCC without cirrhosis.
▪ Describe the blood supply to the liver.	The liver is supplied by the portal vein (75% of blood flow) and hepatic artery. Branches of these vessels divide the liver into the left and right lobes. Efferent blood is carried from the hepatic vein to the inferior vena cava. Portal hypertension occurs when blood flow through the liver is obstructed, often due to cirrhosis.
▪ How does the fetal blood supply to the liver differ from the adult blood supply?	The umbilical vein is the major blood supply to the fetal liver and provides nutrients to the developing fetus. The umbilical vein enters the fetus via the umbilicus, and then joins the left portal vein. A small amount of placental blood perfuses the liver. Most placental blood, however, bypasses the liver via the ductus venosus and joins the left hepatic vein. The left hepatic vein then empties into the inferior vena cava, and ultimately the right atrium. The umbilical vein and ductus venosus disappear 2–5 days after birth, becoming the **ligamentum teres** and **ligamentum venosum**, respectively.
▪ Where is the falciform ligament?	During development, the **falciform ligament** connects the portion of the primitive foregut that will form the liver to the anterior abdomen at the umbilicus. This connection enables the umbilical vein from the placenta to enter its free border at the umbilicus and reach the portal vein at the porta hepatis. The falciform ligament on the anterior surface of the liver divides the liver into the left and right anatomic lobes.
▪ Why does this patient have increased abdominal girth?	The increased abdominal girth is likely due to ascites, or excess peritoneal fluid, resulting from portal hypertension and a failing liver. In liver failure, albumin production falls, decreasing oncotic pressure within vessels. Transudative fluid leaves vessels as a result of the relative increase in hydrostatic pressure (Starling's forces).

A 47-year-old white man is brought to the emergency department by a policeman after being found wandering and incoherent on the streets. He is incontinent with diarrhea. Physical examination reveals a pigmented, scaling rash on his neck, arms, and hands (see Figure 7-11) as well as glossitis.

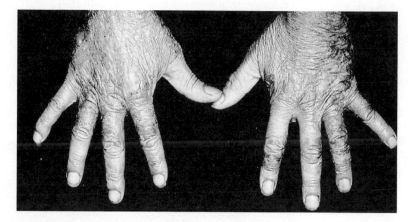

FIGURE 7-11. (Reproduced, with permission, from Wolff K, Johnson RA, Suurmond D. *Fitzpatrick's Color Atlas & Synopsis of Clinical Dermatology*, 5th ed. New York: McGraw-Hill, 2005: 457.)

▪ What is the most likely diagnosis?	Vitamin B₃ (niacin) deficiency. This is also known as **pellagra.**
▪ What is the function of vitamin B₃?	Niacin is a precursor for oxidized nicotinamide adenine dinucleotide (NAD+) and reduced nicotinamide adenine dinucleotide phosphate (NADPH). **NAD** is involved in carrying reducing equivalents away from catabolic processes, such as oxidative phosphorylation. **NADPH** is used as a supply of reducing equivalents in anabolic reactions, such as the biosynthesis of steroids and fatty acids to maintain reduced glutathione, and in the oxygen-dependent respiratory burst of macrophages.
▪ From what amino acid is vitamin B₃ derived?	Tryptophan.
▪ What are the most likely causes of this presentation?	In developed nations, pellagra is seen most commonly in alcoholics (due to malnutrition). It can also be seen in patients with **Hartnup's disease** (a disorder of tryptophan absorption) and carcinoid syndrome (in which there is increased conversion of tryptophan to serotonin). Isoniazid (INH) inhibits the conversion of tryptophan to niacin; thus, patients receiving INH are often prescribed niacin replacement.
▪ What are the symptoms of overdose of vitamin B₃?	Prostaglandin-mediated **flushing** is a symptom seen in overdose. Patients receiving niacin as a treatment for hypertriglyceridemia may experience this adverse side effect. Prophylaxis with aspirin often prevents this reaction.

► **Case 22**

A 56-year-old woman complains of significant pruritus of her skin. She has tried multiple over-the-counter skin lotions and creams, to no effect. On physical examination, there are extensive excoriations on her extremities, slightly jaundiced sclera, and **xanthelasma** (see Figure 7-12). Initial laboratory tests reveal:

Aspartate aminotransferase (AST): 40 IU/L
Alanine aminotransferase (ALT): 40 IU/L
Direct bilirubin: 1 mg/dL
Total bilirubin: 2 mg/dL
Alkaline phosphatase: 540 U/L (normal <230 U/L)
Gamma-glutamyl transferase (GGT): 80 U/L (normal <50 U/L)

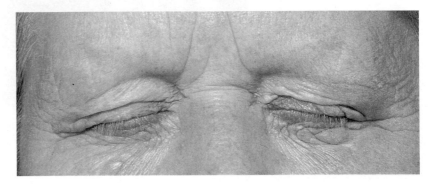

FIGURE 7-12. Xanthelasma. Multiple, longitudinal, creamy-orange, slightly elevated dermal papules on the eyelids of a normolipemic individual. (Reproduced, with permission, from Wolff K, Johnson RA, Suurmond, D. *Fitzpatrick's Color Atlas & Synopsis of Clinical Dermatology*, 5th ed. New York: McGraw-Hill, 2005: 447.)

■ What is the most likely diagnosis?	Primary biliary cirrhosis (PBC), a presumed autoimmune disease with destruction (inflammation and necrosis) of the intrahepatic bile ducts.
■ What are the signs and symptoms of this condition and what laboratory tests confirm the diagnosis?	The most common symptom is fatigue (65%) and pruritus (55%) in a woman 40–60 years old. Jaundice and xanthelasma (see Figure 7-12) are fairly rare (~10%). Most patients are diagnosed on routine lab work: increased alkaline phosphatase, GGT, and bilirubin (total and direct). AST and ALT are characteristically normal.
■ What additional laboratory tests should be ordered?	**Antimitochondrial antibodies** (AMA) should also be ordered. You must know this for the USMLE! There may also be an increase in the erythrocyte sedimentation rate (**ESR**) and serum **IgM** levels.
■ What other conditions may be present in patients with this condition?	Other autoimmune diseases, such as **scleroderma**, **Sjögren's syndrome**, and **rheumatoid arthritis**. Up to 50–75% of patients with PBC present with sicca syndrome—dry eyes (xerophthalmia) and dry mouth (xerostomia)—commonly seen among Sjögren's patients.

■ **What is the most appropriate treatment for the patient's pruritus?**	Antihistamines.
■ **What is the most appropriate treatment for the patient's underlying condition?**	Ursodeoxycholic acid (ursodiol). Methotrexate may be added in more severe cases.
■ **How is this condition distinguished from primary sclerosing cholangitis (PSC)?**	**PSC:** ■ Is more likely in males. ■ Affects both intrahepatic **and** extrahepatic bile ducts. ■ Anti-mitochondrial antibodies are negative. ■ Associated conditions include ulcerative colitis. The classic description of endoscopic retrograde cholangiopancreatography findings of the bile ducts is "pearls on a string" or "bile lakes."

► **Case 23**

An 84-year-old man is hospitalized for a course of intravenous clindamycin to treat an abscess. One week later, he develops profuse heme-positive diarrhea, nausea, and malaise. He is febrile to 38.8°C (101.8°F). Physical examination reveals abdominal tenderness and distention. The WBC count is 19,000/mm^3 with a differential of 91% neutrophils, 7% monocytes, and 2% lymphocytes. Sigmoidoscopy reveals 0.2-2-cm raised, adherent, yellow plaques.

■ What is the most likely diagnosis?	This is a typical presentation of pseudomembranous colitis, which is notorious among hospitalized patients who receive **clindamycin.** Confirmatory findings include the presence of fecal leukocytes, anorexia, and dehydration.
■ What is the causative organism of this condition?	*Clostridium difficile.* This anaerobic gram-positive rod becomes predominant in the bowel after normal flora have been killed off by broad-spectrum antibiotics, such as clindamycin, penicillins (especially ampicillin), and cephalosporins.
■ What is the underlying pathophysiology of this condition?	*C. difficile* releases two exotoxins (**proteins A and B**) that bind to receptors on intestinal epithelial cells. These toxins cause sloughing of epithelial cells into the lumen and mucosal ulceration. A **pseudomembrane** forms, composed of inflammatory cells, proteins, and mucus (see Figure 7-13).
■ What are other manifestations of infections with this organism?	Infection with *C. difficile* can result in a broad spectrum of symptoms, ranging from asymptomatic to fulminant colitis. Antibiotic-associated diarrhea can be mild or profuse and can occur with or without colitis. The colitis itself can appear pathologically nonspecific, or demonstrate pseudomembranes. Fulminant colitis can result in toxic megacolon or even perforation.
■ What are the most appropriate treatments for this condition?	First-line therapy for pseudomembranous colitis is oral metronidazole. Intravenous metronidazole can be used in serious cases. Oral vancomycin can be used to treat *C. difficile* enterocolitis, as it predominantly remains in the gut; however both vancomycin and metronidazole have been implicated as causes of pseudomembranous colitis.

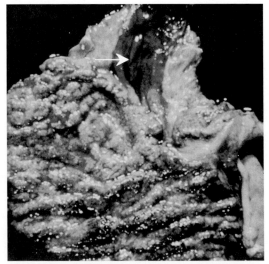

FIGURE 7-13. **Autopsy specimen showing confluent pseudomembranes covering the cecum of a patient with pseudomembranous colitis.** (Reproduced, with permission, from Kasper DL, et al. *Harrison's Principles of Internal Medicine,* 16th ed. New York: McGraw-Hill, 2005: 760.)

► **Case 24**

A 3-week-old white male infant is brought to your clinic by his mother, who complains that the child has intermittent bouts of projectile vomiting food after meals. The mother also states that the child has been more lethargic than usual. On physical examination, the patient appears weak, and has sunken eyes and poor skin turgor. He has fallen to the 25th percentile for weight. An olive-shaped mass is palpated in the right upper quadrant.

▪ What is the most likely diagnosis?	Hypertrophic pyloric stenosis (see Figure 7-14).
▪ What findings are supportive of this diagnosis?	This patient demonstrates the classic presentation of pyloric stenosis, with immediate postprandial, nonbilious, often projectile vomiting ("the hungry vomiter"), and a palpable olive-like mass in the epigastrum. **White males** are more at risk than other populations.
▪ What are the typical laboratory findings in this condition?	Hypochloremic metabolic alkalosis from the loss of large amounts of gastric HCl is seen with pyloric stenosis. Unconjugated hyperbilirubinemia may also be seen.
▪ How is the diagnosis confirmed?	Diagnosis is straightforward when the "olive" is palpable. Otherwise, it may be difficult to distinguish this condition from gastroesophageal reflux without an ultrasound or upper gastrointestinal series. The latter may demonstrate an elongated pylorus (**"string sign"**) with a tapered end (**"beak sign"**).
▪ What is the most appropriate management for this condition?	The definitive management is surgery (pyloromyotomy).
▪ Given appropriate management, what is the patient's expected prognosis?	Patients can be expected to make a complete recovery, including return to normal weight and growth.
▪ What are some other conditions commonly associated with this patient's diagnosis?	Associated conditions include hiatal hernia, midgut volvulus, gastroesophageal reflux, and esophageal atresia.

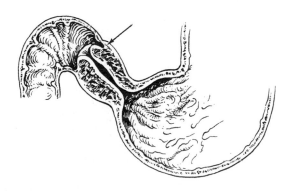

FIGURE 7-14. Hypertrophic pyloric stenosis. (Reproduced, with permission, from Doherty GM, Way LW. *Current Surgical Diagnosis & Treatment*, 12th ed. New York: McGraw-Hill, 2006: 1294.)

▶ **Case 25**

A worried 24-year-old mother brings her 4-year-old daughter to the emergency department (ED). She states the daughter has been ill for the past week with flulike symptoms, including rhinorrhea, cough, headache, and nausea. The child has been increasingly lethargic, and the mother found her barely responsive this morning. The child displays diminished consciousness and sluggish pupils. Kernig's and Brudzinski's signs are negative. She vomits multiple times in the ED and is admitted to the intensive care unit (ICU).

▪ What is the most likely diagnosis?	Reye's syndrome. While extremely rare, this diagnosis is devastating if missed and is a favorite of the USMLE.
▪ What drug did the mother likely administer to the patient?	**Aspirin.** While the USMLE will likely mention that the child was given aspirin, in real life it is often difficult to get the entire history. Therefore, always suspect Reye's syndrome in a child who has altered mental status and vomiting (particularly given a history of a recent viral illness).
▪ What other laboratory findings are expected in this patient?	This patient is at risk for developing hepatic failure, cerebral edema, and death. Characteristic laboratory findings include: ▪ Severe transaminitis (aspartate aminotransferase and alanine aminotransferase >3000 U/L). ▪ Normal or slightly elevated bilirubin. ▪ Hypoglycemia. ▪ Hyperammonemia. ▪ Prolonged prothrombin time and International Normalized Ratio (INR). ▪ Anion gap metabolic acidosis with mixed respiratory alkalosis.
▪ What is the pathophysiology of this condition?	It is thought that salicylate metabolites in the midst of viral infection damage mitochondria, and/or that susceptible individuals have an underlying polymorphism in mitochondrial function. **Mitochondrial dysfunction** leads to increased short-chain fatty acids, hyperammonemia, and cerebral edema, though the exact mechanism is unclear.
▪ What is the association between the patient's recent flulike symptoms and the current presentation?	While the etiology of Reye's syndrome is unknown, the condition typically occurs after a viral infection, particularly an upper respiratory tract infection, influenza, varicella, or gastroenteritis, and is associated with aspirin use during the illness.
▪ What is a possible explanation for the child's change in mental status?	**Cerebral edema.** Interestingly, if cerebral edema can be controlled, the liver usually makes a full recovery. Therefore, ICU management is essential. Options for controlling cerebral edema include: ▪ Mannitol ▪ Hyperventilation ▪ Barbiturates ▪ Ventricular drainage (among others)
▪ Unfortunately, despite treatment, the patient dies. What autopsy findings are expected on pathology of the viscera?	Microvesicular fatty change (**steatosis**) of the liver, kidneys, and brain may be seen on autopsy.

▶ **Case 26**

A 3-month-old female infant born prematurely has been maintained on parenteral nutrition since a length of her bowel was resected secondary to necrotizing enterocolitis when she was 2 weeks old. The removed bowel included the ascending colon, ileum, and distal portion of the jejunum. She is unable to thrive on enteral feeding alone.

▪ **What is the name of this condition?**	Short bowel syndrome.
▪ **After resection of the ileum, which specific molecules will be malabsorbed?**	Vitamin B_{12} and bile salts are absorbed exclusively in the ileum, and thus are deficient in short bowel syndrome.
▪ **The remainder of the patient's jejunum has adapted by increasing the number of cells in the villi, thereby lengthening the villi. What term describes this type of adaptation?**	It is known as **hyperplasia.** Hyperplasia refers to increasing the number of cells within a tissue. This is in contrast to **hypertrophy,** in which the cells increase in size.
▪ **During bowel transplantation, which branch(es) of the aorta must be identified and anastomosed to supply blood to the jejunum, ileum, and ascending colon?**	▪ The **superior mesenteric artery** (SMA). The SMA supplies blood to the intestine from the proximal jejunum to the proximal transverse colon. ▪ The **celiac trunk** supplies the stomach, liver, spleen, and duodenum. ▪ The **inferior mesenteric artery** supplies the distal transverse colon, descending colon, and sigmoid colon.
▪ **How might octreotide be used in this patient?**	As a **somatostatin analog,** octreotide inhibits the release of gastrin, thus reducing gastric secretions that would otherwise be in relative excess compared to the short bowel, and thus further impede absorption.
▪ **How will malabsorption of bile salts affect this patient's prothrombin time (PT) and partial thromboplastin time (PTT)?**	PT and PTT should both increase secondary to depletion of vitamin K, which is due malabsorption of fat and fat-soluble vitamins.

► **Case 27**

A 65-year-old female immigrant from Japan presents with fatigue, weight loss, early satiety, and a gnawing stomach pain. She has been seen by multiple physicians, all of whom suggested that she had peptic ulcer disease and treated her with antacids. However, the pain has not improved for 8 months. She has lost 16 kg (35 lb), and now complains of painful intercourse (dyspareunia) and painful defecation (dyschezia).

■ **What is the most likely diagnosis?**	Stomach cancer. Unfortunately, due to similarities in symptoms with peptic ulcer disease and gastritis, gastric cancer is frequently misdiagnosed. Hence, patients are typically diagnosed at a late stage. Prognosis is poor (5% survival at 5 years).
■ **What risk factors are associated with an increased incidence of this condition?**	■ Infection with *Helicobacter pylori*. ■ Chronic gastritis. ■ Smoking. ■ Diets high in nitrosamines (i.e., smoked, cured, or pickled foods) commonly found in East Asia, the Andes, Scandinavia, and eastern Europe. ■ Pernicious anemia and type A blood (associated with gastritis). ■ Family history. ■ Previous gastric surgery.
■ **What would be seen on biopsy?**	Adenocarcinoma is the most common type of gastric cancer, and its hallmark is **signet-ring cells** on histopathology. Other types include **linitus plastica**, or "**leather-bottle stomach**," which is a diffusely infiltrative cancer and portends a worse prognosis. It is also important to rule out **gastric lymphoma**, which is frequently associated with *H. pylori* and may regress without surgery if the bacteria were to be eradicated.
■ **How does this condition spread?**	Gastric cancer metastasizes by direct extension through the gastric wall, the lymphatic system, and via peritoneal spread.
■ **Why does this patient suffer from dyspareunia and dyschezia?**	It results from metastasis via peritoneal spread to the **pouch of Douglas** (the rectouterine cul-de-sac). This may be felt on rectal examination as an anterior rectal wall mass or a "**Blumer's shelf**." A gastric carcinoma metastasis to the ovary is called a **Krukenberg's tumor**.
■ **What is a Virchow's node?**	An enlarged left supraclavicular lymph node. If this is found on physical examination, there is an increased likelihood of metastatic disease. Additional signs of lymphatic metastasis include a **Sister Mary Joseph's node** (periumbilical nodule) and an **Irish node** (left axillary node).

► **Case 28**

A 45-year-old man presents to the emergency department after vomiting approximately one-half cup of blood. Two days prior, the patient began having nausea and colicky, nonradiating abdominal pain. He has an extensive history of alcohol abuse, and currently drinks 8–10 beers a day. He has a past medical history significant for pancreatitis and hematemesis, and he currently takes no medications. Digital rectal examination reveals dark, heme-positive stool.

■ **What is the most likely diagnosis, and what are its major causes?**	Upper GI bleed. Common causes include: ■ Peptic ulcer disease (55%) ■ Acute hemorrhagic gastritis ■ Esophagitis ■ Esophagogastric varices ■ Mallory-Weiss tears ■ Arteriovenous malformations ■ Tumors Patients with chronic alcohol abuse are particularly prone to developing esophageal varices and **Mallory-Weiss tears.** A history of extensive wretching prior to the onset of hematemesis in an alcoholic is strongly suggestive of a Mallory-Weiss tear.
■ **What anatomic structure distinguishes an upper gastrointestinal (GI) bleed from a lower GI bleed?**	The **ligament of Treitz,** which marks the junction between the duodenum and the jejunum. Bleeding proximal to the ligament of Treitz is defined as an upper GI bleed.
■ **Had this patient presented with bright red blood per rectum rather than dark stool, would the diagnosis change?**	Not necessarily. A brisk upper GI bleed may also present with bright red blood per rectum, in which case there is insufficient transit time for breakdown of heme.
■ **What factors increase the risk of developing peptic ulcer disease?**	■ *Helicobacter pylori* infection ■ Nonsteroidal anti-inflammatory drugs ■ Chronic obstructive pulmonary disease ■ Cirrhosis ■ Smoking ■ Uremia ■ Zollinger-Ellison syndrome
■ **When is nasogastric tube lavage indicated?**	In cases of massive hematemesis, **nasogastric tube lavage** is indicated to prevent aspiration. It is also used to distinguish between upper and lower sources of GI bleeding, and to identify high-risk lesions as sources of bleeding.

ORGAN SYSTEMS

GASTROINTESTINAL

► **Case 29**

A 37-year-old woman with a 20-year history of Crohn's disease presents to her primary care physician complaining of fatigue. Physical examination reveals tachycardia (heart rate 106/min), pale conjunctivae, angular cheilitis, and a beefy red tongue. Relevant laboratory findings include a hematocrit of 21% and an elevated mean corpuscular volume.

■ What is the most likely diagnosis?	Vitamin B_{12} deficiency.
■ What are the functions of this vitamin, and how does its deficiency result in this presentation?	Vitamin B_{12} is a cofactor for methionine synthase, which catalyzes the transfer of a methyl group from N-methyltetrahydrofolate to homocysteine, producing tetrahydrofolate (TH_4) and methionine. Decreased production of TH_4 interferes with DNA synthesis required for hematopoiesis (see Figure 7-15A), resulting in megaloblastic anemia. Vitamin B_{12} is also a cofactor for methylmalonyl CoA mutase (see Figure 7-15B), an enzyme involved in the catabolism of odd-numbered fatty acid chains.
■ What are the possible causes of this patient's condition?	The most common cause of vitamin B_{12} deficiency is **pernicious anemia**, an autoimmune disorder in which **intrinsic factor** producing gastric parietal cells are destroyed. Intrinsic factor is necessary for vitamin B_{12} absorption. Other causes include malabsorption (e.g., celiac sprue, enteritis, or *Diphyllobothrium latum* infection) and absence of the terminal ileum (as in Crohn's disease or surgical resection). Vitamin B_{12} deficiency is rarely due to insufficient dietary intake. However, after several years, strict vegetarians are at risk, because the nutrient is found only in animal products.
■ For what other condition is this patient at risk?	Neurologic problems often manifest as paresthesias and ataxia. Over time, symptoms such as spasticity and paraplegia can develop. The exact role vitamin B_{12} deficiency plays in this pathology is unclear. Neurologic symptoms are often irreversible.
■ What other vitamin deficiency can also cause megaloblastic anemia?	**Folic acid deficiency**. However, this deficiency does not cause neurologic symptoms.

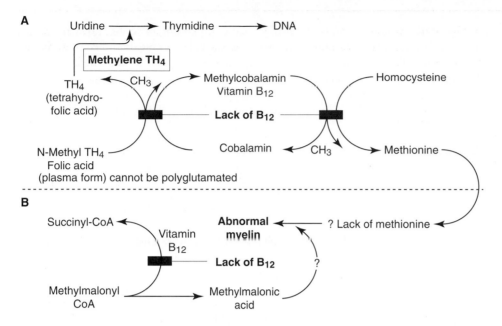

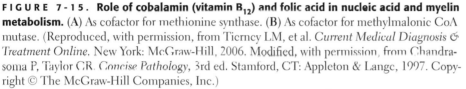

FIGURE 7-15. Role of cobalamin (vitamin B$_{12}$) and folic acid in nucleic acid and myelin metabolism. (A) As cofactor for methionine synthase. (B) As cofactor for methylmalonic CoA mutase. (Reproduced, with permission, from Tierney LM, et al. *Current Medical Diagnosis & Treatment Online.* New York: McGraw-Hill, 2006. Modified, with permission, from Chandrasoma P, Taylor CR. *Concise Pathology*, 3rd ed. Stamford, CT: Appleton & Lange, 1997. Copyright © The McGraw-Hill Companies, Inc.)

▶ **Case 30**

A 35-year-old woman presents to her physician complaining of severe, gnawing epigastric pain of several days' duration. The pain is worse between meals and is somewhat relieved with milk, food, and antacids. She has had three peptic ulcers in the past 2 years. The pain is occasionally accompanied by diarrhea. She denies bloody stools or hematuria, and does not use alcohol or tobacco. Upper endoscopy reveals prominent gastric folds and an erosion in the first portion of the duodenum. The patient's fasting gastrin level is 700 pg/dL.

■ What is the most likely diagnosis?	A history of recurrent peptic ulcers suggests Zollinger-Ellison syndrome, in which there is hypersecretion of gastrin from a gastrinoma, resulting in high gastric acid output.
■ With what endocrine disorder is this condition associated?	Twenty percent of patients with Zollinger-Ellison syndrome have the disease in association with **multiple endocrine neoplasia** type I (Wermer's syndrome). Such patients will also have parathyroid adenomas, resulting in hyperparathyroidism, and/or anterior pituitary tumors.
■ How is secretion of gastric acid regulated?	Gastric acid is secreted by **parietal cells** of the stomach in response to gastrin, acetylcholine (vagal input), and histamine (see Figure 7-16 below). Acid secretion is inhibited by somatostatin.
■ What is the pathophysiology of this patient's diarrhea?	The voluminous acid secretion overwhelms the buffering capacity of pancreatic bicarbonate. Thus, pancreatic enzymes are inactivated in this acidic environment, impeding digestion. Excess acid also interferes with the emulsification of fats, leading to steatorrhea.
■ What are the most appropriate treatments for this condition?	■ Surgical: Resection of the gastrinoma (typically at the head of pancreas) ■ Medical: Proton pump inhibitors to suppress gastric acid secretion

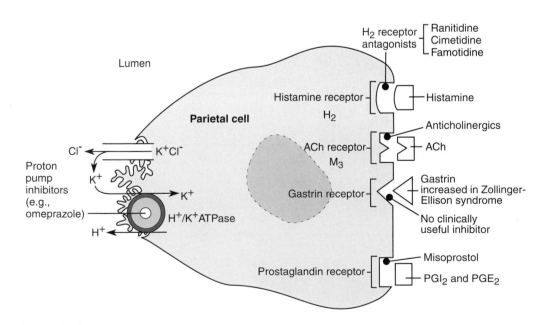

FIGURE 7-16. Regulation of gastric acid secretion. ACh = acetylcholine; PGE_2 = prostaglandin E_2; PGI_2 = prostaglandin I_2. (Reproduced, with permission, from Le T, Bhushan V, Rao DA. *First Aid for the USMLE Step 1: 2008.* New York: McGraw-Hill, 2008: 303.)

Hematology
and Oncology

Case 1   247

Case 2   248

Case 3   250

Case 4   251

Case 5   252

Case 6   254

Case 7   255

Case 8   256

Case 9   258

Case 10   259

Case 11   260

Case 12   261

Case 13   262

Case 14   263

Case 15   264

Case 16   265

Case 17   266

Case 18   268

Case 19   270

Case 20   271

Case 21   27

Case 22   274

Case 23   275

Case 24   276

Case 25   277

Case 26   278

Case 27   280

Case 28   281

Case 29   282

Case 30   283

Case 31   284

Case 32   285

Case 33   286

Case 34   288

Case 35   289

Case 36   290

Case 37   291

Case 38   292

Case 39   293

A 27-year-old woman comes to her physician complaining of severe abdominal pain of 3 days' duration. She says she has had similar attacks in the past, starting in early adolescence. However, she thought the pain was due to menstruation, and did not seek medical attention. Review of systems reveals a history of depression and insomnia. On physical examination, the patient is hyporeflexic in the lower extremities and has generalized weakness, which is worse in the lower extremities than in the upper extremities. Urinalysis reveals the urine color is initially light but darkens on exposure to air and light, and the porphobilinogen level is 110 mg/24 h (normal 0.0–1.5 mg/24 h).

▪ **What is the most likely diagnosis?**	Acute intermittent porphyria (AIP).
▪ **Which biochemical defect is responsible for this condition?**	AIP is caused by a deficiency in **porphobilinogen deaminase,** an enzyme required for hemoglobin production. Virtually all of the porphyrias are autosomal dominant disorders. Typically patients have accumulation of porphobilinogen and present with neuropathy and attacks of abdominal pain. Unlike other porphyrias, cutaneous disease is rarely present in AIP.
▪ **What are the most likely precipitants of this patient's attacks?**	Endogenous and exogenous gonadal steroids, certain drugs (sulfonamides and many antiepileptic agents), alcohol, low-calorie diets, and sunlight can increase α-aminolevulinic acid (ALA) synthase activity, and can precipitate attacks.
▪ **What is the most appropriate treatment for this condition?**	Avoiding common precipitants of attacks (as listed above). IV infusion of dextrose solution can also help abate acute attacks. Heme is a repressor of ALA synthase so an intravenous injection of hemin (intravenous heme) leads to decreased synthesis of ALA synthase, which, in turn, often reduces the severity of symptoms. Hemin is used for refractory cases after failure of carbohydrate loading. Treatment of pain and monitoring for neurologic and respiratory compromise are essential.
▪ **What other condition should be considered if the patient has neurologic manifestations but no abdominal pain?**	Ascending muscle weakness with hyporeflexia or areflexia is the classic presentation of **Guillain-Barré syndrome.** However, the high level of porphobilinogen in the urine is essentially pathognomonic of AIP. If the diagnosis were unclear, a lumbar puncture could be performed, as albumino-cytologic dissociation is seen in the cerebrospinal fluid in patients with Guillain-Barré syndrome.

▶ **Case 2**

A 4-year-old girl is brought to her pediatrician by her parents, who are concerned about a fever that has lasted longer than a week. Her parents have also noticed that she does not seem to have as much energy as she used to, and she now walks with a limp. Physical examination is significant for hepatomegaly, scattered petechiae, and bruising over many surfaces of her body. Relevant laboratory findings are as follows:

Hemoglobin concentration: 6 g/dL
WBC count: $25,000/mm^3$
Platelet count: $39,000/mm^3$
Peripheral smear: Many immature white cells with condensed chromatin, absent nucleoli and scant agranular cytoplasm (see Figure 8-1).

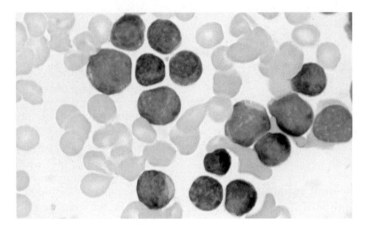

FIGURE 8-1. (Reproduced, with permission, from Lichtman MA et al. *Williams Hematology*, 7th ed. New York: McGraw-Hill, 2005: Figure 91-4.)

▪ **What is the most likely diagnosis?**	Acute lymphoblastic leukemia (ALL), the most common malignancy of childhood. The classic presentation and laboratory findings include fever (the most common sign), fatigue, lethargy, bone pain, arthralgia, and elevated serum lactate dehydrogenase (LDH). Less common symptoms include headache, vomiting, altered mental function, oliguria, and anuria.
▪ **What is the differential diagnosis?**	▪ Idiopathic thrombocytopenic purpura ▪ Aplastic anemia ▪ Infectious mononucleosis ▪ *Bordetella Pertussis*, Epstein-Barr virus ▪ Small, round, blue-cell tumors
▪ **What is the etiology of these physical examination findings?**	Most of the physical examination findings result from leukemic expansion and crowding out of the normal marrow: anemia and thrombocytopenia; bone or joint pain from invasion into the periosteum. Fever results from pyrogenic cytokines released from leukemic cells. Elevated LDH levels are a consequence of increased cellular turnover. Painless enlargement of the scrotum and central nervous system symptoms may also be signs of more extensive extramedullary invasion.

- **To which organs does this condition spread?**

  Liver, spleen, and lymph nodes are the most common sites of extramedullary involvement. Occasionally, an anterior mediastinal (thymic) mass is present which can compress the great vessels and trachea, possibly leading to superior vena cava syndrome (of which symptoms include cough, dyspnea, orthopnea, dysphagia, stridor, and syncope).

- **What is the appropriate treatment for this condition?**

  Complex chemotherapy regimens are standard and divided into induction, consolidation, and maintenance phases. Most regimens involve combinations of cyclophosphamide, doxorubicin, vincristine, dexamethasone/prednisone, methotrexate, asparaginase, and cytarabine. These drugs have been utilized with great effect and >90% of patients achieve disease-free survival after 5 years.

► **Case 3**

A 67-year-old man presents to his physician with a 10-day history of fatigue, bleeding gums, and cellulitis, and a recent weight loss of 9 kg (20 lb). On physical examination, the patient is pale, but has no evidence of lymphadenopathy or hepatosplenomegaly. Results of a blood smear are as follows:

WBC count: 18,300/mm^3 (75% blastocytes, 20% lymphocytes)
Hemoglobin: 9.1 g/dL
Hematocrit: 29%
Platelet count: 98,000/mm^3

■ What is the most likely diagnosis?	Acute myelogenous leukemia (AML).
■ What other symptoms are common at presentation?	■ Epistaxis, skin rash, petechiae, bone pain, and shortness of breath can be seen with AML. ■ Gingival hyperplasia can occur due to leukemic infiltration. ■ Leukemia cutis (skin infiltrates) can also be seen. ■ Monocytic leukemia may be associated with central nervous system involvement. ■ Disseminated intravascular coagulation is often seen with **acute promyelocytic leukemia** (a variant of AML).
■ What are the likely findings on histology?	The proliferation of myeloblasts with characteristic eosinophilic needle-like cytoplasmic inclusions, or **Auer rods**, is pathognomonic for AML (see Figure 8-2).
■ How can genetic testing influence treatment?	A t(15;17) chromosomal translocation indicates acute promyelocytic leukemia (M3 variant) as the specific diagnosis. This can be treated with all-*trans* retinoic acid (ATRA). This agent causes differentiation of promyelocytes into mature neutrophils, thereby inducing apoptosis of the leukemic promyelocytes.
■ Cellulitis is commonly associated with this condition. How does this occur?	Neutropenia caused by replacement of mature WBCs with leukemic cells leads to an increased susceptibility to infection.

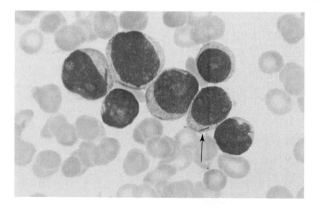

FIGURE 8-2. **Auer rods in acute myelogenous leukemia.** (Reproduced with permission of the Pathology Education Instructional Resource Digital Library [http://peir.net] at the University of Alabama, Birmingham.)

► **Case 4**

A 14-year-old boy presents to his physician with a laceration on his hand that has become badly infected. Upon questioning, the boy mentions he has felt fatigued for some time. Physical examination reveals pallor of the mucous membranes in addition to bleeding on the inside of his cheeks. He has petechiae covering his body, and patches of purpura on his thighs, trunk, and arms. Relevant laboratory findings are as follows:

WBC count: $2,000/mm^3$
Hematocrit: 22%
Platelet count: $48,000/mm^3$

■ **What is the most likely diagnosis?**

Aplastic anemia. This condition results from failure or autoimmune destruction of myeloid stem cells, which leads to pancytopenia. It is characterized by neutropenia (infection), anemia (pallor and fatigue), and thrombocytopenia (petechiae and purpura).

■ **What is the most likely cause of this patient's condition?**

Most cases of aplastic anemia are **idiopathic** (autoimmune). Other possible causes include **viral** agents (parvovirus B19, hepatitis viruses, HIV, and Epstein-Barr virus), **drugs** and **chemicals** (such as alkylating and antimetabolite agents, chloramphenicol, insecticides, and benzene), and **radiation**. Some hereditary cases have been linked to mutations in the telomerase gene (dyskeratosis congenita and aplastic anemia).

■ **What are the typical peripheral blood smear findings in this condition?**

Hypocellularity and pancytopenia would be seen. The visualized cells are morphologically normal. Macrocytosis and dysplastic forms can be seen.

■ **What other test would be useful in confirming the diagnosis?**

Bone marrow biopsy would reveal hypocellular bone marrow with a fatty infiltrate. Figure 8-3A shows a normal bone marrow biopsy, while Figure 8-3B shows a biopsy sample from a patient with aplastic anemia.

■ **What is the most appropriate treatment for this condition?**

Treatment includes RBC and platelet transfusions, allogeneic bone marrow transplant (sibling), granulocyte colony–stimulating factor or granulocyte macrophage colony–stimulating factor, and withdrawal of any toxic agent that may be a cause. If possible, transfusion should be avoided before bone marrow transplantation due to the risks of alloimmunization and graft rejection. Cyclosporine, antithymocyte globulin, and cyclophosphamide are used if no donor can be found.

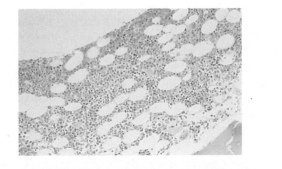
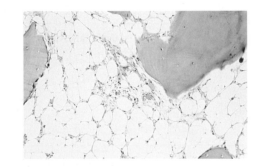

A   **B**

FIGURE 8-3. (A) Normal bone marrow biopsy. (B) Bone marrow biopsy in aplastic anemia. (Reproduced, with permission, from Kasper DL, et al. *Harrison's Principles of Internal Medicine*, 16th ed. New York: McGraw-Hill, 2005: 620.)

► **Case 5**

A 7-month-old Greek boy is brought to his pediatrician by his parents, who have noticed that the baby has been jaundiced and dyspneic for about 2 weeks. The mother claims her son has been healthy up until now, and there were no complications during the pregnancy or delivery. Physical examination reveals tachycardia. Laboratory tests reveal a mean corpuscular volume of 75 fl and a reticulocyte count of 0.3%. The serum iron concentration is within normal limits.

■ **What is the most likely diagnosis?**	β-Thalassemia major, a form of microcytic, hypochromic anemia, is the homozygous form of the genetically transmitted disease, thalassemia. This disease is prevalent in Mediterranean populations. Symptoms emerge after about 6 months of life due to the decline in normal hemoglobin F (α_2/α_2) and rise in hemoglobin A (α_2/β_2).
■ **What is the pathophysiology of this condition?**	In β-thalassemia, the β chain of hemoglobin is either underproduced (**thalassemia minor**) or absent (**thalassemia major**). As a result, the normal α hemoglobin chains build up and form insoluble aggregates that precipitate within the RBCs. This results in either hemolysis of or damage to the RBCs, making them more susceptible to macrophage destruction and splenic sequestration. The result is a hemolytic anemia, in which the microcytic and hypochromic RBCs resemble those seen in severe iron deficiency (see Figure 8-4). The reticulocyte count is low in these patients due to ineffective hematopoiesis. Target cells, nucleated RBCs, and microcytes are commonly seen. **Heinz body** precipitates are the oxidatively destructive α-globin chains in RBCs.
■ **How is this condition diagnosed?**	Gel electrophoresis is used for diagnosis, as it can distinguish mutated and normal forms of hemoglobin. An increased concentration of hemoglobin F (fetal hemoglobin) may also be seen on electrophoresis.
■ **What complications are associated with this condition?**	Complications include pulmonary hypertension, cardiac failure, leg ulcers, folate deficiency, and skeletal abnormalities secondary to ineffective erythropoiesis leading to marrow expansion, extramedullary hematopoiesis and iron overload.
■ **What are the two common forms of this condition?**	The major form of the disease results in severe hemolytic anemia, whereas the minor form of the disease may be completely asymptomatic. Extramedullary hematopoiesis is common in **Cooley's anemia** (thalassemia major).
■ **What is the most appropriate treatment for each form of this condition?**	Thalassemia major causes severe anemia, requiring treatment with repeated blood transfusions. Subsequently, iron chelation for overload (ferritin level >2247 pmol/L) is important. Splenectomy may also be necessary to treat the resultant hypersplenism. Thalassemia minor is usually asymptomatic and its treatment merely requires avoidance of oxidative stressors of RBCs. But beware of *Yersinia enterocolitica* infection, which eats up the free iron.

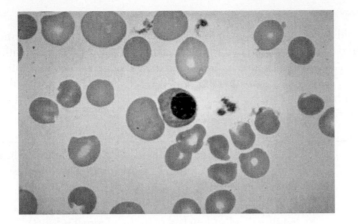

FIGURE 8-4. **Peripheral blood smear in α-thalassemia.** (Reproduced, with permission, from Kasper DL, et al. *Harrison's Principles of Internal Medicine*, 16th ed. New York: McGraw-Hill, 2005: 598.)

▶ **Case 6**

A 32-year-old woman with systemic lupus erythematosus presents to the emergency department reporting increased fatigue and lethargy that has lasted for 3 months. On physical examination, she is afebrile and has mild splenomegaly. Laboratory studies are significant for a hemoglobin concentration of 10.1 g/dL and a hematocrit of 30.6%. The peripheral blood smear shows spherocytes and reticulocytes. The direct and indirect Coombs' test are positive at 37°C but not at 4°C.

■ What is the most likely diagnosis?	Warm autoimmune hemolytic anemia secondary to lupus. However, most cases of this condition are idiopathic or associated with autoimmune processes. The positive Coombs' tests indicate the presence of antibodies on red blood cells (direct) and in the serum (indirect). Since they agglutinate cells at 37°C but not 4°C, this disease is considered warm antibody hemolytic anemia.
■ What are other causes of this condition?	The two most common causes are primary (idiopathic) and secondary due to systemic autoimmune disorders, such as systemic lupus erythematosus. However, medications, lymphomas, and leukemias are also common triggers.
■ What is the pathogenesis of this condition?	This is typically an **IgG**-mediated process. IgG coats RBCs and acts as an opsonin, such that the RBCs are phagocytized by monocytes and splenic macrophages. When medications are the underlying cause, the hapten model has been suggested. RBC-bound drugs are recognized by antibodies and targeted for destruction.
■ What is the significance of the reticulocytes on peripheral smear?	Reticulocytes are immature RBCs. Reticulocytes are seen on the smear because the bone marrow is attempting to compensate for the increased RBC destruction by increasing production.
■ What is the other form of this condition and what are its precipitants?	**Cold agglutinin hemolytic** anemia is the other form, and it occurs when **IgM** antibodies bind, fix complement, and agglutinate RBCs at low temperatures. These antibodies typically appear acutely following certain infections such as **mononucleosis** and *Mycoplasma.* This disease is usually self limited but treatment resistant forms exist. Clinical manifestations include pallor and cyanosis of distal extremities exposed to cold temperatures secondary to vascular obstruction from complement deposition.
■ What is the Coombs' test?	Also known as the direct antiglobulin test, this is used for the detection of autoantibodies bound to the surface of RBCs. RBCs of the patient are washed and incubated with antihuman antibodies (Coombs' reagent). If the test is positive as seen by agglutination, autoantibodies are present on the RBC surface. In this case, cells agglutinated at 37°C but not 4°C, so this disease is considered warm antibody hemolytic anemia.

► **Case 7**

A 57-year-old nulliparous woman presents to her general practitioner concerned about a painless lump she has found in the right upper quadrant of her right breast. Her mother died of breast cancer at the age of 60. Her medical history is significant for mild obesity, an early onset of menarche, and late onset of menopause 3 years previously. She has noted some unilateral pain and dimpling of her right breast but has been scared to make an appointment with her physician. Laboratory tests show a serum calcium level of 9.7 mg/dL.

■ **What is the pathophysiology of this condition?**	Breast cancer results from a transforming, or oncogenic, event that leads to clonal proliferation and survival of breast cancer cells. The events that trigger sporadic breast cancer are often unknown, but abnormalities in cell-cycle pathways, including Her-2, cyclin D1, c-myc, estrogen, and progesterone signaling, have been implicated. *BRCA1* and *BRCA2* genes have been linked to hereditary breast and ovarian cancer and are linked to defects in DNA mismatch repair.
■ **What risk factors are associated with an increased incidence of this condition?**	■ Female gender. ■ Alcohol intake. ■ Breast density. ■ Early menarche or late menopause. ■ Age. ■ Family history (50%–70% of women carrying the *BRCA1* or *BRCA2* genes will develop breast cancer). ■ Hormone replacement therapy. ■ Nulliparity or late first pregnancy. ■ Obesity (in postmenopausal women). ■ Prior breast biopsy, particularly for lesions with atypia. ■ Radiation exposure to the chest.
■ **What are the common forms of this condition?**	Breast cancer is the leading cause of cancer death in women and the most common form of cancer in this group. Most tumors develop in upper/outer quadrants. Types of breast cancer include: ■ Ductal carcinoma in situ (premalignant). ■ Inflammatory carcinoma. ■ Invasive ductal carcinoma (most common form). ■ Invasive lobular carcinoma. ■ Medullary, mucinous, and tubular forms (less common). ■ Paget's disease of the breast. ■ Phylloides tumors, lymphoma, and sarcoma (very rare).
■ **What are the patterns of metastasis in this condition?**	Axillary lymph nodes, lungs, liver, bone, and brain are common sites of metastasis. Metastases to bone are often blastic rather than lytic. Chest wall recurrences are common as well.
■ **What are the most appropriate treatments for this condition?**	The most common treatment is modified mastectomy or lumpectomy with postoperative radiation. Adjuvant tamoxifen or an aromatase inhibitior (such as anastrazole or letrozole) is often added to reduce the risk of recurrence; these drugs are given for 5 years, and often longer. Recently, Herceptin (trastuzumab) has been used in the adjuvant setting to reduce the risk of recurrence in HER-2 overexpressing tumors. Adjuvant chemotherapy (doxorubicin, cyclophosphamide, sometimes with a taxane) is often used for higher-risk patients to reduce the risk of recurrence. Chemotherapy is typically given prior to radiation therapy or hormone therapy.

▶ **Case 8**

A 35-year-old man presents to his primary care physician complaining of watery diarrhea over the past several months. He reports the diarrhea is often "greasy looking," but never bloody. On physical examination, the man's face is flushed, and his neck is covered by a blotchy, violaceous erythema. When asked about this flushing, the man says it has happened several times a day over the past few years, often while he is feeling stressed at work.

■ What is the most likely diagnosis?	Carcinoid syndrome (secretory).
■ What symptoms are most commonly associated with this condition?	Flushing and diarrhea are the two most common presenting symptoms. These symptoms occur in up to 73% of patients initially and up to 89% of patients during the course of disease. Flushing is typically sudden in onset and lasts 2–5 minutes, although it may persist up to an hour with a more advanced disease course. Diarrhea typically occurs with flushing, with steatorrhea present in up to 67% of cases (see Table 8-1).
■ Which laboratory test would be useful to confirm the diagnosis?	Other conditions such as menopause and chronic myelogenous leukemia, as well as reactions to alcohol, glutamate, and calcium channel blockers, may cause flushing. However, flushing in conjunction with an increase in **5-hydroxyindoleacetic acid** (5-HIAA) on urinalysis occurs only in carcinoid syndrome.
■ What is the pathophysiology of this condition?	Carcinoid syndrome occurs only when sufficient concentrations of substances secreted by carcinoid tumors (derived from neuroendocrine cells) reach the circulation. Carcinoid tumors secrete a variety of gastrointestinal peptides, including gastrin, somatostatin, substance P, vasoactive intestinal polypeptide, pancreatic polypeptide, and chromogranin A, as well as serotonin. Diarrhea occurs when the liver can no longer metabolize serotonin due to the presence of metastases. Flushing is thought to be caused by excess histamine release.

TABLE 8-1. **Clinical Characteristics in Patients with Carcinoid Syndrome**

SYMPTOMS/SIGNS	AT PRESENTATION	DURING COURSE OF DISEASE
Diarrhea	32%–73%	68%–84%
Flushing	23%–65%	63%–74%
Pain	10%	34%
Asthma/wheezing	4%–8%	3%–18%
Pellagra	2%	5%
None	12%	22%
Carcinoid heart disease	11%	14%–41%

Modified, with permission, from Kasper DL, et al. *Harrison's Principles of Internal Medicine,* 16th ed. New York: McGraw-Hill, 2005: 2224.

■ **What type of cardiac involvement is typically seen in patients with this condition?**

Right-sided valvular involvement occurs in 11% of patients initially and up to 41% during the course of the disease. Cardiac disease results from serotonin-mediated fibrosis in the endocardium, most commonly in the tricuspid valve. Up to 80% of patients with cardiac involvement develop heart failure. Cardiac involvement can also occur with certain diet drugs that affect serotonin (such as "Phen-Fen").

■ **What is the most appropriate treatment for this condition?**

If localization of a discrete carcinoid tumor is possible, surgical resection is the optimal therapy. However, for all other cases symptomatic management with octreotide is most beneficial.

▶ **Case 9**

A 13-year-old boy is brought to his physician for increasing abdominal distention and pain that has lasted 7 days. Physical examination reveals decreased bowel sounds, tympany, and lower abdominal tenderness. An abdominal CT scan shows a 6-cm mass involving the distal ileum. A biopsy of the mass is taken under radiographic guidance. The histologic sample shows sheets of intermediate-sized lymphoid cells with nonconvoluted nuclei and coarse chromatin along with many macrophages (see Figure 8-5).

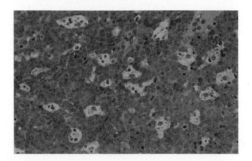

FIGURE 8-5. (Reproduced, with permission, from Lichtman MA, Beutler E, Kipps TJ, et al. *Williams Hematology.* New York, NY: McGraw-Hill, 2006: Plate XIV-7.)

▪ **What is the most likely diagnosis?**	Burkitt's lymphoma, a highly aggressive B-cell non-Hodgkin's lymphoma. The "**starry-sky**" pattern on histology is classic for this condition. Burkitt's lymphoma of the gastrointestinal tract typically involves the ileocecum and peritoneum.
▪ **What are the three forms of this condition?**	The **sporadic** form, as described in this vignette, is the most common form in the developed world and appears in children and young adults.
	The **African/endemic** form, which is closely associated with Epstein-Barr virus (EBV) infection, is another type. The lymphoma will typically present as a maxillary or mandibular mass.
	The **HIV-associated** form is the final type and may stem from reactivation of latent EBV virus in immunosuppressed patients. It typically arises in lymph nodes.
▪ **What is the typical cytogenetic change and what gene does it involve?**	All forms of Burkitt's lymphoma involve the *c-MYC* gene found on chromosome 8. The characteristic translocation is t(8;14) which places the *c-MYC* proto-oncogene adjacent to the immunoglobulin heavy-chain locus on chromosome 14.
▪ **What is tumor lysis syndrome?**	Tumor lysis syndrome is due to the large amount of neoplastic cell death during treatment with chemotherapy. Laboratory analysis shows multiple metabolic complications including hyperphosphatemia, hypocalcemia, hyperuricemia, and hyperkalemia leading to acute renal failure. Allopurinol, aggressive hydration, and diuresis can be used to prevent these consequences.

► **Case 10**

A 55-year-old woman presents to her primary care physician for a routine physical. She reports an unintentional 30-lb (14-kg) weight loss, and chronic fatigue. Abdominal examination reveals an enlarged spleen. Relevant laboratory findings are as follows:

Hemoglobin: 12.9 g/dL
Hematocrit: 38.1%
Mean corpuscular volume: 92 fl
WBC count: 167, 000/mm^3
Platelet count: 625, 000/ mm^3
Blood smear: Many late granulocytic precursor cells, eosinophils and basophils, relatively few metamyelocytes
Cytogenetic analysis: t(9;22) translocation

▪ **What is the most likely diagnosis?**	Chronic myelogenous leukemia (CML), due to the presence of a t(9;22) translocation coupled with the uncontrolled production of maturing granulocytes (neutrophils, eosinophils, and basophils) and platelets (see Figure 8-6). This marked leukocytosis leads to **splenic enlargement.**
▪ **What is this chromosomal abnormality called and what is its product?**	The translocation of the BCR gene on chromosome 9 with the ABL gene on chromosome 22 leads to the *BCR-ABL* fusion product. This abnormality is called a **Philadelphia chromosome** and it is considered pathognomonic for CML.
▪ **What is the pathophysiology of this condition?**	This BCR-Abl fusion protein results in a constitutively active Abl **tyrosine kinase** in the Ras/Raf/MEK/MAPK pathway. This leads to inhibition of apoptosis and unregulated cell division.
▪ **What is the targeted drug treatment for this condition?**	**Imatinib (Gleevec),** a highly specific BCR/Abl tyrosine kinase competitive inhibitor. However, allogeneic bone marrow transplant is still the only potentially curative therapy.
▪ **What is a blast crisis?**	Untreated CML inevitably progresses to an accelerated phase and then a blast crisis in which additional genetic abnormalities accumulate leading to acute myeloid leukemia. Peripheral smears will show a large percentage (>20%) of blast cells.

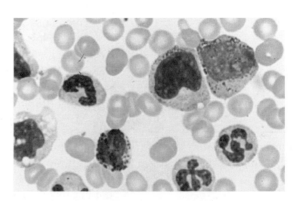

FIGURE 8-6. Chronic myelogenous leukemia. Blood film. Leukemic promyelocytes, a basophilic myelocyte, and segmented neutrophils with increased nuclear material. (Reproduced, with permission, from Lichtman MA, Beutler E, Kipps TJ, et al. *Williams Hematology*, 7th ed. New York, NY: McGraw-Hill, 2006: Plate XIX.)

► **Case 11**

A 52-year-old man visits his primary care physician complaining of constant vague abdominal pain that has been increasing over the past month. He has noted recent weakness and weight loss, which he attributes to recently decreased appetite. His father was diagnosed with colorectal cancer in his late fifties. The patient admits he has never had a colonoscopy and eats a diet high in fat and low in fiber. Rectal examination reveals a palpable mass and occult blood. A CBC reveals the patient's hematocrit is 28%.

■ What is the most likely diagnosis?	Colorectal cancer is the second leading cause of cancer deaths. These malignant polypoid, ulcerating, annular lesions are found in colonic or rectal mucosa. About 15% are mucinous adenocarcinoma, as staged by the Dukes' classification. Spread is via lymphatics and blood to the liver and peritoneal cavity.
■ What risk factors are associated with an increased incidence of this condition?	■ Age >50 years old ■ Family history ■ Lynch syndrome I and II ■ Hereditary nonpolyposis colorectal cancer ■ Long-standing chronic ulcerative pancolitis ■ Tumor suppressor gene and proto-oncogene changes ■ Low-fiber and high-fat diets ■ Male gender
■ What signs and symptoms are commonly associated with this condition?	■ Abdominal pain ■ Anemia ■ Bleeding/mucus per rectum ■ Change in bowel habit ■ Rectal lesions ■ Tenesmus
■ What are the four major locations and associated symptoms of this neoplasm?	■ Left colon (10% of cases): 　■ Altered bowel habits 　■ Bright red blood per rectum ■ Sigmoid colon (20% of cases): 　■ Altered bowel habits 　■ Bright red blood per rectum 　■ Mucus per rectum ■ Right colon (20% of cases): 　■ Anemia 　■ Weight loss 　■ Right iliac fossa mass ■ Rectal (50% of cases): 　■ Polyps (confined to wall) 　■ Ulcer (through bowel wall) 　■ Mass with nodal involvement
■ What are the most appropriate treatments for this condition?	Surgical treatment is indicated. Radiotherapy may be used to shrink tumors preoperatively or for palliative care in inoperable cases. (The benefits of chemotherapy still remain unclear for colon cancer.) There is a 25% survival rate after resections with <5 liver metastases. Carcinoembryonic antigen (CEA) levels can be followed as a marker of response to therapy.

▶ **Case 12**

A 33-year-old African-American woman has been in the intensive care unit of the hospital for 2 days after being admitted for treatment of a severe bacteremia. Her prior medical history is noncontributory. Physical examination now reveals mucosal bleeding, oozing from intravenous access sites, and petechiae on her trunk and extremities. Laboratory tests reveal a prolonged bleeding time, prothrombin time (PT), and activated partial thromboplastin time (aPTT).

■ **What is the most likely diagnosis?**	Disseminated intravascular coagulation (DIC).
■ **What is the pathophysiology of this condition?**	DIC is a systemic process in which there is widespread activation of hemostasis with resultant thrombosis and hemorrhage. Clotting throughout the body, rather than in a localized area, results in a depletion of coagulation factors (see Figure 8-7). Causes of DIC include sepsis, trauma, acute leukemia (especially acute myelogenous leukemia), cavernous hemangiomas (Kasabach-Merritt syndrome), cancer (often found in patients with chronic DIC), amniotic fluid embolism, and snake envenomation.
■ **Which clotting factors are involved in the intrinsic, extrinsic, and common pathways?**	The **intrinsic pathway** involves factors VIII, IX, XI, XII, prekallikrein, and high-molecular weight-kininogen. The **extrinsic pathway** involves factor VII, and the **common pathway** involves factors II, V, and X, and fibrinogen.
■ **Which laboratory tests help differentiate this condition from thrombocytopenia?**	A prolonged bleeding time corresponds to a functional platelet abnormality or thrombocytopenia. An elevated aPTT suggests a problem with the intrinsic pathway, while an elevated PT reveals a defect in the extrinsic pathway. **Thrombocytopenia** and DIC both have prolonged bleeding times, but in DIC, there is also a prolonged PT and aPTT because of the consumption of coagulation factors in addition to platelets.
■ **Which laboratory tests help differentiate this condition from von Willebrand's disease and vitamin K deficiency?**	**von Willebrand's disease** results in ineffective platelet adhesion and functional factor VIII deficiency. Therefore, the bleeding time is prolonged, as is the aPTT. In **vitamin K deficiency**, the activities of factors II, VII, IX, and X are decreased, resulting in a prolonged PT and aPTT and a normal bleeding time.

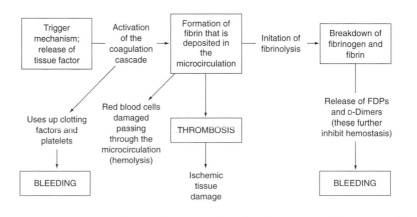

FIGURE 8-7. Pathophysiology of DIC. (Reproduced, with permission, from Tintinalli JE, et al. *Tintinalli's Emergency Medicine: A Comprehensive Study Guide*, 6th ed. New York: McGraw-Hill, 2004: 1328.)

► **Case 13**

A 56-year-old man presents to the emergency department complaining of a 1-day history of nausea and vomiting in the context of significant weight loss over the past few months. Careful questioning reveals he has noticed black specks in his emesis, resembling coffee grounds. On review of systems, he notes early satiety with a decreased appetite, specifically for meat. He attributes his anorexia to a general feeling of fullness after eating. He has no diarrhea, constipation, known sick contacts, or recent travel history, but notes occasional fevers and chills with recent night sweats. Physical examination reveals the patient is afebrile with a nontender, nondistended, soft abdomen remarkable for a firm epigastric mass. Relevant laboratory findings are as follows:

Hematocrit: 28%
Hemoglobin: 9 g/dL
WBC count: 9000/mm^3
Stool test:
  Guaiac positive
  Negative for ova and parasites

▪ What is the most likely diagnosis?	Gastric cancer.
▪ What population is most at risk for this condition?	Men have twice the risk as women. People who consume a diet low in fruits and vegetables and high in starch or nitrites are at increased risk, as are patients with previous gastric operations. The incidence of gastric cancer is decreasing in the United States, but it is still high in Japan.
▪ How is this condition classified?	▪ **Adenocarcinoma** is the most common type of gastric cancer. ▪ Advanced carcinoma develops partly inside the stomach. ▪ Ulcerating carcinoma penetrates all layers of the stomach and may involve neighboring organs. ▪ Polypoid carcinoma involves intraluminal growths that metastasize late in the disease.
▪ What signs and symptoms are commonly associated with this condition?	▪ Anorexia (especially for meat). ▪ Dysphagia (caused by lesions at the cardia of the stomach). ▪ Coffee ground emesis (if bleeding tumor). ▪ Palpable epigastric mass. ▪ Postprandial heaviness. ▪ Vomiting (in cases of pyloric obstruction). ▪ Weight loss. If disease has metastasized: ▪ Intra-abdominal masses. ▪ Virchow's node (left supraclavicular node).
▪ What are the typical laboratory findings in this condition?	Anemia is present in 50% of patients. The stool is guaiac positive. Carcinoembryonic antigen levels are elevated in two-thirds of patients.
▪ What is the most appropriate treatment for this condition?	Diagnosis is via esophagogastroduodenoscopy and biopsy. However, only 50% of patients have resectable lesions, and there has been no proven efficacy of adjuvant chemotherapy.

► **Case 14**

A 56-year-old man who was previously in excellent health is brought to the emergency department after a rapid decline in mental status that began 3 days earlier. His wife notes he has been acting differently and was unable to understand her 2 days earlier. This morning, his wife found him unresponsive and extremely agitated. Currently, the patient is flailing his limbs and is unresponsive to stimuli or to verbal commands. His pupils are equal and reactive. The patient is subsequently sedated, and CT of the head demonstrates a large lesion in the right frontal lobe. MRI establishes the likely diagnosis.

■ **What is the differential diagnosis of a brain lesion?**	The most common brain tumor is a metastatic lesion. Primary brain tumors include gliomas, meningiomas, pituitary adenomas, vestibular schwannomas, and primary central nervous system lymphomas. Brain lesions can be infectious (arising from abscesses, viral processes, progressive multifocal leukoencephalopathy, toxoplasmosis, or cysticercosis), vascular (resulting from cerebral hemorrhage or infarct), or inflammatory (associated with multiple sclerosis or postinfectious encephalopathy).
■ **What is the most likely diagnosis?**	Glioblastoma multiforme (GBM). MRI is the definitive test for a brain mass. Gliomas appear hypointense on T1-weighted imaging and hyperintense on T2-weighted imaging. They also heterogeneously enhance with contrast and can be distinguished from the surrounding edema. The rapidity of onset of this patient's symptoms without signs of infarct also suggests that his symptoms are the result of a highly malignant process.
■ **Where are these tumors typically found?**	GBM is the most commonly diagnosed primary brain tumor. GBM is a grade IV astrocytoma that is most commonly found in adults, in contrast to the peak childhood prevalence of low-grade (pilocytic) astrocytoma. GBM is typically found in the cerebral hemispheres and can cross the corpus callosum to form the characteristic "butterfly glioma."
■ **What are the most common signs and symptoms associated with this tumor?**	The most common symptoms associated with adult GBM are headache (found in 73%–86% of cases) and seizures (found in 26%–32% of cases). The most common neurologic signs are hyperparesis, papilledema, confusion, and aphasia. Symptoms can progress over the course of days to months, but the prognosis of GBM is quite grave, with the majority of patients surviving less than 1 year.
■ **What is the most appropriate treatment for this condition?**	The initial treatment for malignant glioma is resection. Adjuvant radiation therapy along with chemotherapy (with nitrosoureas and Temozolomide) is the current standard of care. Dexamethasone is used to alleviate the vasogenic edema resulting from blood-brain barrier disruption that occurs in the region surrounding many brain tumors. The mechanism of action of dexamethasone is unknown, but it is preferred to other steroids because its relative lack of mineralocorticoid activity decreases the risk of fluid retention.

ORGAN SYSTEMS

HEMATOLOGY & ONCOLOGY

▶ **Case 15**

A 42-year-old African-American man presents to the emergency department with sudden onset of shortness of breath. He complains of feeling fatigued and weak, and notes he saw blood in his urine for the first time this morning. He has no chest pain or palpitations and has no prior history of hypertension, coronary artery disease, or ischemic heart disease. He is being treated with trimethoprim-sulfamethoxazole for a urinary tract infection, but has no other significant medical history. He denies a history of alcohol or drug abuse. Physical examination reveals hepatosplenomegaly, mild scleral icterus, and tachycardia.

■ What is the most likely diagnosis?	Glucose-6-phospate dehydrogenase (G6PD) deficiency.
■ What are the typical peripheral blood smear (PBS) findings in this condition?	PBS will likely reveal bite cells and ghost cells, implying intravascular hemolytic anemia.
■ What is the pathophysiology of this condition?	G6PD protects cells from oxidative damage by converting nicotinamide adenine dinucleotide phosphate (NADP+) to its reduced form (NADPH). Patients with a deficiency in this enzyme are less able to deal with oxidative stresses, such as those that might result from ingestion of a sulfa drug such as sulfamethoxazole.
■ How is this condition acquired?	G6PD deficiency is an X-linked recessive trait and affects males predominantly. Heterozygous females are usually normal. Patients with G6PD deficiency are normal in the absence of oxidative stress. However, exposure to oxidative stress triggers the disease. G6PD in Mediterranean pedigrees results in favism, or hemolysis induced by the ingestion of fava beans.
■ How are anemias classified in terms of cell volume?	■ **Microcytic anemia** (mean corpuscular volume [MCV] <80 fl): Caused by iron deficiency, thalassemia, or lead poisoning. ■ **Normocytic anemia** (MCV 80–100 fl): Caused by enzyme deficiency (such as G6PD or pyruvate kinase), blood loss (as from trauma), anemia of chronic disease, or hemolysis (autoimmune or mechanical). ■ **Macrocytic anemia** (MCV >100 fl): Causes include vitamin B_{12}/folate deficiency, liver disease, drugs that inhibit DNA synthesis, and alcohol.
■ What is the most appropriate treatment for this condition?	Treatment is generally supportive with removal of offending agent.

► **Case 16**

A 67-year-old man presents to his physician with pain on swallowing and hoarseness. He has noted some swelling of the right side of his neck. The patient has smoked one pack of cigarettes per day since he was 15 years old and drinks two beers every night before dinner. Physical examination reveals a palpable neck mass and white plaques in his mouth.

■ **What is the differential diagnosis of a neck mass?**	■ **Congenital:** torticollis, thyroglossal duct cyst, brachial cleft cyst, cystic hygroma, dermoid cyst, carotid body tumor ■ **Acquired:** lymphoma, mononucleosis (Epstein-Barr virus), other causes of lymphadenopathy, cervical lymphadenitis ■ **Thyroid:** goiter (midline) ■ **Malignancy: thyroid cancer** (papillary, medullary, follicular, or anaplastic types), lymphoma, head, or neck malignancy (squamous cell or adenocarinoma)
■ **What is the most likely diagnosis?**	Squamous cell tumor or adenocarcinoma of the head and neck.
■ **Which risk factors increase this patient's likelihood of disease?**	Tobacco and alcohol (for squamous cell carcinomas of the head and neck only).
■ **Which procedures are useful in confirming this diagnosis?**	Diagnostic procedures include biopsy via fine-needle aspiration of the mass, and CT and/or MRI to determine the stage and possible vascular involvement and resectability. If lymphoma is suspected, excisional biopsy should be performed.
■ **Where are these lesions commonly located?**	Head and neck cancers are typically found in the oral cavity, nasopharynx, larynx, oropharynx, and salivary glands.
■ **What are the most appropriate treatments for this condition?**	Localized lesions are removed surgically or via radiotherapy. Palliative radiation is used for larger, more complex lesions. Combined chemotherapy and radiotherapy is the standard of care for advanced lesions.
■ **What is TNM staging?**	This is a classification system used to determine prognosis, treatment strategies, and survival based on disease severity. "T" is used to describe the size of the primary tumor. "N" describes the number of regional lymph nodes with evidence of malignant invasion. "M" classifies distant metastases. Generally the higher ranking indicates larger size of the tumor, more lymph node involvement, and the presence of metastases. These characteristics are also associated with poorer prognosis.

► **Case 17**

A 55-year-old white man is brought to the emergency department after collapsing in a restaurant. He is conscious on arrival and claims he has not seen a doctor for many years. On physical examination, the patient appears jaundiced. An ECG demonstrates he is in atrial fibrillation. Laboratory studies reveal an elevated serum glucose level and the following iron parameters:

Serum iron: 400 µg/dL
Transferrin: 150 µg/dL
Iron saturation: 85%
Ferritin: 1100 ng/mL

■ What is the most likely diagnosis?	Hereditary hemochromatosis (HH), which is an autosomal recessive disease (although with variable penetrance), resulting in excessive iron absorption. Excess iron gradually accumulates at a rate of approximately 0.5–1.0 g/y. Normal body iron content is approximately 3–4 g, and symptoms are noticeable at a body iron content exceeding 20 g. As a result, most men are not diagnosed until after age 40, and women are not diagnosed until after cessation of their menstrual periods. Normal iron loss is 1 mg/d in men and 1.5 mg/d in menstruating women.
■ What is the pathophysiology of this condition?	Normally, iron homeostasis is achieved by regulating iron intake to compensate for losses through the skin, menses, pregnancy, and other processes. However, in hereditary hemochromatosis, an autosomal recessive mutation in chromosome 6 (**HFE gene**) causes excessive iron to be absorbed through the intestine. This iron gradually deposits as hemosiderin throughout the body, particularly in the liver (see Figure 8-8), skin, pancreas, joints, gonads, heart, and pituitary, which eventually leads to oxidative damage to these organs.
■ What signs and symptoms are commonly associated with this condition?	Clinical manifestations correspond to the organs with excessive iron deposits. Patients may present with the classic triad of cirrhosis, diabetes mellitus, and skin pigmentation (hence, the moniker "bronze diabetes"), as well as arthropathy (pseudogout, often of the second and third digits), impotence in men, cardiac enlargement, cardiac conduction defects, and weakness or lethargy (due to pituitary involvement).
■ What are the typical laboratory findings in this condition?	Iron saturation of >60% in men and >50% in women suggests hemochromatosis 90% of the time. A cutoff of 45% for both men and women is typically used, however, for simplicity. Other typical laboratory findings include hyperglycemia, elevated liver enzyme levels, elevated serum iron levels, decreased total iron binding capacity, and elevated ferritin levels.
■ What is the most appropriate treatment for this condition?	Treatment for HH includes serial phlebotomy with the possible use of deferoxamine, an iron-binding agent, especially for those with homozygous *HFE* mutations (C282Y) and iron overload. Compound heterozygotes (e.g., C282Y and H63D) with iron overload should also be treated.

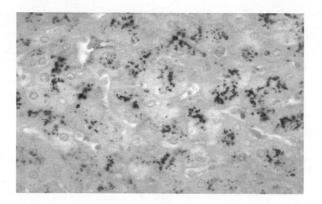

FIGURE 8-8. **Iron deposits in the liver in hemochromatosis.** (Reproduced, with permission, from the Pathology Education Instructional Resource Digital Library [http://peir.net] at the University of Alabama, Birmingham.)

► **Case 18**

A 25-year-old man visits his primary care physician for a routine screening evaluation. He explains that he has been having fevers and drenching night sweats for the past 6 months. Additionally, he has been feeling increasingly tired and itchy over his entire body with no obvious explanation. On physical examination, the patient has lost 11 kg (25 lbs) since his last visit and has a markedly enlarged nontender lymph node in his anterior cervical chain. A biopsy of this node is taken and the photomicrograph is shown below (see Figure 8-9).

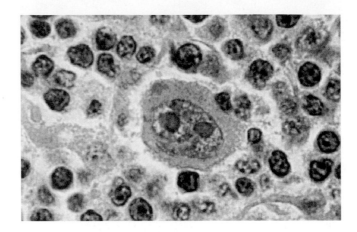

FIGURE 8-9. (Reproduced, with permission, from Lichtman MA, Beutler E, Kipps TJ, et al. *Williams Hematology*, 7th ed. New York: McGraw-Hill, 2006: Plate XXII-32.)

▪ What type of cell is depicted in Figure 8-9?	This is the classic **Reed-Sternberg cell,** with its large size, bilobed nucleus, and nucleolar inclusion bodies ("**owl's eyes**"). Classically these cells also display a common set of markers, including CD15+ and CD30+, and typically lack leukocyte common antigen (CD45), pan-B, and pan-T-cell markers.
▪ What is the most likely diagnosis?	**Hodgkin's lymphoma.** Most patients present with nontender asymptomatic palpable lymphadenopathy, often in the neck and supraclavicular area. Alternatively, many patients will present with a fairly large asymptomatic mediastinal mass on routine x-ray of the chest. Approximately one-third of patients experience fever, night sweats, weight loss, fatigue, and pruritus.
▪ What are B symptoms?	Classic B symptoms are unexplained weight loss, persistent or recurrent fevers, and drenching night sweats. These symptoms generally correlate with an advanced stage of disease and tumor burden.

■ **What are the variants of this condition?**	There are five main classes of Hodgkin's lymphoma (HL): ■ **Nodular sclerosis HL: most common**, especially among younger women. This is defined by fibrous bands dividing a lymph node into nodules, and lacunar cells (Reed-Sternberg variants), carrying a good prognosis. ■ Lymphocyte predominance HL: uncommon and characterized by lymphohistiocytes ("popcorn cells"). ■ Lymphocyte-rich: uncommon with reactive lymphocytes that comprise the infiltrate, there is an association with Epstein-Barr virus (EBV) in 40% of cases. ■ Lymphocyte depleted: least common and characterized by very few lymphocytes, relatively plentiful Reed-Sternberg cells, associated with EBV and HIV, carrying a poor prognosis. ■ Mixed cellularity: common, associated with older age, polymorphic infiltrate with plentiful Reed-Sternberg cells, associated with EBV in 70% of cases.
■ **What is the most appropriate treatment for this condition?**	Over 90% of patients with early stage, localized disease are cured with excision and localized radiotherapy. Patients with more advanced disease typically undergo the ABVD chemotherapy regimen consisting of doxorubicin (Adriamycin), bleomycin, vinblastine, and dacarbazine.

While an 8-month-old boy is brought to his pediatrician by his foster parents, they become concerned that their son has continued to bleed after the heel-stick. The parents also report that during his circumcision, he seemed to bleed for an extended amount of time. Physical examination is significant for multiple bruises on the child's knees and elbows. Relevant laboratory findings include a platelet count of 250,000/mm^3, a normal bleeding time, a prothrombin time of 12 seconds, and a partial thromboplastin time of >120 seconds.

■ **What is the most likely diagnosis?**

Hemophilia. This disease is characterized by normal bleeding time, platelet count and prothrombin time, but an **elevated partial thromboplastin time.**

von Willebrand's disease is the most common hereditary bleeding disorder. It is distinguished from hemophilia by a prolonged bleeding time.

■ **What are the variants of this condition?**

■ Hemophilia A: marked deficiency of factor VIII.
■ Hemophilia B (Christmas disease): marked deficiency of factor IX.
   Hemophilia B is clinically indistinguishable from hemophilia A. However, hemophilia A is 5–10 times more prevalent.

■ **How is this condition inherited?**

Both disease variants are X-linked recessive.

■ **What are the possible complications of this condition?**

Complications include deep and delayed bleeding into joints (hemarthrosis), muscles (hematoma), and the gastrointestinal tract. The most concerning complications are bleeds in the central nervous system and oropharynx.

Mucosal or cutaneous bleeding is uncommon and more characteristic of platelet dysfunction or von Willebrand's disease.

Transmission of blood-borne infection (specifically HIV and hepatitis C) through transfusion has been significantly reduced through modern screening technology and recombinant factors.

■ **What are the most appropriate treatments for this condition?**

Clotting factor concentrate replacements can be used to prevent bleeding and limit existing hemorrhage. Both monoclonal purified and recombinant factor VIII and IX exist.

Fresh frozen plasma and whole blood transfusions are used in the acute setting (but they carry the risk of encouraging the development of inhibitor antibodies to factor VIII).

In mild cases of hemophilia A, desmopressin transiently increases the factor VIII level.

► **Case 20**

A 19-year-old African-American woman presents to her primary physician with pelvic pain and discomfort for the past few months. A bimanual pelvic examination reveals a large left adnexal mass. A subsequent CT scan confirms a 16-cm well-demarcated solid mass in this area. A stereotactic biopsy reveals primitive mesenchymal cells along with tissue suggestive of glands, bone, cartilage, muscle, and neuroepithelial cells (see Figure 8-11).

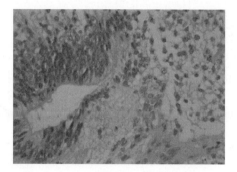

FIGURE 8-11. (Reproduced, with permission, from Kantarjian HM, Wolff RA, Koller CA. *MD Anderson Manual of Medical Oncology*. New York: McGraw-Hill, 2006.)

■ **What is the most likely diagnosis?**	Teratoma, the most common type of germ cell tumor. The component tissues in a teratoma arise from all three germ layers and vary from immature to well-differentiated. Additionally, these tissues are foreign to the anatomic site in which they are found.
■ **What are the three types of this condition?**	■ **Mature (benign dermoid cysts),** which comprise 95% of all ovarian teratomas and are typically lined by epidermis and contain hair, bone, or teeth. These lesions can also be bilateral. ■ **Immature (malignant),** which (as explained in this question) are usually large, rapidly growing tumors with tissue resembling the fetus or embryo rather than the adult. Due to their rapid growth, these tumors also show necrosis and hemorrhage in addition to presenting in younger women. ■ **Monodermal/highly specialized,** which are a rare subset that consists of a predominantly mature histologic cell type, the most common of which are struma ovarii and carcinoid. Remember: most teratomas are benign in women.
■ **How are these masses graded?**	Only malignant teratomas are graded, and the grade of differentiation is based upon the proportion of tissue containing immature neuroepithelium. This is an important prognostic indicator of extraovarian spread.
■ **What is the most appropriate treatment for this condition?**	Complete surgical excision is the standard of care. Higher-grade malignant teratomas are additionally managed with chemotherapy.

► **Case 21**

An 11-year-old girl is brought to her physician because of frequent epistaxis and "purple spots" on her body. She reports no recent history of trauma. Physical examination reveals petechiae and purpura on her arms, outer thighs, and legs (see Figure 8-10). A peripheral blood smear (PBS) shows large platelets, but no helmet cells or schistocytes. Results of a Coombs' test are positive. Relevant laboratory findings are as follows:

Hemoglobin: 12.5 g/dL
Hematocrit: 36%
WBC count: 5000/mm³
Platelet count: 11,000/mm³

Bleeding time: 12 minutes
Prothrombin time (PT): 13 seconds
Partial thromboplastin time (PTT): 25 seconds

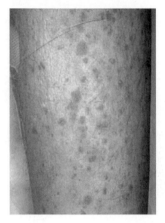

FIGURE 8-10. (Reproduced, with permission, from Bondi EE, Jegasothy BV, Lazarus GS [eds]. *Dermatology: Diagnosis & Treatment.* Norwalk, CT: Appleton & Lange, 1991. Copyright © by The McGraw-Hill Companies, Inc.)

▪ **What is the most likely diagnosis?**	Idiopathic thrombocytopenic purpura (ITP), a disease which is characterized by antiplatelet antibodies.
▪ **What would be the most likely diagnosis if schistocytes were evident on PBS and results of Coombs' test were negative?**	In this case, the likely diagnosis would be thrombotic thrombocytopenic purpura (TTP)/hemolytic-uremic syndrome. This idiopathic disease causes microthrombi to develop in small vessels.
▪ **What are the three main mechanisms of this condition?**	Thrombocytopenia may be caused by: ▪ Splenic sequestration. ▪ Decreased production (due to stem-cell failure, leukemia, aplastic anemia, alcohol, aspirin, clopidogrel). ▪ Increased destruction (due to ITP, TTP, heparin, quinidine).
▪ **What clinical findings are commonly associated with this condition?**	ITP presents with mucous membrane bleeding, petechiae, and purpura (see Figure 8-10). Epistaxis (nosebleed) and easy bruisability are characteristic of bleeding disorders in general. The childhood form of ITP usually develops after a viral infection or immunization and is a self-limited disease. Adult ITP, in contrast, is often a chronic disease.

■ **What additional tests could be used to confirm the diagnosis?**	Bleeding time is increased in ITP, with normal PT and PTT. A PBS reveals large (young) platelets with no schistocytes. Antiplatelet antibodies can be present or absent, and thus are not helpful in making the diagnosis. Bone marrow biopsy would demonstrate increased megakaryocytes.
■ **What are the most appropriate treatments for this condition?**	First-line treatment is high-dose steroids. Second-line treatment includes intravenous immunoglobulin G (IVIG), anti-Rh, splenectomy, or rituximab (anti-CD20). Acute bleeding in ITP is treated with IVIG followed by platelets and pulse methylprednisolone.

▶ **Case 22**

A 60-year-old woman presents to her primary care physician for her annual physical examination. She says she has been feeling "down" and tired lately. Upon questioning, she also admits to some constipation, abdominal pain, joint pain, and muscle aches. Physical examination reveals blue pigmentation in her gum-tooth line. A peripheral blood smear reveals coarse basophilic stippling. Relevant laboratory findings are as follows:

Hemoglobin: 9.0 g/dL
Hematocrit: 26%
Mean corpuscular volume: 76 fl
WBC count: 5000/mm³

■ What is the most likely diagnosis?	Lead poisoning. This is suggested by the blue pigmentation of the gums (**Burton's lines**), the patient's microcytic anemia, and the characteristic basophilic stippling. Additional presenting symptoms include colicky abdominal pain, constipation, irritability, difficulty concentrating, depression/psychosis, decreased short-term memory, arthralgias and myalgias, headache, decreased libido, and anemia. Lead poisoning can also cause peripheral neuropathy, often presenting as extensor weakness (e.g., wrist drop) due to segmental demyelination and degeneration of motor axons.
■ What is the most likely cause of the anemia?	Lead poisoning is an environmental cause of porphyria through inhibition of porphobilinogen synthetase, which converts 5-aminolevulinic acid to porphobilinogen in one of the first steps of heme synthesis. This impairment results in decreased hemoglobin production, and therefore a microcytic, hypochromic anemia.
■ Where does lead distribute in the body?	Lead distributes in the blood, soft tissues, and skeleton, particularly bones and teeth. The vast majority (95%) of the body's lead burden is deposited in the skeleton, where its half-life is approximately 25 years. Therefore, events associated with bone turnover, such as hyperthyroidism, menopause, pregnancy, and breast-feeding, can cause lead to be released into the blood. This can result in acute lead intoxication in the absence of an acute exposure. Lead can also cross the placenta. In children, especially those 1–3 years old, lead can easily enter and harm their developing nervous system because the blood-brain barrier is not completely formed.
■ What do increased serum lead levels and increased free erythrocyte protoporphyrin (FEP) levels indicate about the duration of this condition?	Increased serum lead levels indicate lead exposure within the past 3 weeks. FEP levels are a measure of intoxication in the past 120 days (the average lifetime of an RBC). Chelation therapy with succimer can be useful in severe cases in addition to removing the source of the lead.

A 65-year-old woman presents to her physician with cough, hemoptysis, wheezing, and pleuritic pain. She has noted increased hoarseness of her voice and weight loss over the past few months. She also has noted progressively worsening shortness of breath when ascending or descending one flight of stairs. She has been hospitalized for pneumonia twice during the past 12 months. Sputum analysis reveals atypical cells. A complete blood count reveals her hematocrit is 25% and her WBC count is 12,000/mm^3.

■ What is the most likely diagnosis?	Lung cancer (**Pancoast's syndrome**). This disease is caused by a tumor of the upper lobe of the lung, which causes pain in the ipsilateral arm and Horner's syndrome (ptosis, miosis, and ipsilateral anhidrosis). The tumor is often accompanied by ipsilateral pain or weakness/numbness in the ulnar distribution.
■ What are the major clinical features of this condition?	■ Hoarseness is caused by recurrent laryngeal nerve involvement. ■ Neck or facial swelling is due to superior vena cava obstruction. ■ Diaphragmatic paralysis is due to phrenic nerve involvement. ■ Dyspnea is secondary to airway obstruction and increased ventilation requirements. ■ Metastasis to the liver, adrenal glands, brain, bone, and mediastinal lymph nodes is common. ■ Extrathoracic signs include paraneoplastic syndromes such as Cushing's syndrome, hypercalcemia, the syndrome of inappropriate secretion of ADH (SIADH), clubbing (hypertrophic osteoarthropathy), and Eaton-Lambert syndrome.
■ What are the typical laboratory findings in this condition?	■ Sputum analysis typically reveals atypical cells (not sensitive). ■ Anemia of chronic disease. ■ Chest radiographs and CT scans typically reveal squamous cell carcinomas at the hilum and/or adenocarcinoma at the periphery. ■ Ventilation-perfusion scanning can assess the functional pulmonary reserve. ■ Positron emission tomography may be useful to evaluate lymph node involvement which is critical for staging.
■ What are the primary pathologic types of this condition?	**Non–small cell lung cancer** (which is the most common type) includes the following: ■ **Squamous cell carcinoma** accounts for 30% of lung cancers. It occurs centrally near the hilum; slower growth and cavitation are frequently seen. ■ **Adenocarcinoma** accounts for 30% of lung cancers. These tumors may be mucus-secreting as in acinar adenocarcinoma. ■ **Bronchoalveolar carcinoma** occurs more often in nonsmokers, and is associated with epidermal growth factor receptor (EGFR) mutations. ■ **Large cell carcinoma**, which is rare. **Small cell carcinoma** accounts for 25% of lung cancers. These tumors occur centrally and are early to metastasize. They are very sensitive to chemotherapy but frequently relapse.
■ What are the most appropriate treatments for this condition?	Surgery is considered for lesions without distant metastasis, if the patient has sufficient cardiopulmonary reserve. Radiotherapy is used to treat unresectable tumors. Adjuvant chemotherapy is also used with some patients undergoing surgery; patients with stage Ib disease or higher require chemotherapy. For patients with metastatic disease, chemotherapy is often used palliatively, often with biological agents (such as antiangiogenic agents and EGFR inhibitors).

► **Case 24**

A 45-year-old man presents to his physician for a regular checkup. He has no previous medical or surgical history. As part of the checkup, the physician orders routine laboratory tests; relevant findings are as follows:

Hemoglobin: 11 g/dL
Hematocrit: 33%
Reticulocyte count: 0.2%
Mean corpuscular volume: 120 fl

■ What is the most likely diagnosis?	The tests are indicative of a macrocytic anemia. However, one must remember that macrocytic anemia is not a diagnosis in itself, and a cause for the anemia must always be pursued.
■ What other test could be used to confirm the diagnosis?	In megaloblastic anemias, a peripheral blood smear would reveal the presence of hypersegmented neutrophils (>5 nuclei) (see Figure 8-12).
■ What are some possible etiologies for this condition?	■ Alcoholism. ■ Folate deficiency. ■ Vitamin B_{12} deficiency. ■ Hypothyroidism. ■ Mild aplastic anemia. ■ Myelodysplastic syndrome. ■ Pharmaceutical agents (especially antimetabolites such as methotrexate or chemotherapeutic agents).
■ What diagnosis should be considered if the patient also had decreased vibration sensation in his feet?	This neuropathy would indicate a vitamin B_{12} deficiency (subacute combined degeneration). Historically, a **Schilling test** would be helpful in excluding other possible causes, such as pellagra or celiac sprue. The Schilling test involves administering radiolabeled vitamin B_{12} and measuring urinary excretion of radioisotope before and after the administration of intrinsic factor. Beware, however, that bacterial overgrowth can cause false-positive results. Now there are more simple direct tests for vitamin B_{12} and folate levels.

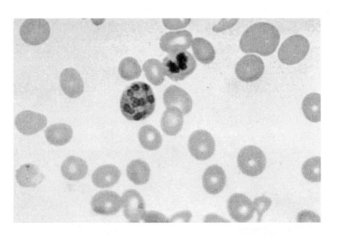

FIGURE 8-12. Multilobed PMNs characteristic of megaloblastic anemias. (Reproduced, with permission, from Kasper DL, et al. *Harrison's Principles of Internal Medicine*, 16th ed. New York: McGraw-Hill, 2005: 605.)

► **Case 25**

A 66-year-old postmenopausal woman presents to her physician with complaints of fatigue, dyspnea, dizziness, and tachycardia. She also says she craves chewing on ice cubes. Physical examination reveals pallor of the mucous membranes of her mouth. The cells on a peripheral blood smear are microcytic and hypochromic (see Figure 8-13). Relevant laboratory findings are as follows:

Hemoglobin: 11 g/dL
Hematocrit: 30%
Reticulocyte count: 0.2%
Mean corpuscular volume: 74 fl

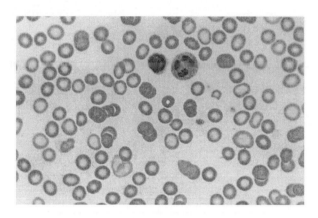

FIGURE 8-13. (Reproduced, with permission, from Le T, Bhushan V, Rao DA. *First Aid for the USMLE Step 1: 2008.* New York: McGraw-Hill, 2008: Color Image 20.)

▪ **What is the most likely diagnosis?**	Iron deficiency anemia. This diagnosis would be further supported by laboratory studies demonstrating a decreased iron concentration, *increased* total iron binding capacity, and *decreased* ferritin levels. The cause for a patient's iron deficiency however needs to be further pursued. In addition, comorbid inflammatory conditions can raise serum ferritin, resulting in values within the normal range.
▪ **What factors can lead to this disease?**	▪ Chronic blood loss (especially gastrointestinal blood loss secondary to colon cancer). ▪ Dietary deficiency (increased demand or decreased absorption). ▪ Increased iron requirement (as in pregnancy or childhood growth). ▪ Intestinal hookworm infection (this is the most common cause worldwide, and should be considered in patients who have immigrated from developing countries).
▪ **Why are measurements of the total iron binding capacity important?**	Total iron binding capacity is high in iron deficiency anemia and low in anemia of chronic disease. Both illnesses have decreased serum iron levels.
▪ **What other conditions is this patient at a greatly increased risk for developing?**	**Plummer-Vinson syndrome**, due to an extreme lack of iron. This syndrome is characterized by atrophic glossitis, esophageal webs, and anemia.
▪ **What are the common causes of microcytic, hypochromic anemia?**	Microcytic anemia results from either decreased hemoglobin production or faulty hemoglobin function. Iron deficiency, thalassemia, sideroblastic anemia, and lead poisoning are the four possible etiologies of microcytic, hypochromic anemia.

► **Case 26**

A mother brings her 4-month-old infant to the pediatrician because the child has had watery diarrhea almost daily for the past month. Previously a good eater, the baby is now refusing to feed and is irritable most of the time. While holding the baby, the mother also calls attention to a mass in his belly that has not resolved in several days.

■ **What is the most common tumor occurring in infants?**	Neuroblastoma.
■ **What is the origin of this tumor?**	Neuroblastoma is a malignancy of the sympathetic nervous system that arises during embryonic development. In the embryo, **neuroblasts** (pluripotent sympathetic stem cells) invaginate and migrate along the neuraxis to the adrenal medulla, the sympathetic ganglia, and various other sites. Figure 8-14 shows a large neuroblastoma occupying the left flank in an older child. The site of disease presentation depends on the area to which the neuroblasts migrate.
■ **What are the types of small, round, blue-cell tumors?**	■ Neuroblastoma ■ Ewing's sarcoma ■ Wilms' tumor ■ Acute leukemia ■ Mesothelioma ■ Rhabdomyosarcoma ■ Medulloblastoma ■ Retinoblastoma ■ Primitive neuroectodermal tumor
■ **What prognostic factors are important in this tumor?**	Tumor stage and the patient's age at diagnosis are the two most important prognostic factors. Patients with localized disease, regardless of age, have a favorable prognosis (80%–90% 5-year survival). Overall, younger age at diagnosis carries a more favorable prognosis. The 5-year survival rate is 83% for infants, 55%–60% for children 1–5 years old, and 40% for children older than 5 years.
■ **What are the likely findings on biopsy of this tumor?**	Histologically, neuroblastoma presents as dense nests of small, round, blue-tumor cells with hyperchromatic nuclei. **Homer-Wright pseudorosettes** are seen in 10%–15% of cases. These pseudorosettes are composed of neuroblasts surrounding neuritic processes and are pathognomonic of neuroblastoma.
■ **What are the most appropriate treatments for this tumor?**	For patients with localized disease, surgical excision is curative. For more advanced disease, treatment consists of surgical excision followed by chemotherapy. Chemotherapy for neuroblastoma consists of combination regimens, typically vincristine, cyclophosphamide, and doxorubicin. Other regimens include etoposide in combination with either cisplatin or carboplatin.

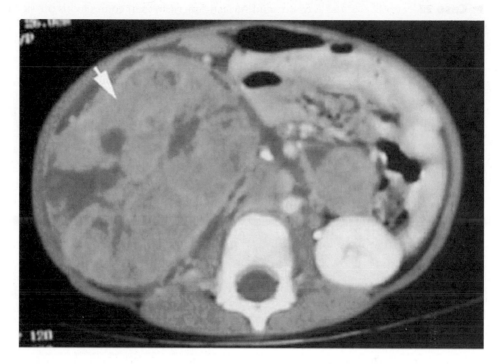

FIGURE 8-14. **Abdominal neuroblastoma arising from the right retroperitoneium (arrow).** (Reproduced, with permission, from Brunicardi FC, Andersen DK, et al. *Schwarts's Principles of Surgery*, 8th ed. New York: McGraw-Hill, 2005.)

► **Case 27**

A 62-year-old African-American man comes to his physician complaining of lower back pain of recent onset. His past medical history is unremarkable except for two recent attacks of pneumonia that were successfully treated. Relevant laboratory values are as follows:

Sodium: 140 mEq/L
Bicarbonate: 25 mEq/L
Magnesium: 1.8 mg/dL
Potassium: 4.0 mEq/L
Calcium: 14 mg/dL

Phosphate: 3.6 mg/dL
Chloride: 106 mEq/L
Blood urea nitrogen: 15 mg/dL
Creatinine: 2.0 mg/dL

■ **What is the most likely diagnosis?**

Back pain, increased recent susceptibility to infection, and elevated serum calcium and creatinine levels strongly suggest multiple myeloma.

■ **What is the pathophysiology of this condition?**

Multiple myeloma is a clonal proliferation of B cells that have then differentiated into plasma cells. These mature B cells cause lytic lesions in the bones, called **punched-out lesions.** These cells produce massive quantities of identical immunoglobulin molecules, usually IgG or IgA, that are either κ or λ light chain (κ more common than λ). Rarely, IgD or nonsecretory myeloma can be diagnosed.

■ **What aspects of the condition are responsible for this patient's symptoms?**

The abnormal lymphocytes are incapable of mounting a normal immunologic response, which explains the patient's recent susceptibility to infection. The elevated serum calcium level and back pain are the result of bone breakdown and osteoclast-activating factor. Finally, the increased creatinine level indicates renal involvement.

■ **What renal complications are associated with this condition?**

The large amount of **Bence Jones proteins** (free immunoglobulin light chains) found in the urine of patients with multiple myeloma causes azotemia. Other renal complications include inflammation with potential giant cell formation and metastatic calcification. The differential diagnosis of renal failure in myeloma includes amyloid kidney, myeloma kidney, light chain deposition disease, uric acid stones, hypercalcemia, sepsis with acute tubular necrosis, and obstruction.

■ **What other tests could be used to confirm the diagnosis?**

A complete blood count should be ordered. Patients with multiple myeloma may be anemic as a result of tumor cells overcrowding myeloid precursor cells. Electrophoresis with immunofixation will demonstrate **M protein**, the term given to the massively produced immunoglobulin. **Monoclonal gammopathy of undetermined significance** (MGUS) is the precursor lesion here if the M protein level is <3 g/dL, there are <10% plasma cells in the bone marrow, and if no clinical manifestations are present. Urinalysis of a 24-hour collection may reveal the presence of a Bence Jones protein. Bone marrow biopsy shows a two- to four fold increase in plasma cells. Additionally, the total immunoglobulin levels may be low. Finally, as a result of the marked hyperglobulinemia, RBCs on peripheral blood smear will clump in a formation that resembles poker chips. This pattern is called **rouleaux formation.**

► **Case 28**

A 30-year-old woman comes to her physician complaining of a headache that has affected her intermittently for the past 6 months. The frontally located headache occurs on most days and is typically dull but sometimes piercing. Over the same time period, the woman has also had profound weakness in her right arm to the point at which she is sometimes unable to hold her 1-year-old daughter or to comb her hair. She also reports an intermittent sensation of "pins and needles" in her right hand.

■ **What is the most likely diagnosis?**

Oligodendroglioma. These relatively rare, slow-growing tumors occur at a rate of 0.3 per 100,000 individuals and are responsible for 2%–4% of primary brain tumors and 4%–15% of all intracranial gliomas. They occur with equal incidence in women and men, and the peak age incidence is 42 years. Primary brain tumors represent approximately 2% of all cancers.

■ **Where do these tumors typically occur?**

Oligodendrogliomas almost always (92% of cases) occur supratentorially and are most often found in the frontal lobes. Lesions are typically peripheral. Most oligodendrogliomas arise in the cortex and extend into the white matter of the cerebral hemispheres.

■ **What symptoms are typically associated with these tumors?**

As with most primary brain tumors, the clinical presentation of oligodendrogliomas is typically attributable to compression of adjacent structures by the tumor. Oligodendrogliomas often cause headache, mental status changes, and paresis. Seizures may also occur. Because they are slow-growing, these tumors may have a more insidious presentation, while the anaplastic forms present with more rapid neurologic decline.

■ **What are the likely findings on histology?**

"Fried egg" cells are typically seen on histologic section. These cells have characteristic round nuclei with clear cytoplasm (see Figure 8-15). The tumors often calcify (30% of cases), and calcifications may be apparent on histologic section.

■ **What is the prognosis for patients with this tumor?**

About 50% of patients with oligodendrogliomas survive longer than 5 years, and there is a 25%–34% 10-year survival rate. Mortality increases with features of increasing nuclear atypia, necrosis, and mitosis. Some oligodendrogliomas contain astrocytic components and are termed **mixed gliomas.** Patients with highly anaplastic oligodendrogliomas have a median survival of <2 years.

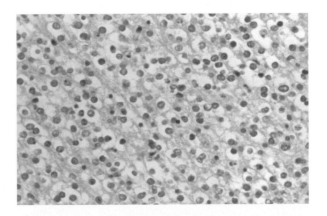

FIGURE 8-15. **"Fried egg" cells on histologic exam in oligodendroglioma.** (Reproduced, with permission, from the Pathology Education Instructional Resource Digital Library [http://peir.net] at the University of Alabama, Birmingham.)

▶ **Case 29**

A 49-year-old woman presents to her gynecologist because her menstrual periods have become irregular. The patient also reports she has hair growing on her face and has developed mild acne, which she hasn't had since she was a teenager. On physical examination, the patient's abdomen is somewhat distended and there is a palpable mass on the left adnexum.

■ What is the most likely diagnosis?	A palpable adnexal mass in conjunction with abdominal swelling is suggestive of ovarian cancer, which is often accompanied by ascites. The patient's irregular periods may simply be normal menopause, but the triad of irregular periods, facial hair, and acne suggest androgen excess. The **Sertoli-Leydig ovarian tumor**, also known as an androgenoma, is an androgen-producing neoplasm that presents with hirsutism in 50% of patients.
■ From what cell line does this tumor originate?	The Sertoli-Leydig cell tumor is of sex cord–stromal origin. Tumors from this origin are relatively rare, and account for only 5% of ovarian neoplasms. They consist of mixtures of stromal fibroblasts, granulosa cells, theca cells, and cells that resemble testicular Sertoli cells and Leydig cells.
■ What other tumors have the same origin?	Other stromal ovarian tumors include: ■ **Fibromas**, solid tumors consisting of cells that resemble fibroblasts. ■ **Thecoma** tumors, which contain fibroblasts plus lipid-containing cells. ■ **Granulosa cell** tumors, which consist of estrogen-secreting granulosa cells and may present with abnormal vaginal bleeding or endometrial hyperplasia.
■ What are the likely findings on histology?	The Sertoli-Leydig cell tumor typically is composed of large cells with large amounts of eosinophilic cytoplasm arranged into tubules and surrounded by a fibrous stroma. Sertoli cells are found lining the tubules, and Leydig cells may be found in the stroma.
■ What is the lymphatic drainage of the ovaries?	Like that of the testicles, the ovaries' lymphatic drainage is to the lumbar and para-aortic lymph nodes. The lymph vessels from the ovaries travel with the venous drainage in the broad ligament.

► **Case 30**

A 36-year-old diabetic African-American man presents to his primary care physician after his wife noted scleral icterus and a recent, unintentional, 11.4-kg (25-lb) weight loss. The patient denies abdominal pain. Physical examination reveals a mass in the right upper quadrant of the abdomen. Relevant laboratory findings are as follows:

Alkaline phosphatase: 127 U/L
Bilirubin: 2 mg/dL
Calcium: 10.6 mg/dL

▪ **What is the pathophysiology of this condition?**	Pancreatic tumors form mostly in the head and neck of the pancreas from the endocrine and exocrine portions of the pancreas. The majority of pancreatic cancers are exocrine and originate in the ductal epithelium, acinar cells, connective tissue, and lymphatic tissue.
▪ **What risk factors are associated with an increased incidence of this condition?**	▪ African-American race ▪ Cigarette smoking ▪ History of chronic pancreatitis ▪ History of diabetes mellitus ▪ Male gender
▪ **What are the common sites of invasion for this condition?**	Pancreatic cancer can invade the duodenum, the ampulla of Vater, and the common bile duct. As a result, pancreatic cancer can often cause biliary obstruction. Figure 8-16 shows a pancreatic adenocarcinoma, which appears as a large, heterogeneously enhancing mass at the neck of the pancreas. In this case, the mass is compressing the common bile duct, portal vein, splenic vein, superior mesenteric vein, and the inferior vena cava.
▪ **What is the most common form/location for this condition?**	Ninety percent of pancreatic tumors are adenocarcinomas, with 60% found in the head of the pancreas.
▪ **What are the common sites of metastasis?**	Metastasis often begins in the regional lymph nodes and spreads to the liver, or less often to the lungs. Pancreatic cancer can also directly invade the duodenum, stomach, and colon.

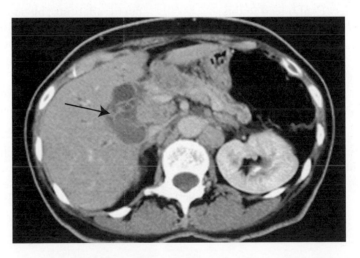

FIGURE 8-16. CT of pancreatic cancer. (Reproduced, with permission, from the Pathology Education Instructional Resource Digital Library [http://peir.net] at the University of Alabama, Birmingham.)

► **Case 31**

During the course of an annual physical examination, a previously healthy 70-year-old man mentions he has recently noted weakness and rib pain. His appetite has been good, and he has not experienced fevers, nausea, vomiting, or changes in bowel habits. Physical examination reveals splenomegaly. Results of a complete blood count are as follows:

WBC count: 10,000/mm^3
Hemoglobin: 22 g/dL
Hematocrit: 62%
Platelet count: 425,000/mm^3

▪ What is the most likely diagnosis?	Polycythemia rubra vera, also known as **primary erythrocytosis**. This patient's elevated hemoglobin concentration is a sign of increased RBC count. An increased RBC mass (>32 mL/kg in women and >36 mL/kg in men) is diagnostic of polycythemia in the absence of secondary causes of primary eythrocytosis. (Greater than 95% of patients with polycythemia have an activating mutation of JAK2).
▪ Levels of which hormone should be measured to establish the diagnosis?	**Erythropoietin** can help the physician distinguish between primary and secondary causes of polycythemia. Erythropoietin levels will be decreased or normal in primary polycythemia (**polycythemia vera**). In secondary polycythemia, increased erythropoiesis results from increased erythropoietin stimulation (e.g., erythropoietin-secreting tumor, hypoxemia, altitude, or erythropoietin receptor mutations).
▪ Which two types of carcinoma are associated with this condition?	**Renal cell carcinoma** and **hepatocellular carcinoma**. In a healthy adult, the kidneys produce a majority of the body's erythropoietin, and the liver is a secondary source.
▪ What mature cells descend from a myeloid progenitor cell?	Erythrocytes, platelets, basophils, eosinophils, neutrophils, and macrophages. Disorders of myeloid stem cell multiplication, as in polycythemia vera, can present with elevated cell counts of multiple myeloid descendants.
▪ How can an uncorrected ventricular septal defect (VSD) lead to this condition?	In patients with uncorrected VSD, atrial septal defect, or patent ductus arteriosus, blood is shunted from the left side of the heart to the right side, which exposes the pulmonary vasculature to systemic blood pressures. Over time, the pulmonary vasculature adapts by increasing pulmonary resistance, and blood flow through the shunt is reversed to flow from right-to-left. This reversal of flow is known as **Eisenmenger's syndrome**. Right-to-left shunts cause hypoxemia and cyanosis, a potent stimulus for erythropoietin secretion and a cause of secondary polycythemia.
▪ What are the most appropriate treatments for this condition?	Phlebotomy can reduce the risk of blood clots in patients with polycythemia to that of the normal population. In high-risk patients (the elderly or those with a history of clots), hydroxyurea may be useful for controlling the hematocrit; caution is advised, however, as this may be leukemogenic. Low-dose aspirin should be taken as primary prevention of arterial thrombosis.

▶ **Case 32**

A 3-year-old boy is brought to the pediatrician by his parents, who noticed that his right eye has turned "white" (see Figure 8-17). When they referred back to earlier photographs, the child's eyes were normally colored. The boy denies any pain or irritation in his eyes, and he does not complain of loss of vision. The parents deny any trauma to the area and there is no family history of ocular disease. On physician examination, the boy's extraocular movements are intact and symmetrical, his pupillary light reflexes are normal, and he has intact central and peripheral vision in both eyes. However, when he is asked to fixate at a point in the distance, the boy's right eye deviates toward his nose (esotropia). Funduscopic examination reveals a chalky, white-gray retinal mass in the right eye.

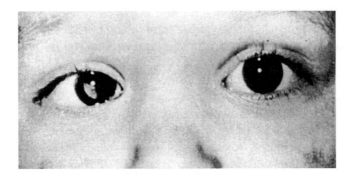

FIGURE 8-17. (Reproduced, with permission, from Riordan-Eva P, Whitcher JP. *Vaughan & Asbury's General Ophthalmology*, 16th ed. New York: McGraw-Hill, 2004: Figure 10-32.)

■ **What is the most likely diagnosis?**	Retinoblastoma. Other causes of leukocoria ("white pupil") include congenital cataracts, developmental anomalies of the vitreous and retina, and inflammatory conditions.
■ **What is the pathogenesis of this condition?**	Retinoblastoma results from mutations of both alleles of the *Rb* **gene**, on chromosome 13q14, which codes for a tumor suppressor protein. The Rb protein binds and sequesters transcription factors of the E2F family, to prevent the G1-to-S phase transition. Loss of this tumor suppressor protein promotes unregulated growth.
■ **What is the "two-hit hypothesis"?**	The **two-hit hypothesis** (Knudsen's hypothesis) suggests that two separate mutations are required for tumorigenesis involving a suppressor gene. In heritable disease, patients inherit a mutated germline allele from a parent, and acquire a second somatic mutation later in development. This often gives rise to binocular and multifocal disease. In noninherited disease, two spontaneous mutations arise in a single retinal cell during development, giving rise to uniocular, unifocal disease.
■ **What secondary malignancies is this patient at risk of developing?**	Osteogenic sarcoma, soft tissue sarcoma, and malignant melanoma commonly develop in patients with retinoblastoma. Metastatic spread occurs rapidly through direct infiltration or via the subarachnoid space, blood, and lymphatics.
■ **What is the most appropriate treatment for this condition?**	The treatment of choice for retinoblastoma is enucleation of the affected eye, with an effort to remove a large portion of the optic nerve, as this is the most common path for metastasis to the brain. Other treatment options include external beam radiation therapy, cryotherapy, and chemotherapy.

► **Case 33**

A 20-year-old African-American woman visits her physician complaining of episodes of extreme pain and discomfort in her legs and lower back. She has been experiencing these recurrent episodes, accompanied by extreme fatigue, since she was a child. On physical examination, she appears jaundiced and has a hematocrit of 23% and a hemoglobin level of 7 g/dL. She reports she has family members who experienced the same symptoms.

■ **What is the most likely diagnosis?**	Sickle cell anemia.
■ **What is the pathophysiology of this condition?**	Sickle cell anemia develops at around 6 months of age when hemoglobin S (HbS) replaces hemoglobin F (HbF). The course of disease is punctuated by episodes of painful crises, which are believed to be a result of hypoxic tissue injury from microvascular occlusions. HbS is the result of a single missense mutation in the β-globin gene of hemoglobin. This causes hemoglobin to be susceptible to polymerization in conditions of low oxygen or dehydration (see Figure 8-18), dramatically reducing the flexibility of the RBC membrane. Sickled cells, microcytosis, and high reticulocyte counts are seen. Any organ can be affected by the vascular congestion, thrombosis, and infarction caused by sickling cells, so these patients tend to have multiple health problems. The combination of sickle cell anemia and β-thalassemia is common and can also result in sickle crises.
■ **What complications are common in patients with this condition?**	Complications include painful (vaso-occlusive) crisis, aplastic crisis (cessation of erythropoiesis due to parvovirus B19 infection), and splenic sequestration crisis. Splenic sequestration eventually leads to autosplenectomy, which results in increased susceptibility to encapsulated organisms, including *Pneumococcus*. Other complications include increased susceptibility to *Salmonella* osteomyelitis for reasons not understood. Priapism, stroke, leg ulcers, acute chest syndrome (fat emboli, infection, and vaso-occlusion), and dactylitis are important complications.
■ **How prevalent is this condition among African-Americans?**	Sickle cell anemia is an autosomal recessive disease with an 8% carrier rate in African-Americans. An estimated 0.2% of African-Americans have this disease.
■ **What are the typical radiologic findings in this condition?**	Erythropoiesis must increase in order to compensate for the decreased life span of RBCs (from 120 days to approximately 20 days). The resultant marrow expansion can lead to resorption of bone and subsequent new bone formation on the external aspect of the skull. This leads to a "crew cut" appearance on skull radiographs.
■ **What is the most appropriate treatment for this condition?**	Appropriate supportive care, including pain control for sickle complications is the mainstay of therapy. Medical therapy includes hydroxyurea, which acts to increase HbF production, thereby reducing the number of cells with the potential to sickle. Exchange transfusion with normal RBCs may reduce the sickle RBC percentage and is used to treat the life-threatening complications of acute chest syndrome, stroke, and splenic sequestration.

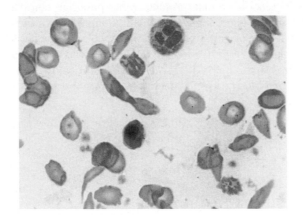

FIGURE 8-18. **Peripheral blood smear of sickle cell anemia.** (Reproduced, with permission, from the Pathology Education Instructional Resource Digital Library [http://peir.ne] at the University of Alabama, Birmingham.)

► **Case 34**

A 55-year-old woman presents to her physician complaining of a 2- to 3-month history of cough. The cough was initially nonproductive but has become progressively more productive of sputum and occasionally blood. She has a 50-pack-year history of cigarette smoking. Physical examination reveals marked wheezing, and an x-ray of the chest demonstrates hilar enlargement and a perihilar mass on the right side. The mass is biopsied, and the histologic specimen is shown in Figure 8-19.

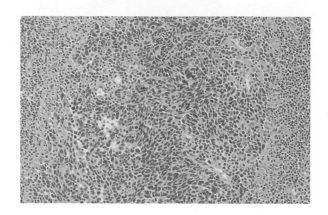

FIGURE 8-19. (Reproduced, with permission, from the Pathology Education Instructional Resource Digital Library [http://peir.net] at the University of Alabama, Birmingham.)

■ **What is the most likely diagnosis?**	Small cell lung carcinoma (SCLC). SCLC often presents as a hilar or mediastinal mass.
■ **What risk factors are associated with increased incidence of this condition?**	**Smoking** is the major risk factor for the development of most lung cancers, including small cell, squamous cell, and adenocarcinoma of the lung. Large cell lung cancer and bronchoalveolar carcinoma, however, are not thought to be related to smoking. Exposure to other substances, including asbestos, polycyclic aromatic hydrocarbons, and ionizing radiation, also increases the risk of certain lung cancers.
■ **What other syndrome is this patient at greatly increased risk for developing?**	She is at risk for developing **Lambert-Eaton myasthenic syndrome**. This condition, which is very similar to myasthenia gravis, is caused by autoantibodies against the P/Q-type calcium channels in the presynaptic neuromuscular junction. It causes weakness of the proximal musculature, especially of the lower limbs. Cranial nerves are commonly affected, which often manifests as ptosis of the eyelids and diplopia.
■ **What are the most common sites of metastasis for this tumor?**	Lung cancers metastasize to virtually every organ in the body. Brain metastases are common, with resulting neurologic deficits. Bone metastases result in bone pain or fractures and can cause spinal cord compression. Liver, supraclavicular lymph nodes, and adrenal metastases are also common.
■ **What are the most appropriate treatments for this tumor?**	Most patients with SCLC have unresectable disease at the time of presentation. In patients with small peripheral lesions and no metastases, surgical resection may be an option. Treatment for SCLC involves chemotherapy, typically etoposide plus cisplatin, with or without radiotherapy. In patients who do not receive chemotherapy or radiation, mean survival ranges from 6 to 17 months.

Upon presentation to his family physician, an 8-month-old boy is noted to have jaundice and dyspnea. Physical examination reveals tachycardia and splenomegaly. The mother recalls a long family history of "blood disease." A Coombs' test is negative. Relevant laboratory findings are as follows:

Hemoglobin: 8.5 g/dL
Hematocrit: 29%
Mean corpuscular volume (MCV): 85 fl
Mean corpuscular hemoglobin concentration (MCHC): 400 g/L

▪ What is the most likely diagnosis?	Hereditary spherocytosis, an autosomal dominant form of hemolytic anemia.
▪ What protein defect causes this condition?	RBC membrane defects are the result of mutations in **spectrin** or **ankyrin** (erythrocyte skeletal proteins). This results in a decreased membrane:volume ratio, which makes the cells more fragile. Thus, a positive result on osmotic fragility testing is virtually pathognomonic for the disease. Cells are trapped in the spleen, where they are destroyed.
▪ What are the typical peripheral blood smear findings in this condition?	Small RBCs without central pallor (**spherocytes**) (see Figure 8-20) are seen on a peripheral blood smear.
▪ What blood test would be useful in establishing the diagnosis?	An osmotic fragility test may confirm the presence of fragile sphere-shaped RBCs. The MCHC is increased due to a reduction in membrane surface area in the setting of a constant hemoglobin concentration. MCV remains normal because the overall volume remains stable. High reticulocyte counts (5%–10%) with elevated indirect bilirubin levels are also seen.
▪ What test could be used to differentiate this condition from autoimmune etiologies?	A direct Coombs' test is used to distinguish hereditary spherocytosis from warm antibody hemolysis: Hereditary spherocytosis is Coombs'-negative, while warm antibody hemolysis is Coombs'-positive. A positive result on a direct Coombs' test indicates the presence of antibodies on RBCs. A positive result on an indirect Coombs' test indicates the presence of antibodies in the serum.
▪ What are the most appropriate treatments for this condition?	Splenectomy is curative and should be considered in patients with more severe disease. Surgery also helps prevent gallstone (bilirubin) formation. Folate supplementation may also be useful.

ORGAN SYSTEMS

HEMATOLOGY & ONCOLOGY

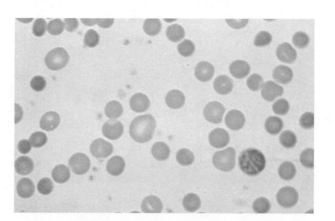

FIGURE 8-20. Histology of spherocytosis. (Reproduced, with permission, from Kasper DL, et al. *Harrison's Principles of Internal Medicine*, 16th ed. New York: McGraw-Hill, 2005: 609.)

▶ **Case 36**

A 27-year-old man is brought to the emergency department via ambulance after a motor vehicle accident. He was a restrained passenger in a two-car collision. He is complaining of left upper quadrant pain. On physical examination he appears restless and agitated, and he is noted to be tachycardic and tachypneic.

■ **Damage to what organ is most likely involved in this case?**

The spleen. It is an important organ in immune function and hematopoiesis. The primary function of the spleen is clearance of abnormal RBCs, microorganisms, and particulate matter from the bloodstream. Additionally, it is involved in hematopoiesis (extramedullary hematopoiesis) and synthesis of IgG, properdin, and tuftsin.

■ **What is the normal size of this organ?**

A normal spleen weighs 150 g and is nonpalpable. Spleens that are prominent below the costal margin typically weigh 750–1000 g. Figure 8-21A is a CT scan of a man with splenic injury due to blunt trauma. This scan, obtained soon after contrast administration, shows multiple large lacerations of the spleen, hematoma, and perihepatic free fluid. Figure 8-21B, obtained after the contrast had cleared, more clearly shows a large laceration on the posterior surface of the spleen extending anteriorly to the hilum.

■ **Where is the injured organ located?**

The spleen is located under the rib cage in the left upper quadrant of the abdomen, below the diaphragm. Therefore, during palpation, descent of an enlarged spleen is felt on inspiration.

■ **Where is the most common site of referred pain in this injury?**

Left shoulder and trapezius ridge tenderness (C3–C5 dermatomes, same as the roots of the phrenic nerve) may also be present as a result of subdiaphragmatic phrenic nerve irritation; referred pain is due to subdiaphragmatic pooling of blood.

■ **Why is a blunt injury to this organ so concerning?**

The spleen is a very vascular organ that filters up to 15% of the total blood volume per minute. The spleen can hold an average of 40–50 mL of RBCs in reserve and can pool significantly more blood.

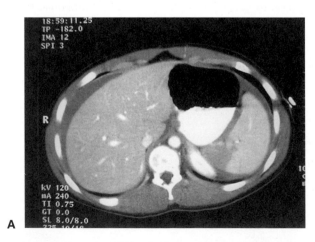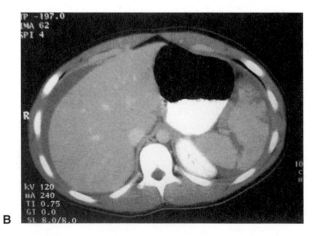

FIGURE 8-21. (A) CT of spleen early after contrast administration in a patient with blunt trauma to the spleen. (B) CT of spleen after contrast clears more clearly shows splenic laceration. (Reproduced, with permission, from Stone CK, Humphries RL. *Current Emergency Diagnosis & Treatment*, 5th ed. New York: McGraw-Hill, 2004: 471.)

A 36-year-old sexually active man goes to his doctor after noticing that his left testicle has been swollen for the past few weeks. The patient has noticed a dull, achy sensation in this testicle, but no acute pain. On physical examination, the left testicle is larger than the right, and a nontender, round, firm, rubbery mass is palpated. Transillumination with a penlight reveals an opaque mass. Laboratory tests reveals a normal chemistry panel, normal complete blood count, an elevated lactate dehydrogenase (LDH) level, a normal serum human chorionic gonadotropin (hCG) level, and a normal α-fetoprotein (AFP) level.

■ **What is the most likely diagnosis?**	This is a testicular tumor, as suggested by the presence of a painless, nontransilluminating testicular mass. In a young man, the most likely diagnosis is a **seminoma**, which has a peak incidence of age 35 years and accounts for 40% of testicular tumors. This diagnosis is further supported by the elevated LDH level, normal hCG level (is elevated in 20% of seminomas), and normal AFP level. Seminoma can be differentiated from epididymitis or orchitis, which present with a painful testicle and an elevated WBC count. Elevated AFP levels would suggest a nonseminomatous germ cell cancer. A hydrocele would transilluminate.
■ **What is the pathology of this tumor?**	Seminoma cells resemble primary spermatocytes, and have large, vesicular nuclei and pale cytoplasm. The tumor cells occur in clusters, with a surrounding lymphoid infiltrate.
■ **What is the analogous tumor in women?**	The analogous ovarian tumor is the **dysgerminoma**, the most common germ cell tumor in women. It is usually malignant, and more common in younger patients. Like seminomas, they can produce LDH. They can also produce alkaline phosphatase.
■ **What is the lymphatic drainage of this tumor?**	Understanding the lymphatic drainage of the testicles is important in considering metastases. Because the testicles descend from the abdomen during development, the lymph vessels ascend to the lumbar and preaortic lymph nodes. Contrast this to the lymph drainage of the scrotum, which is an outpouching of skin. The lymph vessels of the scrotum drain to the superficial inguinal nodes.
■ **What other tumors are characterized by an elevated hCG level?**	Only 10%–20% of seminomas present with elevated hCG levels. Tumors in women that are likely to present with an elevated hCG level include hydatidiform moles, choriocarcinomas, and gestational trophoblastic tumors.

► **Case 38**

A 45-year-old woman presents to the emergency department with the sudden onset of confusion, severe headaches, and blurred vision. These symptoms have been progressive over the past week. On physical examination, she is febrile and disoriented with diffuse petechial hemorrhages throughout her body. Relevant laboratory studies include:

Serum blood urea nitrogen: 42 mg/dL
Serum creatinine: 4.0 mg/dL
Hemoglobin: 10.8 g/dL
Hematocrit: 33%
Mean corpuscular volume: 90 fl
WBC count: 7800/mm^3 with a normal differential
Platelet count: 36,000/mm^3
Peripheral blood smear shows schistocytes and reticulocytes

▪ **What is the most likely diagnosis?**	Thrombotic thrombocytopenic purpura/hemolytic-uremic syndrome (TTP/HUS).
▪ **What are the five cardinal symptoms of this condition?**	▪ Transient neurological problems ▪ Fever ▪ Thrombocytopenia ▪ Microangiopathic hemolytic anemia ▪ Acute renal insufficiency
▪ **What is the pathogenesis of these symptoms?**	TTP/HUS involves the widespread development of hyaline thrombi composed of platelet aggregates in the microcirculation. This consumption of platelets leads to thrombocytopenia and microangiopathic hemolytic anemia which can cause widespread organ dysfunction.
▪ **What would coagulation studies show in this patient?**	Coagulation studies will be within **normal** limits. This is predominantly a thrombocytopenic disease with no coagulation cascade abnormalities.
▪ **Which inherited risk factor predisposes patients to this condition?**	A deficiency of the **von Willebrand metalloproteinase** (ADAMTS-13) is the inherited factor which results in very large von Willenbrand factor multimers that accumulate in the plasma and promote clot formation.
▪ **What management is most appropriate for this condition?**	**Plasma exchange** reverses the platelet consumption that is responsible for the thrombus formation. Severe cases may also require adjunctive **immunosuppressive treatment** with prednisone. Platelet transfusion is contraindicated because it may lead to new or worsening thrombosis and subsequent neurologic symptoms. Prompt initiation of treatment is essential to avoid irreversible renal failure, and possibly death.
▪ **What is a common cause of this condition in children?**	Typically, TTP/HUS is preceded by severe bloody diarrhea due most often to enterohemorrhagic *Escherichia coli* O157:H7 infection. This is thought to be due to systemic absorption of a Shiga-like toxin that binds to and damages endothelial cells, inciting platelet activation and thrombosis.

A 2-year-old boy is brought to his family physician by his parents, who are concerned about the multiple bruises on the boy's shins and hands. They report the child seems to get large bruises with minimal injury, and bleeds profusely when his teeth are brushed. They also relate that a month ago, he fell and hit his head on a coffee table and they could not stop the bleeding for hours. On questioning, they reveal the child has a grandmother with a bleeding disorder. The physician is concerned about child abuse, but orders laboratory tests; relevant findings are as follows:

Bleeding time: 14 minutes
Prothrombin time (PT): 12 seconds
Partial thromboplastin time (PTT): 41 seconds

▪ **What is the most likely diagnosis?**	von Willebrand's disease (vWD) is the most common inherited bleeding disorder. It is the result of a quantitative (type 1 or 3) or qualitative (type 2) defect in **von Willebrand factor** (vWF). vWF is a large protein made by endothelial cells and megakaryocytes. It is a carrier for factor VIII and is a cofactor for platelet adhesion. There are now more specific tests which measure vWF antigen levels and activity (ristocetin cofactor assay) directly.
▪ **What clinical findings are commonly associated with this condition?**	vWD disturbs both primary and secondary hemostasis. Its role in adhesion of platelets to exposed subendothelium leads to **increased bleeding time** and an overall clinical picture of platelet dysfunction (mucous membrane bleeding, petechiae, and purpura) with vWF defects. The role of vWF as a carrier protein for factor VIII means that its deficiency leads to a clinical picture similar to a coagulation factor deficit: "deep bleeds" such as hemarthroses (bleeding into joints), easy bruising, and macro-hemorrhages. Patients often have a positive family history.
▪ **What do the PT and PTT values reflect?**	The PT reflects changes in factor II, V, VII, or X. The PTT reflects changes in any of the coagulation factors except factors VII and XIII and it can be elevated in vWD.
▪ **How would the PT and PTT values differ with the administration of warfarin versus heparin?**	**Heparin** affects the intrinsic pathway, causing increased PTT. **Warfarin** affects the extrinsic pathway, increasing PTT and PT. PT should always be monitored with patients taking warfarin. A useful mnemonic is **"WEPT"**: Warfarin, Extrinsic, **PT.**
▪ **Which coagulation factors require vitamin K for synthesis?**	Factors II, VII, IX, and X and proteins C and S require vitamin K for synthesis. Warfarin interferes with vitamin K, leading to a similar clinical picture as vitamin K deficiency. The liver is important in the synthesis and metabolism of vitamin K and the coagulation factors (except VIII). Therefore, liver disease can also result in a similar clinical picture.
▪ **What are the most appropriate treatments for this condition?**	Treatment for mild bleeding in type 1 disease involves the use of desmopressin, which causes release of vWF from endothelial stores. Severe disease may be treated with Factor VIII concentrates which contain high vWF Ag. Cryoprecipitate is no longer used as viruses cannot be inactivated (high infection risk).

Musculoskeletal

Case 1	296
Case 2	297
Case 3	298
Case 4	300
Case 5	301
Case 6	302
Case 7	303
Case 8	304
Case 9	305
Case 10	306
Case 11	308
Case 12	309
Case 13	310
Case 14	312
Case 15	313
Case 16	314
Case 17	316
Case 18	317

► **Case 1**

A 62-year-old woman presents to her physician with a 2-day history of right-sided chest pain. She describes a sharp, nagging pressure lateral to her right breast. Physical examination reveals the chest wall is tender, and the pain is exacerbated by movement of her trunk and deep inspiration.

■ **What is the pathophysiology of this condition?**	Costochondritis, the inflammation of the costochondral or costosternal joints, causes localized pain and tenderness. Often more than one of the seven costochondral joints is affected, especially between the second and fifth joints. Repetitive minor trauma is the most likely cause, but bacterial and fungal infections can lead to costochondritis, as can thoracic surgery.
■ **What is the innervation of the intercostal space?**	The intercostal nerves (thoracic spinal and ventral rami) supply general sensory innervation to the skin of the thoracic and anterior abdominal walls. The dermatomes follow a girdle-like distribution. The sensory nerves also supply the parietal pleura and parietal peritoneum. The intercostal nerves also have motor innervation through the ventral rami of T1–T12. Intercostal nerve 1 participates in the brachial plexus, nerves 2–6 innervate the thorax, and nerves 7–12 innervate the anterior abdominal wall.
■ **What are the three types of intercostal muscles?**	The intercostal muscles are divided into three groups of muscular and tendinous fibers running between the 11 intercostal spaces: ■ External intercostal muscles ■ Internal intercostal muscles ■ Innermost intercostal complex (transversus thoracis, innermost intercostals, subcostalis)
■ **How many ribs are there in the human body?**	The thoracic cage consists of 12 pairs of ribs. The first seven are true ribs because their cartilage articulates with the sternum, and the last five pairs are false ribs. The eleventh and twelfth ribs are floating ribs.
■ **What is the blood supply of the intercostal space?**	At each space there is a posterior and anterior set of arteries. The posterior artery originates from the descending thoracic aorta. Anterior intercostal arteries are smaller and include the supreme thoracic artery. The posterior intercostal vein, artery, and nerve run together as a neurovascular bundle along the lower border of each rib. Thus, it is important during thoracentesis that the needle is inserted above the lower rib in the intercostal space to avoid injury to the vessels and nerve.

► **Case 2**

A 63-year-old farmer has noticed an area of discoloration on her cheek which seems to have dramatically grown over the past 2 years. On physical examination, there is a well demarcated 1.5-cm rough, scaly, erythematous patch. A biopsy of the lesion is taken which reveals hyperkeratosis and atypical keratinocytes and basal cells that invade through the basement membrane.

■ What is the most likely diagnosis?	Cutaneous squamous cell carcinoma is the second most common tumor of the skin (after basal cell carcinoma). It arises from the malignant proliferation of epidermal keratinocytes. The condition typically presents as a firm, well demarcated, scaling, crusting, or ulcerated lesion. Histologic examination is necessary to make a diagnosis. In this vignette, the patient's carcinoma displays invasive properties, as it has invaded the basement membrane.
■ What precursor lesion leads to this condition?	**Actinic keratosis**, a dysplastic lesion of the epidermis. These lesions have a "stuck on" appearance, and some may present as a "cutaneous horn."
■ What risk factors are associated with an increased incidence of this condition?	The most important risk factor is **sunlight exposure** with ultraviolet (UV) rays causing DNA damage. Other exogenous factors include ionizing radiation, immunosuppression, chronic inflammation (from burns, scars, or ulcers), and arsenic exposure.
■ What inherited disorders predispose development of this condition?	**Xeroderma pigmentosum** displays a defect in DNA excision repair that results in an impaired ability to repair UV-induced DNA damage. **Albinism** is also associated with squamous cell carcinoma due to generalized pigment loss due to dysfunction and deficiency of melanocytes.
■ What is the prognosis for patients with this condition?	Even though cutaneous squamous cell carcinoma can be locally invasive, it rarely metastasizes (1%–5% of cases). Therefore, more than 90% of patients can be cured with local excision.

▶ **Case 3**

A 17-year-old boy is brought to the emergency department by ambulance after a gunshot wound to the left flank. On survey, one entry site is noted with no exit wound; x-rays of the chest and abdomen indicate that the bullet has lodged in the left flank. During assessment, the patient begins to go into hypovolemic shock with a steadily decreasing blood pressure. Because of his condition, the patient is rushed to the operating room for exploratory laparotomy. Relevant laboratory findings are as follows:

Hematocrit: 22%
WBC count: 17,000/mm^3
Blood pressure: 60/35 mm Hg

▪ What retroperitoneal structures of the abdomen could the bullet have hit?	▪ Ascending/descending colon ▪ Great vessels ▪ Kidneys ▪ Sympathetic trunk ▪ Adrenal glands ▪ Ureters
▪ What layers of the skin did the bullet pass through?	The **epidermis** is the thin outer layer; it contains: ▪ Stratum corneum ▪ Keratinocytes (squamous cells) ▪ Basal layer The **dermis** is the middle layer; it is held together by collagen and contains ▪ Blood vessels ▪ Lymph vessels ▪ Hair follicles ▪ Sweat glands The **subcutaneous** is the deepest layer; it contains mesh of collagen and adipocytes. See Figure 9-1 for a schematic drawing of the layers of the skin.
▪ What is the blood supply to the kidney?	Renal artery → segmental artery → lobar artery → arcuate artery → afferent arteriole → glomerulus → efferent arteriole → vasa recta → segmental vein → renal vein.
▪ What is the blood supply to the spleen?	The main arterial blood supply is provided by the splenic artery, which is a branch of the celiac trunk. Branches of the splenic artery are the left gastro-omental and the short gastric arteries.
▪ What organs supply the splenic vein?	The splenic vein starts at the hilus of the spleen and receives blood from the stomach, pancreas, and inferior mesenteric vein.

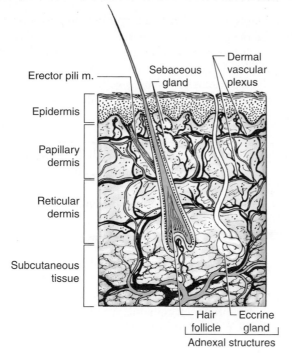

FIGURE 9-1. Schematic drawing of the layers of the skin. (Reproduced, with permission, from Brunicardi FC, et al. *Schwartz's Principles of Surgery*, 8th ed. New York: McGraw-Hill, 2005: 430.)

► **Case 4**

A 12-year-old girl complains of 6 weeks of pain and swelling over her right mid-thigh, particularly at night. She denies any trauma or recent illness. Physical examination reveals a firmly attached soft tissue mass in the right leg with overlying tenderness and warmth. Erythema is absent. X-ray of the leg shows a large poorly demarcated "moth-eaten" lytic lesion in the right femoral diaphysis with extension to the soft tissue (see Figure 9-2). A biopsy of the mass reveals sheets of primitive round cells with small uniform nuclei and scant cytoplasm.

■ What is the most likely diagnosis?

Ewing's sarcoma (see Figure 9-2). The young age at clinical presentation with tenderness, warmth, and swelling without any systemic signs of infection suggests Ewing's. Additionally, this lesion's location and histologic appearance (small, round, blue-neuroectodermal cells) are characteristic of this neoplasm.

■ What conditions should be included in the differential diagnosis?

■ Infectious causes, including acute osteomyelitis.
■ Benign lesions such as eosinophilic granuloma and giant cell tumor of bone.
■ Other common solid tumors of childhood such as osteosarcoma, primary lymphoma, spindle cell sarcoma, acute leukemia, and metastasis from a neuroblastoma.

■ What is the most likely chromosomal aberration?

Eighty-five percent of cases demonstrate a **t(11;22) translocation.**

■ What is the most appropriate treatment for this condition?

Ewing's sarcoma is a systemic disease due to the high relapse rate (80%–90%) seen in patients undergoing only local therapy. Therefore it is believed that most patients have subclinical microscopic metastatic disease at the time of diagnosis, which needs to be treated with chemotherapy.

■ What percentage of patients have metastatic disease at the time of diagnosis?

Only 25% of patients have overt metastases at the time of diagnosis.

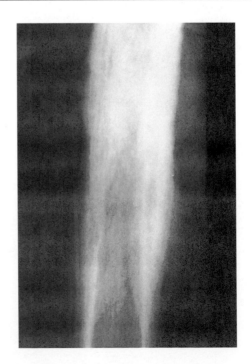

FIGURE 9-2. Radiograph of periosteal response in Ewing's sarcoma of the femur in a 15-year-old boy. (Reproduced, with permission, from Skinner HB. *Current Diagnosis & Treatment in Orthopedics*, 4th ed. New York: McGraw-Hill, 2006: 336.)

► **Case 5**

A 72-year-old woman with a history of osteoporosis presents to her primary care physician after having fallen 2 days earlier on a slippery sidewalk and landing on her left side. Since the fall, she has been unable to walk due to severe pain in her left hip that is worse when she tries to move it. When asked to walk for assessment of her gait, she refuses, saying that it is too painful. Physical examination reveals extreme pain with both external and internal rotation of the hip, as well as tenderness over the anterolateral portion of the left hip.

■ **What is the most likely diagnosis?**	This is most likely a fracture of the neck of the femur, which is the portion of the femur that lies between the intertrochanteric line anteriorly and the intertrochanteric crest posteriorly (these run between the greater and lesser trochanter). Femoral neck fractures can be either incomplete or complete with either no, partial, or total displacement.
■ **What is a potential complication of this type of injury?**	Fracture of the neck of the femur may disrupt blood supply to the head of the femur. The major arterial supply to the head of the femur is the medial and lateral circumflex femoral arteries (branches of the deep femoral artery or femoral artery), and the artery of the ligament of the head of the femur (branch of the obturator artery). The circumflex arteries may be disrupted by a fracture of the femoral neck, leaving only the artery of the ligament (a branch of the obturator) as a supply. Disruption of the blood supply may result in **avascular necrosis** of the femoral head.
■ **What bones form the hip joint?**	The hip joint consists of the head of the femur articulating with the acetabulum. The acetabulum is formed by the ilium, the ischium, and the pubis. The fibrocartilaginous rim, the acetabular labrum, attaches to the acetabular margin and deepens the acetabular cup.
■ **Six weeks later, an x-ray taken of this patient shows a callus. Where did the cells that form the callus originate?**	The osteoprogenitor cells that form the callus are from the inner surface of the periosteum, not from the marrow or the epiphyseal plate.

ORGAN SYSTEMS

MUSCULOSKELETAL

► **Case 6**

A 2-week-old term boy is brought to his pediatrician because his parents have noticed he has a large, full right scrotum. The left scrotum and testicle are normal. On physical examination, the right scrotum appears to be filled with a volume of fluid that can be reduced by applying pressure. A small reducible bulging mass is also seen in the inguinal area on the right.

■ What is the most likely diagnosis?	Right communicating hydrocele and right inguinal hernia. The fluid in the scrotum is a **hydrocele** that results from communication with the intraperitoneal fluid.
■ What structures define Hesselbach's triangle?	**Hesselbach's triangle** is formed by the lateral border of the rectus abdominis muscle, the inguinal ligament, and the inferior epigastric vessels.
■ How is this condition classified?	**Direct hernias** protrude through a weakness in the floor of the inguinal canal within Hesselbach's triangle (directly through the triangle) medial to the inferior epigastric vessels to enter the external ring into the scrotal sac. **Indirect hernias** enter the inguinal canal lateral to Hesselbach's triangle (lateral to the inferior epigastric vessels) indirectly through the internal inguinal ring (located in the fascia transversalis), then via the inguinal canal to the external inguinal ring located above and lateral to the pubic tubercle, and finally into the scrotal sac (see Figure 9-3).
■ Which type of this condition is more common in infants and children?	Indirect inguinal hernias are more common in children, as they result from a congenital failure of the processus vaginalis to close.
■ What are the contents of the normal spermatic cord?	The spermatic cord in the inguinal canal contains the testicular artery and veins, lymphatic vessels, and the vas deferens. The sheath of the cord is formed by the internal spermatic fascia, the cremasteric muscle, and the external spermatic fascia. The ilioinguinal nerve is in the sheath and exits at the external ring; it is vulnerable to injury in surgical repairs of hernias. The genital branch of the genitofemoral nerve supplies the cremaster muscle. The processus vaginalis is an extension of peritoneum that normally obliterates spontaneously between the upper pole of the testes and the internal inguinal ring. In some cases, however, this structure remains patent, increasing the risk of hydrocele and indirect hernia.

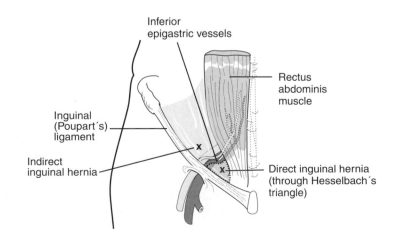

FIGURE 9-3. Direct and indirect inguinal hernia. (Reproduced, with permission, from Le T, Bhushan V, Rao DA. *First Aid for the USMLE Step 1: 2008.* New York: McGraw-Hill, 2008: 299.)

► **Case 7**

A 19-year-old woman comes to the emergency department accompanied by her coach after the student injured her left knee during sports practice. She says she had made a quick turn when she developed a sharp pain on the lateral side of her knee, heard a "pop," and her leg "collapsed."

▪ **What are the intracapsular ligaments in the knee?**	The **anterior cruciate ligament** extends from the anterior intercondylar area of the tibial plateau and traverses superior and lateral to the medial surface of the lateral femoral condyle. The **posterior cruciate ligament** extends from the posterior intercondylar area of the tibial plateau and traverses superior and medial to the lateral surface of the medial condyle of the femur (see Figure 9-4).
▪ **What is the blood supply to the knee?**	It consists of genicular branches of the following blood vessels: ▪ Anterior recurrent tibial artery ▪ Anterior tibial artery ▪ Descending branch of the lateral circumflex artery ▪ Femoral artery ▪ Patellar plexus ▪ Popliteal artery ▪ Posterior tibial artery
▪ **What is the role of the meniscus?**	The **meniscus** is cartilage in a half-moon shape that is found between the femur and tibia. The meniscus is responsible for absorbing the impact load of the joint and is involved in stability. The meniscus is mostly avascular and is divided into the anterior horn, body, and posterior horn.
▪ **How do the collateral and cruciate ligaments differ in function?**	The cruciate ligaments remain tight in flexion and extension and relax at 30° of flexion. The collateral ligaments are tight in extension and relaxed in flexion. Also, the cruciate ligaments prevent anterior and posterior displacement of the tibia. The collateral ligaments prevent abduction/adduction of the knee.
▪ **Which ligament of the knee is most often injured?**	The medial collateral ligament is weaker than the anterior or the posterior cruciate ligaments, so medial collateral ligament injuries are more common.
▪ **What is the terrible or unhappy triad?**	This is a common injury in contact sports that occurs to the knee when lateral trauma is applied to the knee joint while the foot is fixed to the ground. Subsequently, the medial collateral ligament, medial meniscus and the anterior cruciate ligament are damaged.

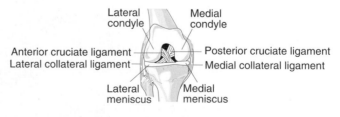

FIGURE 9-4. Anatomy of the knee. (Reproduced, with permission, from Le T, Bhushan V, Rao DA. *First Aid for the USMLE Step 1: 2008.* New York: McGraw-Hill, 2008: 343.)

► **Case 8**

A 47-year-old man presents to his primary care physician concerned about a suspicious lesion on his shoulder that has increased in size over the past 2 years. He reports no other associated signs or symptoms. Physical examination reveals an 11-cm asymmetric, irregularly colored lesion with notched borders that is slightly tender to palpation. Several other nevi are noted to be scattered over his chest and back.

▪ **What is the most likely diagnosis?**	Malignant melanoma. The **ABCD** rules can be applied to distinguish melanoma from other lesions (see Figure 9-5): ▪ **Asymmetry.** Malignant lesions are usually asymmetric. ▪ **Border irregularity.** Most melanomas lack smooth, round, uniform boundaries. ▪ **Color variegation.** Malignant lesions usually have variations in pigmentation, and occasionally lose pigmentation. ▪ **Diameter.** A diameter >6 mm greatly increases the chances of malignancy, and most lesions are >10 mm.
▪ **Which cells are responsible for this lesion and what is their origin?**	Melanocytes, which are derived from neural crest tissue and reside in the epidermis or, less frequently, in the dermis.
▪ **What is the etiology of this lesion?**	**Sun exposure** is the likely etiology. Malignant melanomas are more likely to appear in sun-exposed areas. Other risk factors include atypical/dysplastic nevi, hereditary factors, and exposure to certain carcinogens.
▪ **What is the most important prognostic factor for this condition?**	Vertical invasion, with deeper lesions having a worse prognosis.
▪ **What is the natural history of this lesion?**	Initial lesions usually spread superficially and horizontally across the skin and then enter a vertical growth phase into the deeper layers of the skin. Melanomas may then spread either lymphatically or hematogenously, with the earliest detectable metastases occurring to regional lymph nodes. Classic sites of hematogenous spread include brain, lung, liver, and bone.
▪ **What is the most appropriate treatment for this condition?**	Surgical excision with optional regional node dissection for more advanced disease remains the first-line treatment. However, metastatic malignant melanoma is deemed incurable, with survival in patients with visceral metastases generally <1 year.

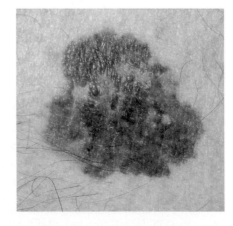

FIGURE 9-5. Malignant melanoma that demonstrates the ABCD criteria. (Reproduced, with permission, from Wolff K, et al. *Fitzpatrick's Dermatology in General Medicine,* 7th ed. New York: McGraw-Hill, 2008: 1138.)

▶ **Case 9**

A 3-year-old boy is brought to the pediatrician by his parents because he has been having trouble getting up from a sitting or lying position, although he had previously done so with ease. His developmental history is notable for delayed motor skills; he began to walk at 18 months. The boy has a waddling gait, and when sitting he uses his arms to push himself into the upright position (Gower's sign; see Figure 9-6). Physical examination shows marked muscle weakness of the extremities, particularly of the proximal muscle groups, and hypertrophy of his calf muscles. Notably, the patient's maternal uncle, who died at age 16 years, suffered from similar symptoms when he was younger.

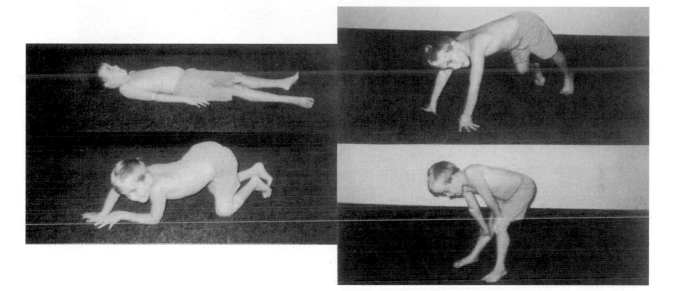

FIGURE 9-6. (Reproduced, with permission, from Kasper DL, et al. *Harrison's Principles of Internal Medicine*, 16th ed. New York: McGraw-Hill, 2005: 2526.)

■ **What is the most likely diagnosis?**	Duchenne's muscular dystrophy (DMD). DMD is an X-linked recessive (Xp21) disorder in which there is a deficiency of functional **dystrophin**, a 23,000-kB protein involved in stabilization of muscle fibers. About one-third of cases are sporadic, due to spontaneous mutations (noninherited) that arise most commonly by a misalignment of chromosomes during a recombination event.
■ **What is the prognosis for patients with this condition?**	Patients with DMD are usually unable to walk by the end of the first decade, and are confined to a wheelchair by age 12 years. Sadly, most afflicted patients die by the end of their second decade, usually due to extreme weakness of respiratory muscles or cardiomyopathy.
■ **What are the typical findings on muscle biopsy?**	■ Atrophic muscle fibers of various sizes in disarray ■ Degeneration and necrosis of individual muscle fibers with fibrous replacement ■ Inflammation
■ **The patient's parents have a second son who is now 6 months old. What is the chance that he too will develop this condition?**	The chances are 50%. Because the mother is a carrier of this disorder, each son has a 50% chance of inheriting the X chromosome with the mutated allele from her.
■ **Which band(s) in a sarcomere stay constant in length during muscle contraction?**	The A band, which corresponds to the length of the thick myosin filaments.

▶ **Case 10**

A 65-year-old man presents to his primary care physician complaining of a 10-year history of increasing morning stiffness and dull pain in his lower back and left hip. The pain is typically exacerbated by activity and relieved by rest. Physical examination reveals limited range of motion in the affected joints and tenderness on palpation without warmth or erythema. X-ray of the pelvis and lower spine show joint space narrowing, subchondral sclerosis, and osteophyte formation (see Figure 9-7).

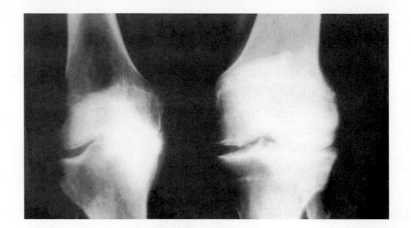

FIGURE 9-7. (Reproduced, with permission, from South-Paul JE, Matheny SC, Lewis EL. *Current Diagnosis & Treatment in Family Medicine,* 2nd ed. New York: McGraw-Hill, 2008: 235.)

■ **What is the most likely diagnosis?**	Osteoarthritis. This case presents a typical history with asymmetric gradually progressive joint pain and stiffness. Physical examination findings typically include tenderness to palpation without signs of inflammation, along with joint effusions, crepitus, and osteophytes of the affected joints. Plain radiographs also confirm the typical changes seen in this disease, as described in the vignette.
■ **What is the characteristic distribution of this condition?**	Osteoarthritis most often affects large weight-bearing joints including the knees, hip, and spine, as well as the interphalangeal joints, and only rarely affects the elbows, wrists, and ankles.
■ **What is the pathophysiology of this condition?**	Osteoarthritis is characterized by degenerative noninflammatory changes in articular cartilage secondary to chondrocyte dysfunction. These changes may be the result of a complex interaction between metabolic, biochemical, and biomechanical factors with secondary components of inflammation. This results in progressive mechanical damage to the joint and bone eburnation, particularly in weight-bearing joints. This degeneration results in reactive bone formation subchondrally and at the margins of affected joints.
■ **What would be the results of arthrocentesis (tapping of the joint)?**	Arthrocentesis is likely to show mild pleocytosis, normal viscosity, and modestly elevated protein. This test would be effective in ruling out a septic joint, which would show infective organisms as well as plentiful leukocytes.

■ **What is the most appropriate treatment for this condition?**	Acetaminophen and nonsteroidal anti-inflammatory drugs remain the mainstays for analgesia. In a patient with a history of gastroduodenal disease, a selective cyclooxygenase-2 (COX-2) inhibitor would be preferred in addition to a gastroprotective agent. Occasionally, intra-articular glucocorticoids are utilized when there are persistent symptoms in a few joints. Surgery may be required for refractory cases (joint replacement or fusion).
■ **What risk factors are associated with an increased incidence of this condition?**	■ Age ■ Obesity ■ Female gender ■ Lack of osteoporosis ■ Physically demanding occupations ■ Previous injury ■ Genetic diseases such as Wilson's disease and hemochromatosis.

ORGAN SYSTEMS

MUSCULOSKELETAL

► **Case 11**

A young Caucasian couple seeks genetic counseling prior to conceiving their first child. The man is concerned because he has had bilateral tumors removed from his acoustic nerves. His mother suffered from similar tumors, but his father did not. The woman reports two previous surgeries for the removal of spinal cord tumors; her father and sister have had similar tumors. The woman's physical examination is significant for axillary freckles and approximately 15 light brown patches of skin averaging 3 cm in diameter.

■ **What genetic syndromes do this man and woman have?**	The woman has neurofibromatosis type 1 (NF1, or von Recklinghausen's neurofibromatosis), and the man has neurofibromatosis type 2 (NF2). NF1 is characterized by café-au-lait spots, meningiomas, **neurofibromas** (subcutaneous nodules), and axillary freckling. NF2 presents with bilateral acoustic neuromas.
■ **What is their probability of having an asymptomatic child?**	The probability is 25%. NF1 and NF2 are both autosomal dominant genes. On the basis of their family histories, the man and woman must be heterozygous for NF2 and NF1, respectively. Thus, each mutant gene has a 50% chance of being inherited by the child. NF1 is on chromosome 17, and NF2 is on chromosome 22; thus, the inheritance of each mutant gene occurs independently of the other. The probability of two independent events occurring at once is the product of the probability of each event: 50% × 50% = 25%.
■ **Which cell line is implicated in the formation of the woman's lesions?**	**Neural crest cells** are involved. Most clinical signs of NF1 are related to abnormal descendants of neural crest cells.
■ **What is the mechanism of tumor formation for the woman?**	The *NF1* gene is a tumor suppressor gene. Multiple loss-of-function mutations in this gene lead to tumor growth.
■ **Describe the path of the eighth cranial nerve (CN VIII) from the periphery to its site of entry into the central nervous system.**	From the cochlea and vestibular canals in the petrous bone, CN VIII enters the cranial vault through the internal acoustic meatus to enter the brain stem at the junction of the pons and the medulla.

An 8-year-old girl is brought to the pediatrician for evaluation of recurrent skeletal fractures. Although she avoids contact sports, she has already suffered three fractures of her femur, tibia, and elbow following seemingly minor trauma. The pediatrician notes the girl is short for her age and has mild scoliosis and blue sclerae. The girl's mother has blue sclerae as well.

▪ **What is the differential diagnosis for recurrent fractures in children?**	▪ Accidental injury ▪ Birth trauma ▪ Bone fragility (including osteogenesis imperfecta and rickets) ▪ Child abuse (which accounts for the vast majority of cases)
▪ **What is the most likely diagnosis?**	Osteogenesis imperfecta, which is an inherited disorder involving defects in type I collagen. It is also known as **brittle bone disease**, and its most common form has autosomal dominant inheritance. This disease is also associated with cardiac insufficiency and mitral valve prolapse. The most severe form is lethal in utero or soon after birth because of multiple fractures and pulmonary failure. Severe forms are inherited in a recessive fashion.
▪ **What are the four major types of collagen, and where are they predominantly found?**	▪ **Type I:** bone, skin, tendon ▪ **Type II:** cartilage ▪ **Type III:** reticular, arterial walls, uterus ▪ **Type IV:** basement membrane
▪ **What steps are involved in collagen synthesis?**	Procollagen strands containing a repeating Gly-Pro-X sequence are synthesized in the ribosome, hydrolyzed by prolyl hydrolase, and glycosylated in the rough endoplasmic reticulum and Golgi complex. Three procollagen strands associate in a triple helix and are secreted into the extracellular space, where the propeptides are cleaved, allowing for polymerization with other collagen molecules to form collagen fibrils.
▪ **What enzymes in collagen synthesis are dependent on ascorbic acid?**	Proline hydroxylase (which hydroxylates prolyl and lysyl residues) cross-links collagen and is dependent on ascorbic acid. Vitamin C deficiency can lead to **scurvy**, which causes ulceration of the gums, bruising, anemia, poor wound healing, and hemorrhage due to deficient collagen synthesis.

▶ **Case 13**

A 62-year-old woman presents to her clinician with joint pain and morning stiffness for the past few years. The joint pain is present in both hands and feet bilaterally and has resulted in significant deformity and weakness. On physical examination, these joints are tender to palpation, warm, and swollen with no erythema. Her metacarpal joints display ulnar deviation bilaterally and subcutaneous nodules can be palpated at the elbow.

■ What is the most likely diagnosis?	Rheumatoid arthritis (RA). Clinical features of RA include: ■ Morning stiffness >1 hour and present for >6 weeks ■ Arthritis in three joints or more for >6 weeks ■ Arthritis of hand joints for >6 weeks ■ Symmetric joint swelling and involvement ■ Rheumatoid cutaneous nodules ■ Positive serum rheumatoid factor ■ Typical radiographic changes
■ What is the pathophysiology of this condition?	RA is a chronic **systemic autoimmune inflammatory disorder** that destroys articular cartilage. While the etiology is unclear, the autoimmune reaction is mediated by CD4+ T cells and macrophages along with cytokines (tumor necrosis factor and interleukin-1) which promote the inflammatory response. Together these elements form a **pannus** that gradually erodes and disfigures joints.
■ What test could be used to confirm the diagnosis?	Although no specific laboratory test is diagnostic of rheumatoid arthritis, most patients have a **positive serum rheumatoid factor** and antibodies to citrullinated proteins. The former is an IgM antibody that reacts with the Fc portion of the patient's own IgG. Radiographic changes of RA are shown in Figure 9-8.
■ What is the characteristic distribution of this condition?	Symptoms usually develop symmetrically in the small joints of the hands and feet (metacarpophalangeal [MCP], proximal interphalangeal [PIP], metatarsophalangeal [MTP], and interphalangeal [IP] joints) as well as wrist, elbows, knees, and ankles. The cervical spine may also be involved. Involvement of axial and central joints, such as the shoulders and hips, is less common.
■ What are the characteristic joint deformities seen in this condition?	Ulnar deviation/drift, swan-neck and Boutonniere deformities of the fingers and the "bow-string" sign (prominence of the tendons in the extensor compartment of the hand) are all characteristic of RA. Occasionally patients present with synovial cysts from increased intra-articular pressure and eventual tendon rupture.
■ What are the primary pharmacologic therapies for this condition?	■ Analgesics including acetaminophen ■ Nonsteroidal anti-inflammatory drugs ■ Glucocorticoids ■ Disease-modifying antirheumatic drugs such as hydroxychloroquine, sulfasalazine, or methotrexate ■ Anticytokine therapies such as etanercept, infliximab and adalimumab ■ Other biologic agents such as abatacept and rituximab

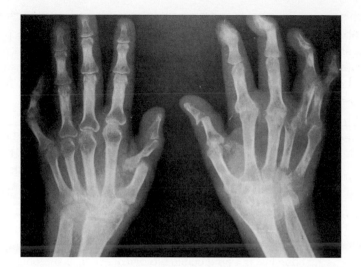

FIGURE 9-8. Radiographic changes in rheumatoid arthritis. Severe destruction of radio-carpal articulation with subluxation and ulnar deviation at the wrist; loss of ulnar styloid bilaterally; dislocation of the proximal interphalangeal joint of the left thumb and dislocation of the right fourth and fifth finger metacarpophalangeal joints and left metacarpophalangeal joint; diffuse joint space narrowing of many interphalangeal joints. (Reproduced, with permission, from Brunicardi FC, Andersen DK, Billiar TR, et al. *Schwartz's Principles of Surgery*, 8th ed. New York: McGraw-Hill, 2005: 1679.)

► **Case 14**

A 65-year-old woman presents to the emergency department with sharp pain in her lower back after lifting some heavy objects in the course of moving into a new home. The pain radiates to the anterior abdomen and is exacerbated by sitting and moving. On physical examination, she appears kyphotic with a "dowager hump." A plain film radiograph reveals multiple vertebral compression fractures.

■ What underlying condition contributed to this fracture?	Osteoporosis. This disease is characterized by reduced bone mass with microarchitectural disruption, porosity, and skeletal fragility, resulting in an increased risk of fracture. However, osteoporosis is difficult to diagnose, as there are often no clinical manifestations until there is a fracture.
■ What two primary factors contribute most to this condition?	The majority of postmenopausal women with osteoporosis have bone loss related to **age** and/or **estrogen deficiency**. Age-related bone loss is a predictable biological event, as osteoblasts lose replicative and biosynthetic ability with age. Estrogen naturally suppresses cytokines and RANKL (both potent stimulators of osteoclast function); therefore, estrogen deficiency results in unopposed osteoclast activity.
■ What secondary factors increase the likelihood of this condition?	■ Physical inactivity ■ Genetic factors ■ Calcium deficiency ■ Prolonged glucocorticoid therapy ■ Hyperparathyroidism ■ Hyperthyroidism
■ What sites of fracture are most common in this disease?	**Vertebral compression fractures** are the most common clinical manifestation of osteoporosis. Most fractures are asymptomatic and usually an incidental finding on x-ray of the chest or abdomen. However, they may manifest as spinal deformity and shortened stature. **Hip** and **distal radius fractures** also should raise clinical suspicion of osteoporosis.
■ What tests and/or imaging tools could be useful in testing bone density?	Osteoporosis cannot be reliably detected in plain radiographs until a significant percentage of bone mass is lost. Laboratory tests typically reveal normal calcium, phosphorus, and alkaline phosphatase levels. Therefore, dual-energy x-ray absorptiometry (**DEXA**) scans are used to compare bone density to an age-matched reference population. Density more than two standard deviations below the expected range confirms the diagnosis of osteoporosis.
■ What is the most appropriate treatment for this condition?	The mainstay of treatment and prevention of osteoporosis is **bisphosphonates** such as alendronate and risedronate. These agents act by decreasing osteoclastic bone resorption. Raloxifene, a **selective estrogen receptor modulator (SERM)** is also used. Intermittent administration of recombinant parathyroid hormone is also shown to be effective. Calcitonin and calcitriol have limited efficacy in osteoporosis.

► **Case 15**

A 15-year-old is brought to the emergency department via ambulance after a knife fight with his cousin. He has two stab wounds, one on the left immediately below his clavicle and the second on his right between the fifth and sixth ribs. Physical examination reveals the patient is tachypneic and hypotensive. X-ray of the chest shows a hemothorax, and thus a chest tube is placed on the right.

■ **What major structures are at risk in wounds of this nature?**	Left lung, aorta, or right atrium, depending on how low the stab wound is found.
■ **What nerves are at risk in wounds of this nature?**	■ Cardiac plexus ■ Recurrent laryngeal nerve ■ Phrenic nerve ■ Pulmonary plexus (contiguous with the cardiac plexus) ■ Vagus nerve
■ **What vessels supply blood to this region?**	**Arterial supply:** ■ Aortic arch ■ Brachiocephalic trunk ■ Common carotid ■ Internal thoracic ■ Left bronchial ■ Subclavian **Venous supply:** ■ Azygos ■ Brachiocephalic ■ Internal thoracic ■ Jugular
■ **How is the lymphatic system organized in the thoracic cavity?**	The lymphatics in the lung arise from the superficial lymphatic plexus (located below the visceral pleura) and the deep lymphatic plexus (located along the bronchial tree except the alveoli). Both of the plexuses drain into hilar nodes (bronchopulmonary nodes). Lymph from the hilar nodes drains first into the carinal (tracheobronchial) nodes, then into the tracheal nodes. The tracheal nodes also receive lymph from the trachea, upper esophagus, and inferior larynx. Lymph from the tracheal nodes finally enters the bronchomediastinal lymph trunks.
■ **What is the difference between the left and right main-stem bronchi?**	The main-stem bronchus passes inferolaterally from the bifurcation of the trachea at the sternal angle to the hilum. The **right main bronchus** is shorter and wider and runs more vertically, allowing for passage of aspirates more easily than the left bronchus. The **left main bronchus** is longer and travels anterior to the esophagus between the thoracic aorta and the left pulmonary artery.

► **Case 16**

A 63-year-old woman goes to her primary care physician complaining that, since falling on her outstretched hands 3 weeks ago, she can no longer use her right arm to remove books from the overhead shelves in her office. Further questioning reveals that she also has pain in her right shoulder at night that occasionally wakes her up, and that she now avoids sleeping on her right side. Physical examination reveals tenderness to palpation below the right acromion; also, the patient has pain at 60° as she abducts her right arm, and is unable to abduct with resistance. When the patient is asked to hold her right arm abducted at 45° and laterally rotate her forearm against resistance, she is unable to do so.

▪ What is the most likely diagnosis?	Rotator cuff tear, which presents with both pain and weakness. The subacromial bursa may also be involved, in which case pain is also felt at the insertion of the deltoid muscle in the middle of the upper arm. This is because the subacromial bursa is continuous with the subdeltoid bursa. Rotator cuff tendinitis would present with pain, but not weakness. A nerve injury would present with weakness, but not pain.
▪ The tendons of which two muscles are most likely involved?	The supraspinatus and infraspinatus are likely to be involved.
▪ What events commonly precipitate such an injury?	Rotator cuff tears are rare in patients <40 years old, but quite common in patients >50 years with shoulder pain. However, sports injuries with rotator cuff tears are seen in young athletes. Other common causes of rotator cuff tears include: ▪ Direct blow to the affected shoulder ▪ Falling onto an outstretched hand (as this patient did) ▪ History of recurrent rotator cuff tendinitis ▪ Lifting a heavy object ▪ Shoulder dislocation
▪ What other tendons are likely involved in this injury?	The rotator cuff is made up of the tendons of the "SITS" muscles: the Supraspinatus, Infraspinatus, and Teres minor insert on the greater tuberosity, and the Subscapularis inserts on the lesser tuberosity (see Figure 9-9).
▪ What are the innervations and actions of these muscles?	▪ Supraspinatus: the suprascapular nerve (C4–C6), abduction of the arm beyond the initial 20° (the deltoid abducts the arm for the initial 20°) ▪ Infraspinatus: the suprascapular nerve (C4–C6), external rotation of the arm ▪ Teres minor: the axillary nerve (C5–C6), help in external rotation of the arm ▪ Subscapularis: the upper and lower subscapular nerves (C5–C7), help with median rotation and adduction of the arm

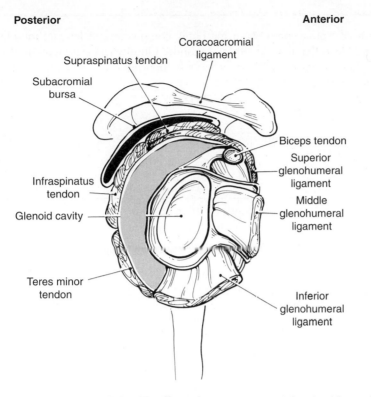

Posterior

Anterior

Coracoacromial ligament

Supraspinatus tendon

Subacromial bursa

Biceps tendon

Superior glenohumeral ligament

Infraspinatus tendon

Middle glenohumeral ligament

Glenoid cavity

Teres minor tendon

Inferior glenohumeral ligament

FIGURE 9-9. Lateral view of shoulder illustrating coracoacromial arch with rotator cuff and subacromial bursa. (Reproduced, with permission, from Tintinalli JE, et al. *Tintinalli's Emergency Medicine: A Comprehensive Study Guide,* 6th ed. New York: McGraw-Hill, 2004: 1780.)

ORGAN SYSTEMS

MUSCULOSKELETAL

► **Case 17**

A 24-year-old woman presents to the clinic complaining of fatigue, muscle and joint aches, and fevers that have lasted for 2 months. On physical examination, she displays a rash over her cheeks and nose as well as a friction rub on cardiac auscultation. Laboratory studies show the following:

Hemoglobin: 10.8 g/dL
Hematocrit: 32.8%
Platelet count: 145,000/mm^3
WBC count: 4350/mm^3
Urinalysis: 3+ proteinuria

■ **What is the most likely diagnosis?**

Systemic lupus erythematosus (SLE). SLE is a multisystem autoimmune connective tissue disease with a variable clinical presentation that most commonly affects young women in their 20s and 30s. Most manifestations of SLE are secondary to immune complex deposition.

■ **What laboratory tests could be used to confirm the diagnosis?**

Antibody testing including antinuclear antibodies (ANA), antiphospholipid antibodies, antibodies to double-stranded DNA (dsDNA), and anti-Smith (Sm) antibodies would all be useful in diagnosing SLE. Positive anti-dsDNA and anti-Sm test results are specific for SLE. A positive ANA test is sensitive, but not specific.

High-yield fact: antiphospholipid antibodies also bind the cardiolipin antigen used in syphilis testing; therefore lupus patients have a false-positive test.

■ **What would a positive anti-histone antibody suggest?**

It would suggest **drug-induced lupus,** but the reason for this correlation is unknown. Common medications that can cause drug-induced lupus include hydralazine, procainamide, minocycline, penicillamine, and isoniazid.

■ **What are the 11 classification criteria for this diagnosis?**

Remember *SOAP BRAIN MD*: **S**erositis, **O**ral ulcers, **A**rthritis, **P**hotosensitivity, **B**lood changes, **R**enal involvement (proteinuria or casts), **A**NA, **I**mmunological changes, **N**eurological signs (seizures, frank psychosis), **M**alar Rash, **D**iscoid Rash.

For the diagnosis of SLE, a patient must display a minimum of 4 out of 11 characteristics.

■ **This condition has significant impact on renal function. What are the typical findings in this condition?**

There are six different classes of renal disease in SLE, which are usually differentiated with a renal biopsy. Immune complex–mediated glomerular diseases are most common. SLE nephropathy typically displays a nephrotic syndrome pattern with "**wire loop**" lesions and subepithelial or subendothelial deposits with inflammation.

A 54-year-old woman presents to the clinic with tightness in her fingers. Additionally, she explains that her fingers occasionally become pale and painful when she forgets to wear her gloves on cold days. On physical examination, her skin is very taut and thickened over her hands and face. Her hands appear claw-like and have decreased motion at all of the small joints symmetrically.

■ **What is the most likely diagnosis and what are the two forms?**

Systemic sclerosis (scleroderma), an autoimmune connective tissue disorder (see Figure 9-10). Scleroderma exists in two forms, limited and diffuse, both of which occur in the setting of Raynaud's phenomenon. This patient displays the limited form in which the skin of the fingers, forearms, and face are often affected with distinctive thickening.

Diffuse systemic sclerosis will eventually involve visceral organs as well as including the gastrointestinal tract (particularly the esophagus), heart, muscles, lungs, and kidneys. This results in dysphagia, respiratory difficulty, arrhythmias, and mild proteinuria. The most concerning manifestation of this disease is malignant hypertension leading to renal failure.

■ **What serologic marker is used to test for this disease?**

Anti-DNA topoisomerase I (**Anti-Scl-70**) antibody is highly specific for systemic sclerosis. Positive antinuclear along with anti-centromere antibodies are characteristic of CREST syndrome.

■ **What is the pathogenesis of this condition?**

The etiology for this condition is unknown: however, symptoms begin with vascular damage and are due to excessive synthesis of extracellular matrix, increased deposition of collagen in normal tissue, fibrosis, immune activation, and vascular damage.

■ **What is CREST syndrome?**

CREST is an acronym for the five findings in individuals with limited systemic sclerosis: calcinosis, Raynaud's phenomenon, esophageal dysmotility, sclerodactyly, and telangiectasia.

■ **What is the recommended treatment for this condition?**

Most therapies are supportive with skin softening agents and gloves used to help skin sclerosis and Raynaud's phenomenon. Bosentan and prostacyclin analogs might also be useful in pulmonary hypertension. Additionally, cytotoxics have a role in treating inflammatory lung disease.

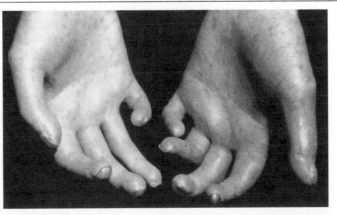

FIGURE 9-10. **Flexion deformities of the fingers and sclerodactyly.** The skin over the fingers and hands is taut and indurated. There is shortening and bony resorption of distal phalanges of the second and third fingers. Ulcers may develop over the distal phalanges and dorsal surfaces of the metacarpophalangeal and proximal interphalangeal joints. (Reproduced, with permission, from Kasper DL, Braunwald E, Fauci AS, et al. *Harrison's Principles of Internal Medicine*, 16th ed. New York: McGraw-Hill, 2005: 1984.)

Neurology

Case 1	321
Case 2	322
Case 3	324
Case 4	325
Case 5	326
Case 6	328
Case 7	329
Case 8	330
Case 9	331
Case 10	332
Case 11	334
Case 12	336
Case 13	338
Case 14	340
Case 15	341
Case 16	342
Case 17	344
Case 18	345
Case 19	346
Case 20	348
Case 21	349
Case 22	350
Case 23	352
Case 24	354
Case 25	355
Case 26	356
Case 27	358

Case 28   359

Case 29   360

Case 30   362

Case 31   363

Case 32   364

Case 33   366

Case 34   367

Case 35   368

Case 36   370

Case 37   372

Case 38   373

Case 39   374

Case 40   376

Case 41   378

Case 42   379

► **Case 1**

A 73-year-old well-educated woman is brought to the physician by her daughter, who has become concerned about her mother's behavior. The mother volunteers at the local library shelving books, but for the past few months she has had trouble remembering where the books go. In addition, she often forgets to turn the stove off after cooking her family's long-time favorite dishes.

■ What is the most likely diagnosis?	This history is consistent with Alzheimer's disease, which is characterized by loss of short-term memory and general preservation of long-term memory.
■ What risk factors are associated with the development of this condition?	Advancing age and a family history of Alzheimer's disease are two well-known risk factors. Additionally, because the amyloid precursor protein (APP) is located on chromosome 21, patients with Down syndrome (trisomy 21) have increased APP levels; these patients often develop Alzheimer's disease at 30–40 years old.
■ What are the likely gross pathology findings in this condition?	Neurofibrillary **tangles** and amyloid **plaques** (Figure 10-1A; arrows point to tangles) are commonly seen on autopsy. A high degree of cerebral atrophy in the frontal, temporal, and parietal regions is also present, as can be seen in Figure 10-1B.
■ What biochemical mechanism is believed to be involved in the pathogenesis of this condition?	A preferential loss of acetylcholine and choline acetyltransferase in the cerebral cortex may play a role in the development of clinical disease. The acetylcholinesterase inhibitor class of medications, including tacrine, donepezil, rivastigmine, and galantamine, have been shown to slow the progress of memory loss. Memantine, an N-methyl-D-aspartate (NMDA) receptor antagonist, may protect from Alzheimer's disease by blocking the excitotoxic effects of glutamate, independently of the effects of acetylcholinesterase inhibitors.
■ What is the most appropriate treatment for this condition?	Tacrine, which is an acetylcholinesterase inhibitor, is the only drug that is known to slow the progress of Alzheimer's-related memory loss.
■ What is the prognosis for the patient's daughter?	The familial form of Alzheimer's disease, which affects approximately 10% of patients with the disease, usually has an onset between the ages of 30 and 60 years. Given the mother's age and current symptoms, the mother likely does not have the familial form, and the daughter should not have an increased risk on the basis of family history alone.

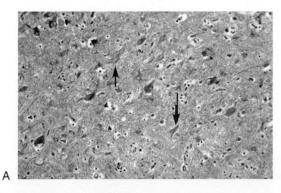
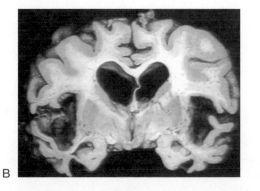

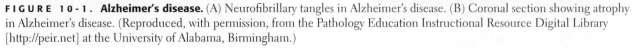

FIGURE 10-1. Alzheimer's disease. (A) Neurofibrillary tangles in Alzheimer's disease. (B) Coronal section showing atrophy in Alzheimer's disease. (Reproduced, with permission, from the Pathology Education Instructional Resource Digital Library [http://peir.net] at the University of Alabama, Birmingham.)

▶ **Case 2**

A 35-year-old construction worker is taken to the emergency department following an accident in which a piece of metal became lodged in his back. In addition to experiencing excruciating pain at the site of his injury, the patient is unable to move his right leg. In the emergency department, a neurologic examination reveals the man's right leg is paralyzed, with an ipsilateral hyperactive patellar reflex and a positive Babinski's sign. The patient can move his left leg without difficulty and has a normal patellar reflex and no Babinski's sign. However, sensory testing reveals loss of temperature and pinprick sensation on the left leg up to the navel, along with loss of vibration sensation on the right leg up to the navel.

■ **What is the most likely diagnosis?**	Brown-Séquard syndrome due to a hemicord lesion. Brown-Séquard syndrome is characterized by ipsilateral spastic (upper motor neuron–type) paralysis (1 in Figure 10-2), ipsilateral loss of vibration and position sensation (2 in Figure 10-2), and contralateral loss of pain and temperature sensation (3 in Figure 10-2).
■ **At what level is the lesion?**	The loss of sensation up to the navel suggests that the lesion is near T10, because the dermatome that includes the navel is supplied by T10.
■ **Damage to which tracts is causing the ipsilateral deficits in this case?**	The motor deficits are due to damage to the **lateral corticospinal tract** (see Figure 10-3), which carries motor neurons from the cortex that have decussated in the pyramids. The loss of vibration and position sense is due to damage to the **dorsal columns**, which carry information from sensory nerves that enter through the dorsal root, ascend to the caudal medulla (where the primary neuron synapses), and then cross to ascend to the contralateral sensory cortex. These deficits are ipsilateral because the tracts cross the midline high in the spinal cord.
■ **Damage to which tracts is causing the contralateral deficits in this case?**	The loss of pain and temperature sensation is due to damage to the **spinothalamic tract** (see Figure 10-3). The sensory neurons that travel in the anterolateral tract enter the spinal cord through the dorsal root, synapse almost immediately, and cross the midline (within one or two levels) via the anterior commissure to ascend to the cortex.
■ **If the lesion were above T1, how would the presentation differ?**	A hemicord lesion above T1, in addition to the findings above, will present as **Horner's syndrome**, which consists of ptosis, miosis, and anhidrosis (droopy eyelid, constricted pupil, and decreased sweating).

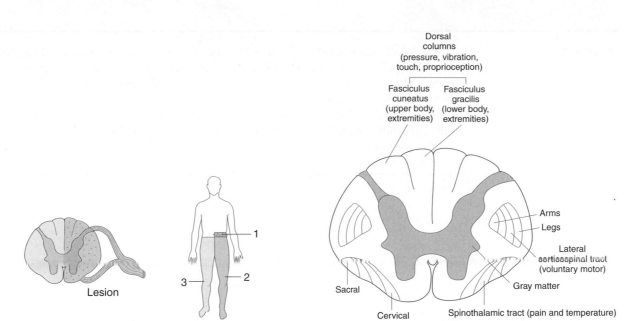

ORGAN SYSTEMS

NEUROLOGY

► **Case 3**

A 38-year-old man presents to his primary care physician with a complaint of progressive weakness in his hands and feet. The patients states that these symptoms have slowly progressed over the last few months. Initially, he was unable to manipulate small objects such as picking up a coin or buttoning his shirt. Now he complains of difficulty grasping a gallon of milk and notices the muscles in his hands twitching. He often trips while walking because he feels he can't lift his toes up and lacks coordination. In addition, he says that the muscles in his leg occasionally cramp or spasm.

▪ What is the most likely diagnosis?	**Amyotrophic lateral sclerosis (ALS)**, or Lou Gehrig's disease, is a neurodegenerative disorder that causes progressive muscle weakness.
▪ What is the pathogenesis and epidemiology of this condition?	The etiology of ALS is unknown with a yearly incidence of approximately 5000 new cases per year in the United States with almost all cases being sporadic. Incidence increases with age, although people in their twenties and thirties can be affected.
▪ Where are the lesions located and how does this explain the hallmark findings?	The hallmark of this disorder is the presence of **both upper motor neuron (UMN) and lower motor neuron (LMN)** lesions. ALS affects **anterior horn motor neurons** in the spinal cord (LMN) and the lateral corticospinal tracts carrying UMNs from the cortex. Sensory and cognitive functions are generally preserved.

▪ What distinguishes UMN signs from LMN signs?	▪ UMN findings:
	  ▪ Hyperreflexivity
	  ▪ Increased tone
	  ▪ Positive Babinski sign
	  ▪ Muscle spasm
	▪ LMN findings:
	  ▪ Weakness
	  ▪ Muscle atrophy
	  ▪ Muscle fasciculations

▪ What is the natural history of this disease?	ALS is currently an untreatable disease with progressive neurodegeneration and muscle weakness resulting in death within 3–5 years after diagnosis. Neuromuscular respiratory failure is the primary cause of death.

▶ **Case 4**

A 16-year-old high school student goes to see the school nurse because of severe eye pain and a feeling that there is something "stuck" in his right eye. He does not wear contact lenses. He reports he was recently working with machines in shop class without wearing protective goggles. Ophthalmologic examination reveals no visible foreign body in the eye; visual acuity is slightly decreased at 20/30; pupils are equal, round, and reactive to light bilaterally; corneal reflex is intact; and extraocular muscles are intact, although the student says his right eye hurts when he moves it.

▪ **What is the most likely diagnosis?**	The student has a corneal abrasion, which typically presents with significant eye pain and a foreign body sensation. The patient will also have photophobia. This patient also has a history suggestive of a source for his eye injury: working with machinery without wearing protective eyewear.
▪ **What is the pathway of the corneal blink reflex?**	The excruciating pain being experienced by this patient is due to the rich innervation of the cornea by the ophthalmic branch of cranial nerve (CN) V, (V1). It is this same nerve that constitutes the afferent portion of the corneal blink reflex. After synapsing in the sensory nucleus of CN V, there is bilateral projection to the nucleus of CN VII. From there, motor neurons project to the orbicularis oculi muscles, causing a consensual blink response.
▪ **What space lies between the cornea and the lens?**	The space between the cornea and the lens is the anterior compartment, which is subdivided by the iris into the anterior chamber and the posterior chamber (see Figure 10-4). The entire anterior compartment is filled with aqueous humor, which is secreted by the ciliary body.
▪ **What space lies behind the lens?**	Behind the lens is the posterior compartment (see Figure 10-4), which is filled with vitreous humor, a gelatinous substance. At the anterior aspect of the posterior compartment, the lens is held in place by the suspensory ligament, which extends from the ciliary body of the choroid to the lens.
▪ **From what embryologic structures do the cornea, iris, ciliary body, lens, and retina develop?**	The optic cup is an embryologic structure derived from neuroectoderm that gives rise to the retina, iris, and ciliary body. The lens is derived from surface ectoderm. The inner layers of the cornea are derived from mesenchyme, and the outer layer is from the surface ectoderm.

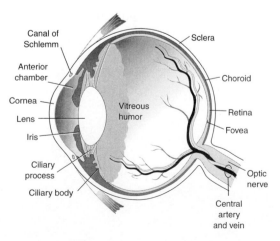

FIGURE 10-4. The eye and retina. (Reproduced, with permission, from Le T, Bhushan V, Rao DA. *First Aid for the USMLE Step 1: 2008.* New York: McGraw-Hill, 2008: 379.)

▶ **Case 5**

A 70-year-old man with a history of rheumatoid arthritis comes to his physician complaining of weakness 1 day after a motor vehicle accident. Physical examination reveals intact sensation and strength in the lower extremities along with bilateral upper extremity weakness. The patient is able to move his arms parallel to the ground but is unable to lift his arms, forearms, or hands upward against gravity; strength is rated 2/5. A cervical CT scan rules out the presence of a cervical spine fracture, and MRI demonstrates traumatic C6 disc herniation, buckling of the ligamentum flavum, and edema within the cervical cord in that area.

■ What is the most likely diagnosis?	Central cord syndrome. This syndrome is characterized by upper extremity weakness that exceeds lower extremity weakness, along with varying degrees of sensory loss below the level of the lesion.
■ What is the arterial supply to the cervical spinal cord?	The spinal cord is supplied by an anterior spinal artery (which is supplied by the vertebral arteries) that supplies the anterior two-thirds of the cord, and by two posterior spinal arteries (which are supplied by the vertebral posterior inferior cerebellar arteries) that supply the dorsal columns and part of the posterior horns.
■ What is a vascular watershed zone?	A **watershed zone** is an area between two major arteries in which small branches of the arteries form anastomoses. Important watershed zones lie between the cerebral arteries (e.g., between the middle and anterior cerebral arteries) and in the central spinal cord. These areas are particularly susceptible to infarction during times of hypotension or hypoperfusion. In this case, edema and trauma impair blood flow to the cervical cord, and the predominant symptoms result from damage within the central cord watershed zone.
■ What is supplied by the long tracts in the areas labeled "region A" in Figure 10-5?	Region A in Figure 10-5 indicates the most medial portions of the corticospinal tracts. These fibers supply the muscles of the upper extremity. Because they are medial structures, motor impairment of the upper extremities can occur following a smaller central cord lesion. The cross-hatched pattern in Figure 10-6 indicates the area of impairment that would be associated with a central cord lesion.
■ What changes in the biceps, triceps, and brachioradialis reflexes would one expect to see following damage to the anterior horn cells supplying the C6 nerve root?	The biceps reflex, which is regulated by fibers from C5 and C6, will be moderately diminished secondary to diminished lower motor neuron input. The triceps reflex is regulated primarily by C7 and should thus be unaffected by a C6 lesion. The brachioradialis reflex is primarily regulated by C6 and will thus be markedly diminished following a C6 lesion.

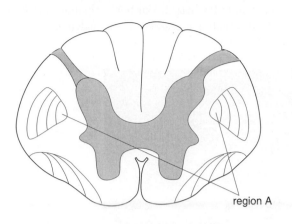
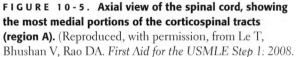

region A

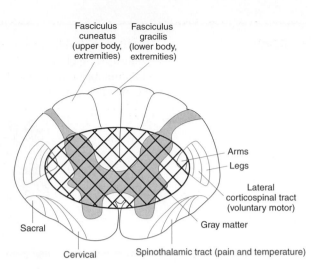

Fasciculus cuneatus (upper body, extremities)

Fasciculus gracilis (lower body, extremities)

Arms

Legs

Lateral corticospinal tract (voluntary motor)

Gray matter

Sacral

Cervical

Spinothalamic tract (pain and temperature)

ORGAN SYSTEMS

NEUROLOGY

► **Case 6**

A 10-year-old boy is brought to the pediatrician by his parents for evaluation of short stature. The child is below the 10th percentile for height. Further evaluation reveals a bitemporal hemianopia. MRI of the head reveals a suprasellar cystic, calcified mass as seen below in Figure 10-7.

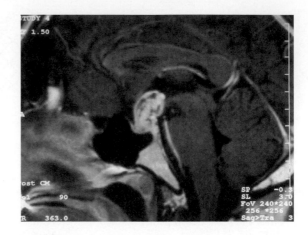

FIGURE 10-7. (Reproduced, with permission, from Riordan-Eva P, et al. *Vaughn & Asbury's General Ophthalmology*, 17th ed. New York: McGraw-Hill, 2008: 281.)

■ What is the likely diagnosis?	The hallmark lesion for **craniopharyngioma** is a **suprasellar, cystic, calcified** mass. The differential diagnosis for a suprasellar mass includes optic gliomas, meningiomas, pituitary adenomas, and metastases.
■ From what tissue does this tumor derive?	Craniopharyngiomas are very rare tumors derived from Rathke's pouch. Rathke's pouch is an invagination of **ectoderm** lining the primitive mouth that develops into the adenohypophysis.
■ What tests or imaging tools may be used to confirm the diagnosis?	CT scan or MRI of the head can visualize the cystic calcified suprasellar mass characteristic of craniopharyngioma. Plain radiographs of the skull can pick up advanced cases. Testing of the pituitary axis and optic pathways can determine if tumor has affected these structures.
■ What is the epidemiology of this condition?	Craniopharyngiomas exhibit a bimodal distribution, with one peak among children and the second among patients 55–65 years of age. It is the third most common intracranial tumor in children.
■ What are the clinical manifestations of this condition?	Craniopharyngiomas are slow-growing tumors with a highly variable clinical presentation. Symptoms occur as the tumor involves the pituitary gland or the optic chiasm. Patients may present with growth hormone deficiency, hypothyroidism, or central diabetes insipidus. Visual disturbances and headaches are common.

A 45-year-old woman presents to her physician with a 3-month history of anxiety, tremor, hyperreflexia, hair thinning, and an unintentional weight loss of 4.5 kg (10 lb). She is treated surgically. After surgery, her symptoms have resolved, but the patient now complains of hoarseness.

■ **What is the cause of the patient's hoarseness?**	Damage to the recurrent laryngeal nerve may occur as the surgeon is ligating the inferior thyroid artery, which is adjacent to the nerve.
■ **What cranial nerve is involved in this patient?**	The recurrent laryngeal nerve is a branch of the vagus nerve (cranial nerve [CN] X).
■ **This nerve provides motor innervation to which structures?**	The recurrent laryngeal nerve innervates all intrinsic muscles of the larynx except for the cricothyroid, which is innervated by the external laryngeal nerve (also a branch of CN X).
■ **Describe the course of this nerve.**	The left recurrent laryngeal nerve branches off the vagus nerve at the level of the aortic arch, wraps posteriorly around the aorta, and ascends superiorly to the larynx (see Figure 10-8). The right recurrent laryngeal nerve branches off the vagus at the level of the right subclavian artery and vein, and wraps around the artery to ascend posteriorly to the larynx. Because the left recurrent laryngeal nerve has a long course arising from the vagus in the superior mediastinum, it is prone to injury from abnormal structures, such as enlarged lymph nodes, aneurysm of the arch of the aorta, a retrosternal goiter, or a thymoma.
■ **What are other scenarios by which this nerve may be injured?**	Left atrial enlargement (e.g., from mitral regurgitation) and tumor in the apex of the right upper lobe of the lung can impinge on and injure the recurrent laryngeal nerve. Injury of the left recurrent laryngeal nerve may also result in compression by abnormal structures in the superior mediastinum (see above).

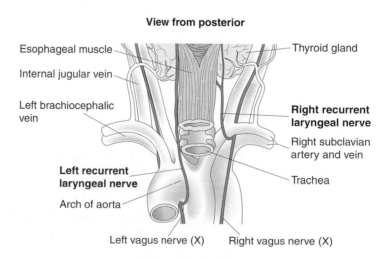

View from posterior

Esophageal muscle
Internal jugular vein
Left brachiocephalic vein
Left recurrent laryngeal nerve
Arch of aorta
Left vagus nerve (X)

Thyroid gland
Right recurrent laryngeal nerve
Right subclavian artery and vein
Trachea
Right vagus nerve (X)

FIGURE 10-8. Course of the recurrent laryngeal nerve. (Reproduced, with permission, from Bhushan V, Le T, et al. *First Aid for the USMLE Step 1: 2005*. New York: McGraw-Hill, 2005: 83.)

► **Case 8**   A 72-year-old woman falls while at home and lands face down. She is unable to get up and remains prone on the floor overnight, until a neighbor notices her missing and calls 911. She is taken to the emergency department (ED), where she is noted to have several hematomas on her face and a large hematoma on her right upper thigh. On physical examination, the ED resident discovers that the patient is unable to flex her right hip or extend her right lower leg. The resident cannot elicit a patellar reflex on the right. Leg adduction and abduction are intact bilaterally.

■ **What is the most likely diagnosis?**	The patient has femoral neuropathy (L2–L4), as suggested by weakness of the quadriceps muscles and hip flexors (which are innervated by the femoral nerve) and lack of patellar reflex. The cause of the neuropathy in this case is a hematoma (secondary to trauma) compressing the nerve. Because both the hip flexors (L2–L3) and the quadriceps muscles (L3–L4) are involved, the nerve is being affected above the inguinal ligament.
■ **What sensory defects would be expected in this patient?**	The femoral nerve innervates the skin of the anterior and medial thigh; thus, light touch sensation would be decreased in these areas. The lateral aspect of the thigh is innervated by the lateral femoral cutaneous nerve (L2–L3), and would be spared in an isolated femoral neuropathy. The **saphenous nerve** is a cutaneous branch of the femoral nerve that arises from the femoral nerve in the femoral triangle. It innervates the skin of the anteromedial knee, leg, and foot to the medial side of the big toe. Because this lesion is above the femoral ligament, the saphenous nerve distribution will also be involved.
■ **What other structures are found with this nerve in the femoral triangle?**	The femoral nerve is the largest branch of the lumbar plexus and, after forming in the abdomen, runs posterolaterally to the inguinal ligament. It crosses under the inguinal ligament lateral to the psoas muscle and enters the femoral triangle. In the **femoral triangle** (which is bounded by the sartorius muscle, inguinal ligament, and adductor longus), it runs lateral to the femoral artery, which in turn is lateral to the femoral vein. The vessels are enclosed within the femoral sheath and the nerve is outside it.
■ **Why is thigh adduction spared in this patient?**	The major muscles responsible for thigh adduction are the adductor longus, adductor brevis, adductor magnus, and the gracilis, which are innervated by the obturator nerve (L2–L4). Because this is a peripheral neuropathy, not pathology of the nerve root, the obturator nerve is spared, and so is thigh adduction.
■ **What other clinical scenarios can be associated with this condition?**	■ Diabetic vasculitic damage ■ Direct penetrating trauma ■ Hip fracture ■ Iliac aneurysms ■ Incorrect placement of the femoral line ■ Prolonged hip flexion during gynecologic or urologic procedures ■ Tumor

► **Case 9**

A 70-year-old man with a history of hypertension goes to his ophthalmologist for a routine eye examination. He has needed to wear eyeglasses while driving since he was 18 years old. Ocular examination reveals increased intraocular pressure in both of the patient's eyes. On a field test, there is significant loss of peripheral vision, and a funduscopic examination reveals cupping.

■ **What is the most likely diagnosis?**	Open-angle glaucoma.
■ **What is the pathophysiology of this condition?**	Open-angle glaucoma is caused by elevated intraocular pressure resulting from obstruction of flow of aqueous humor through the normal outflow channels.
■ **What are the most appropriate treatments for this condition?**	Pilocarpine and carbachol are the most appropriate drugs for the treatment of open-angle glaucoma. These direct cholinergic agonists act by stimulating ciliary muscle contraction, thereby relieving tension in the suspensory ligament. Cholinomimetics will also stimulate the sphincter pupillae of the iris, resulting in widening of the canal of Schlemm and pupillary constriction (miosis). Adverse effects include nausea, vomiting, diarrhea, salivation, sweating, vasodilation, and bronchoconstriction.
■ **What effect does pilocarpine have on cardiac muscle?**	Pilocarpine is an M3/M2 muscarinic receptor agonist. Cardiac cells have M2 receptors that, when activated, stimulate a G protein that inhibits adenyl cyclase and increases potassium conductance. Pilocarpine stimulation thus results in a decrease in heart rate and decreased force of contraction (**negative inotrope**).
■ **What additional classes of drugs are useful in treating this condition?**	■ Adrenergic agonists such as epinephrine ■ β-Blockers and acetazolamide (a carbonic anhydrase inhibitor), which decrease aqueous humor secretion ■ Prostaglandins, which increase the outflow of aqueous humor

► **Case 10**   A 52-year-old man is brought to the emergency department after sustaining his first tonic-clonic seizure. The patient states he has had a bitemporal dull, constant headache for the last 2 weeks. MRI of the head is shown in Figure 10-9.

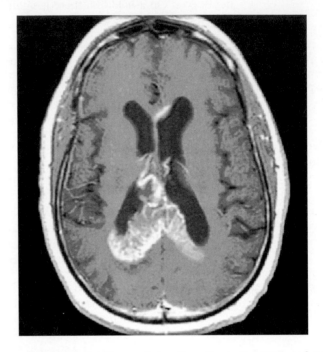

FIGURE 10-9. (Reproduced, with permission, from Kantarjian HM, et al. *MD Anderson Manual of Medical Oncology.* New York: McGraw-Hill, 2006: 796.)

■ What is the likely diagnosis?	Glioblastoma multiforme (GBM), the most common primary brain tumor. GBM represents almost 20% of all primary intracranial tumors.
■ Where are these lesions typically located?	Glioblastomas are found supratentorially in the cerebral hemispheres and often cross hemispheres via the corpus callosum ("butterfly glioma") as seen above.
■ What are the histologic findings in this condition?	Glioblastomas are composed of highly malignant astrocytes that are visualized with a glial fibrillary acidic protein (GFAP) stain. Histology of glioblastomas shows pseudopalisading tumor cells surrounding focal areas of necrosis (see Figure 10-10).
■ What is the treatment for this condition?	Treatment is largely palliative and only moderately increases survival time. Treatment may include surgical resection, radiation, and chemotherapy.
■ What is the natural history of this condition?	Glioblastoma is a very aggressive tumor and without treatment most patients die within 3 months of diagnosis. With treatment the median survival time is 1 year, and less than 10% of patients survive 5 years.

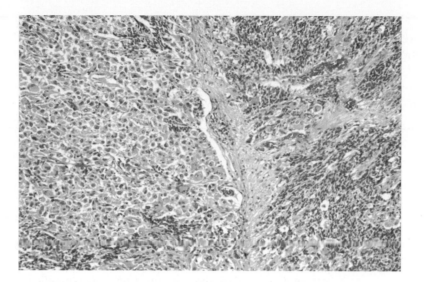

FIGURE 10-10. This slide shows pseudopalisading tumor cells on the right with focal areas of necrosis from a patient with glioblastoma multiforme (hematoxylin and eosin). (Reproduced, with permission, from the Pathology Education Instructional Resource Digital Library [http://peir.net] at the University of Alabama, Birmingham.)

▶ **Case 11**

A 27-year-old man comes to his physician complaining of a tingling sensation in his toes and progressive weakness in both of his legs. On questioning, he recalls he had a minor cold 3 weeks ago that lasted for a few days. He has not traveled recently and has not eaten anything out of the ordinary. Physical examination reveals markedly decreased patellar and Achilles tendon reflexes bilaterally.

▪ What is the most likely diagnosis?	Guillain-Barré syndrome (GBS). GBS, or acute inflammatory demyelinating polyradiculoneuropathy, is characterized by symmetric ascending muscle weakness or paralysis that begins in the lower extremities. Hyporeflexia or areflexia is invariable but may not be present early in the course of disease.
▪ What physical findings are commonly associated with this condition?	Associated findings in GBS include ascending paresthesias, cranial nerve deficits leading to dysphagia, dysarthria, facial weakness, papilledema, autonomic dysfunction, and in extreme cases, respiratory muscle paralysis. Figure 10-11 shows papilledema of the optic nerve head in GBS, along with the vascular congestion, elevation of the nerve head, and blurred disc margins often seen in papilledema, papillitis, and compressive lesions of the optic nerve.
▪ In what settings does this condition usually occur?	GBS often occurs 1–3 weeks after a gastrointestinal or upper respiratory tract infection, vaccination, or allergic reaction. Common associated infections include *Campylobacter jejuni* and herpesvirus. Although a preceding event is present in most patients, about one-third of patients with GBS report no such events during the preceding 1–4 weeks.
▪ What is the etiology of this condition?	GBS is thought to be an autoimmune reaction that develops in response to a previous infection or other medical condition. This process results in aberrant demyelination of peripheral nerves and ventral motor nerve roots. Cranial nerve roots can also be affected.
▪ What laboratory finding is likely in this condition?	The cerebrospinal fluid (CSF) reveals a markedly elevated protein concentration with a normal cell count, commonly referred to as **albuminocytologic dissociation.** This is in contrast to the increased cell counts typical of central nervous system infection. An increased CSF protein level can lead to papilledema.
▪ If this patient's symptoms were to worsen over the next few months with no signs of improvement, what alternative diagnosis might be considered?	**Chronic inflammatory demyelinating polyradiculopathy** is a chronic progressive counterpart of GBS that often presents with similar symptoms.

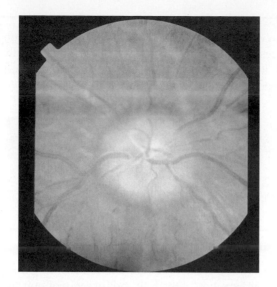

FIGURE 10-11. Papilledema of the optic nerve. (Reproduced, with permission, from Tintinalli JE, et al. *Tintinalli's Emergency Medicine: A Comprehensive Study Guide*, 6th ed. New York: McGraw-Hill, 2004: 1464.)

▶ **Case 12**

A 45-year-old man comes to the physician for a routine visit. On physical examination, his left eye appears abnormal (see Figure 10-12). In addition, his left pupil is constricted, although it reacts normally to light and accommodation. On questioning, he states the left side of his face has become abnormally dry.

FIGURE 10-12. (Reproduced, with permission, from Tintinalli JE, et al. *Tintinalli's Emergency Medicine: A Comprehensive Study Guide*, 6th ed. New York: McGraw-Hill, 2004: 1463.)

▪ What is the most likely diagnosis?	Horner's syndrome.
▪ What is the pathophysiology of this condition?	Horner's syndrome results from a disruption in the sympathetic innervation of the face and subsequent uninhibited parasympathetic activity, producing the classic symptoms of ipsilateral **P**tosis (slight drooping of the eyelid), **A**nhidrosis (absence of sweating), and **M**iosis (pupillary constriction) (remember the mnemonic **PAM**).
▪ What nerve pathway is disrupted in this condition?	The first neuron of the sympathetic pathway begins in the hypothalamus and synapses in the intermediolateral column of the spinal cord near T1 (see Figure 10-13). The second, preganglionic neuron travels to the superior cervical ganglion. The third and final neuron of the pathway then innervates the pupil, the sweat glands of the face, and the smooth muscle of the eyelid.
▪ If this patient presented with nystagmus to the left side and frequent falling, what acute condition should be considered?	**Wallenberg's syndrome**, which results from a stroke in the lateral medullary region supplied by the posterior inferior cerebellar artery, can present with ipsilateral Horner's syndrome, nystagmus to the side of the lesion, ipsilateral limb ataxia, and vertigo. Another distinguishing feature is impaired pain and temperature sensation in the ipsilateral face and contralateral hemibody.
▪ What are other common causes of this condition?	Any pathology that causes interruption of the described pathway can cause Horner's syndrome. These include Pancoast's tumor, neck trauma, carotid dissection, cervical cord lesions, and multiple sclerosis. Additionally, many cases of Horner's syndrome are idiopathic.
▪ What is Pancoast's tumor?	**Pancoast's tumor** is a carcinoma that usually affects the lung, occurring in the apex of the lung. It can cause Horner's syndrome and ulnar nerve pain.

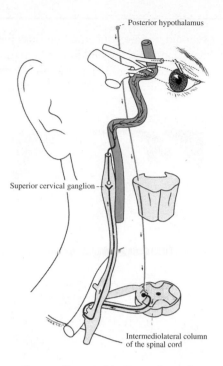

Posterior hypothalamus

Superior cervical ganglion

Intermediolateral column
of the spinal cord

FIGURE 10-13. **Nerve pathways disrupted in Horner's syndrome.** (Reproduced, with permission, from Tintinalli JE, et al. *Tintinalli's Emergency Medicine: A Comprehensive Study Guide,* 6th ed. New York: McGraw-Hill, 2004: 1463.)

▶ **Case 13**   The parents of a term, 1-year-old girl are concerned because the child's head seems abnormally large. Their pediatrician notes the child's head circumference has accelerated beyond her established growth curve over the past month. An axial CT of her head (see Figure 10-14) demonstrates dilated atria of the lateral ventricles and a rounded third ventricle.

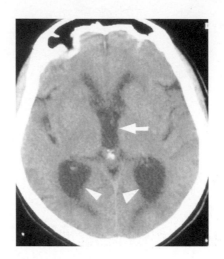

FIGURE 10-14. (Reproduced, with permission, from Brunicardi FC, et al. *Schwartz's Principles of Surgery*, 8th ed. New York: McGraw-Hill, 2005: 1650.)

■ **What is the most likely diagnosis?**	Hydrocephalus, which is defined as an excessive volume of cerebrospinal fluid (CSF) within the ventricles of the brain. Because CSF is trapped within the ventricular system in this case, this is an example of a **noncommunicating hydrocephalus. A communicating hydrocephalus** can occur in states of excess CSF production. In this CT image showing a dilated ventricular system (Figure 10-14), note the dilated atria of the lateral ventricles (arrowheads) and rounded third ventricle (arrow).
■ **Where is CSF produced?**	CSF is produced by the choroid plexus epithelium within the cerebral ventricles. The anatomy of the ventricular system is shown in Figure 10-15. The lateral ventricle communicates with the third ventricle via the foramen of Monro. The third ventricle communicates with the fourth ventricle via the aqueduct of Sylvius. The fourth ventricle communicates with the subarachnoid space via the foramen of Luschka (laterally) and the foramen of Magendie (medially).
■ **How is CSF reabsorbed?**	Arachnoid villus cells, which are located in the superior sagittal sinus, return CSF to the bloodstream within vacuoles (via a process called **pinocytosis**).

■ What forms the blood–brain barrier?	Capillary and choroid endothelium form the **blood-brain barrier**. Tight junctions of capillary endothelium within the brain impede the passage of water and solutes. Within the choroid plexus, the choroid endothelium regulates the transport of water and solutes.
■ What is the pathophysiology of this condition?	Hydrocephalus results from a mismatch of CSF production and reabsorption in which the rate of production exceeds reabsorption. Thus, causes of the condition include: ■ Excess CSF production (e.g., choroid plexus papilloma) ■ Impaired CSF reabsorption (due to obstruction or disruption of arachnoid villi) ■ Blockage of the flow of CSF

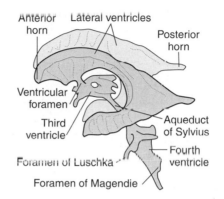

FIGURE 10-15. Anatomy of the ventricular system. (Reproduced, with permission, from Le T, Bhushan V, Rao DA. *First Aid for the USMLE Step 1: 2008.* New York: McGraw-Hill, 2008; 370.)

▶ **Case 14**

A 39-year-old man is concerned about his health because his father died at the age of 45 years after several years of dementia, uncontrollable twitching, and dance-like movements in his extremities. On further questioning, the patient reports many members of his family have had similar symptoms. The patient's knowledge of his family history allows the physician to construct a detailed family tree (see Figure 10-16; the asterisk represents the patient).

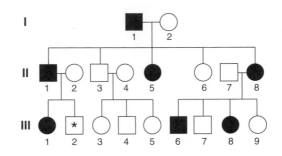

FIGURE 10-16.

■ What condition is the patient at risk for developing?	Huntington's disease, which is characterized by dementia, choreoathetoid movements of the face and extremities, and early death. Huntington's disease has an autosomal dominant inheritance.
■ What is the genetic basis of this condition?	A mutation in chromosome 4 results in expansion of trinucleotide CAG repeats, which may result in decreased transcription of a striatal neurotrophic factor, brain-derived neurotrophic factor.
■ What neuronal pathology in patients with this condition makes CT imaging useful?	Patients with Huntington's disease have marked atrophy of the striatum, including the caudate and putamen, representing degeneration and loss of γ-aminobutyric acid (GABA)-ergic and cholinergic neurons.
■ What other conditions often present with similar movement abnormalities?	Sydenham's chorea in rheumatic fever, tardive dyskinesia, and Wilson's disease are among other diseases associated with choreoathetoid movements.
■ What is the prognosis for this patient?	Expansion of trinucleotide repeats over successive generations leads to earlier manifestations of disease in offspring; this is called **anticipation**. The patient's father died at age 45 years and likely developed Huntington's disease many years earlier. If this patient had the genetic mutation, then he might already be expected to show symptoms.
■ What other conditions are associated with trinucleotide repeats?	Fragile X syndrome, myotonic dystrophy, and spinocerebellar ataxia types I and II are also associated with trinucleotide repeats.

► **Case 15**

A 75-year-old woman visits an ophthalmologist because she has noticed a gradual decline in both her distance and near vision over the past 2 years. In particular, she has difficulty reading, focusing on objects in front of her, and has trouble adjusting her vision to the dark. She denies pain in her eye or any associated trauma. Funduscopic examination reveals deposits in the macula (see Figure 10-17) and abnormal vision as assessed by the Amsler grid (see Figure 10-18). Her peripheral vision and extraocular movements are intact.

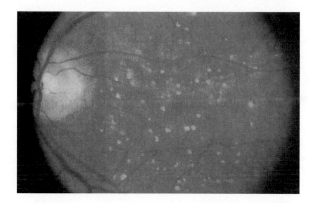

FIGURE 10-17. (Courtesy of Richard E. Wyszynski, MD, as published in Knoop KJ. Stack LB, Storrow AB. *Atlas of Emergency Medicine*, 2nd ed. New York: McGraw-Hill, 2002: 77.)

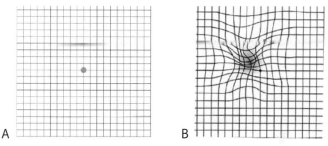

FIGURE 10-18. Normal grid (A), patient's view (B).

▪ **What is the abnormality in this patient's vision as assessed by the Amsler grid?**	The **Amsler grid** assesses the degree of central vision loss (see Figure 10-18A). Patients are asked to cover one eye, and with the open eye, focus on the dot at the center of the grid. Patients with vision deficits in their macula will see a distortion of the grid (see Figure 10-18B).
▪ **What is the most likely diagnosis?**	The most likely diagnosis is age-related macular degeneration (ARMD), a significant cause of vision loss in the elderly, in which central vision is blurred. In contrast, glaucoma typically affects peripheral vision while sparing central vision.
▪ **What are the two variants of this condition?**	There are dry and wet forms of macular degeneration. The **dry form** (representing 85% of cases) typically progresses more slowly and occurs earlier in the disease process. The **wet form**, although rarer (representing 15% of cases), causes the vast majority of significant blindness in patients.
▪ **What are the histologic features of the retina in this condition?**	**Drusen** are extracellular protein and lipid deposits in the retina, which appear on funduscopic examination as yellow or white spots in the eye (see Figure 10-19). Irregularity, and in later stages atrophy of the retinal pigmented epithelium, also occur. In wet ARMD, new vessels from the choroid may grow into the subretinal space, causing **metamorphopsia** (a wavy distortion of vision), hemorrhage, and scarring.
▪ **What is the macula?**	The **macula**, which is located temporal to the optic disc, is the area of the retina that is specialized for fine-detail vision. The center of the macula is the **fovea**, which has the highest density of cone photoreceptor cells in the retina and the smallest amount of convergence to bipolar cells. This provides for exquisite detail in visual perception.

► **Case 16**

A 67-year-old man with a history of hypertension and coronary artery disease presents to the ophthalmologist with a complaint of decreased vision on his right. For the past month, he has noticed that two or three times a week he has had decreased vision on his right. Each episode lasts about 20 minutes and is accompanied by a severe retro-orbital headache. During the episodes, he is unable to read and bumps into objects on his right. Yesterday, he experienced the same visual loss which has not resolved. Automated perimetry visual field testing reveals the pattern shown in Figure 10-19, with areas of visual loss in black.

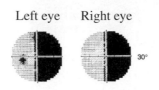

Left eye   Right eye

30°

FIGURE 10-19.

■ What is this visual field defect?	The defect is a **right homonymous hemianopia** likely caused by a stroke. His symptoms suggest he experienced a number of transient ischemic attacks previously.
■ What is the pathway from photoreceptors in the retina to the visual cortex?	**Photoreceptors** (rods and cones), synapse on **bipolar cells** that synapse on **ganglion** cells in the retina, which form the **optic nerve.**
	The optic nerve travels posteriorly and merges to form the **optic chiasm** where nasal (medial) retinal fibers from both eyes cross. The nasal hemiretina fibers are responsible for the temporal visual fields. Once past the chiasm it is known as the **optic tract,** which then synapses on the lateral geniculate nucleus (**LGN**) of the thalamus.
	Axons exiting the LGN fan out posteriorly through the white matter. The inferior radiations carry information from the **inferior retina** or **superior visual field**, travel through the temporal lobe, and are known as Meyer's loop. The superior radiations carry information from the superior retina or inferior visual field and travel through the parietal lobe.
	The **optic radiations** synapse in the **visual cortex** of the occipital lobe near the calcarine fissure. The superior radiations synapse superior to the calcarine fissure, and the inferior radiations inferior to the fissure (see Figure 10-20).
■ Where along the optic pathway may a lesion be located to give this visual field defect?	A lesion in the left optic tract, posterior to the chiasm and anterior to the lateral geniculate nucleus may be the cause, as may a large lesion affecting the upper and lower optic radiations or a lesion in the left visual cortex.
■ What visual field defect would a lesion in the right temporal lobe show?	The inferior optic radiations (Meyer's loop) travel through the temporal lobe. A lesion to this area would show a left upper quadrantic anopia ("pie in the sky") as indicated by lesion **J** in Figure 10-20.

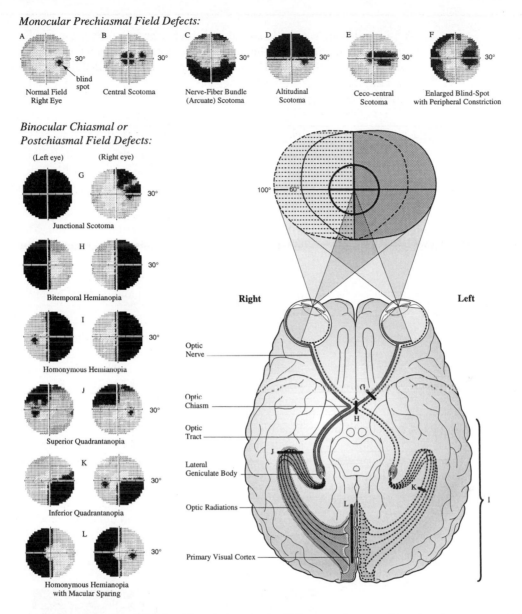

Monocular Prechiasmal Field Defects:

A
Normal Field
Right Eye
— blind spot
30°

B
Central Scotoma
30°

C
Nerve-Fiber Bundle
(Arcuate) Scotoma
30°

D
Altitudinal
Scotoma
30°

E
Ceco-central
Scotoma
30°

F
Enlarged Blind-Spot
with Peripheral Constriction
30°

Binocular Chiasmal or Postchiasmal Field Defects:

(Left eye)   (Right eye)

G
Junctional Scotoma
30°

H
Bitemporal Hemianopia
30°

I
Homonymous Hemianopia
30°

J
Superior Quadrantanopia
30°

K
Inferior Quadrantanopia
30°

L
Homonymous Hemianopia
with Macular Sparing
30°

Right   Left

100°   60°

Optic Nerve

Optic Chiasm

Optic Tract

Lateral Geniculate Body

Optic Radiations

Primary Visual Cortex

FIGURE 10-20. View of the visual fields and pathways. Lesion **I** illustrates the area affected in this patient with lesions possible in the left optic tract, the optic radiations, or the primary visual cortex. (Modified, with permission, from Kasper DL, et al. *Harrison's Principles of Internal Medicine*, 16th ed. New York: McGraw-Hill, 2005: 165.)

ORGAN SYSTEMS

NEUROLOGY

► **Case 17**

A 5-year-old boy is brought to the pediatrician by his mother for a follow-up appointment. Two months ago, the patient was seen for a chief complaint of morning headaches, vomiting, and decreased energy. A gastrointestinal illness was suspected. At this visit, the mother reports that her son continues to have worsened symptoms as well as new-onset falling and a stumbling gait.

■ What is the likely diagnosis?	The history is suggestive of a **medulloblastoma**, a highly malignant tumor most often found in the cerebellum. The majority of patients are between 4 and 8 years of age, with males being affected more than females. In children, 70% of intracranial tumors are infratentorial, while in adults 70% are supratentorial.
■ What tests or imaging tools may be used to confirm the diagnosis?	MRI is used to visualize the extent of the tumor. Medulloblastomas are seen as heterogenous enhancements in the cerebellum, often with invasion of the fourth ventricle. This can cause obstructive hydrocephalus. Figure 10-21 shows an MRI with tumor involvement of the cerebellum and destruction of the fourth ventricle.
■ This condition may present with what other syndrome?	The association of inherited colonic syndromes with brain tumors is named Turcot's syndrome. Patients with autosomal dominant familial adenomatous polyposis (FAP) are at risk for medulloblastomas and gliomas. Patients with hereditary nonpolyposis colorectal cancer (HNPCC) are at risk for development of gliomas only.
■ What is the morphology of this condition?	Medulloblastomas are rapidly-growing, well circumscribed, friable tumors found exclusively in the cerebellum. Microscopically, **Homer-Wright rosettes,** described as circular patterns of tumor cells surrounding a center of neutrophils, can be seen.
■ What is the most appropriate treatment for this condition?	Treatment consists of complete or near complete surgical excision followed by radiation and chemotherapy. Current treatment protocols are designed to minimize damage to adjacent structures and prolong survival.

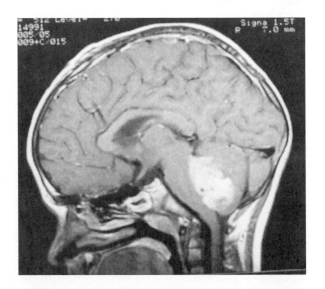

FIGURE 10-21. **Sagittal MRI illustrates medulloblastoma involving the cerebellum and fourth ventricle.** (Reproduced, with permission, from Ropper AH, et al. *Adams and Victor's Principles of Neurology,* 8th ed. New York: McGraw-Hill, 2005: 567.)

A 47-year-old woman is brought to the emergency department following a minor car accident. CT scan of the head with contrast reveals no intracranial hemorrhage. However, a spherical, 3-cm, bright enhancement abutting the falx cerebri is found incidentally. On physical examination, the patient has no neurologic deficits and denies headache, nausea, vomiting, and visual changes. MRI of the head is shown below in Figure 10-22.

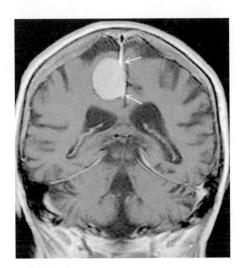

FIGURE 10-22. (Reproduced, with permission, from Kasper DL, et al. *Harrison's Principles of Internal Medicine*, 16th ed. New York: McGraw-Hill, 2005: 2456.)

■ What is the likely diagnosis?	The location of the lesion on MRI scan is typical for a **meningioma**. Meningiomas are usually benign slow-growing tumors arising from the arachnoid cells penetrating the dura. It is the second most common primary brain tumor.
■ Where are the lesions with this disease typically located?	Meningiomas are found along the dura, most often in the sylvian region, superior parasagittal region, and cerebellopontine angle. Other diseases also have a predilection for involving the dura, such as lymphoma, metastatic carcinoma, and tuberculosis.
■ What are the histologic findings in this condition?	Meningiomas display elongated spindle cells arranged concentrically in a whorled pattern, as well as psammoma bodies. Psammoma bodies are laminated, concentric calcified concretions formed by meningiomas (**head**), papillary adenocarcinomas of the thyroid (**neck**), malignant mesothelioma (**thorax**), and serous papillary cystadenocarcinoma of the ovary (**pelvis**).
■ What is the most appropriate treatment for this condition?	For small, slow-growing, and asymptomatic tumors, careful observation is appropriate. Surgical resection is indicated for symptomatic tumors or quickly growing tumors. Complete resection is often curative; however, tumors can recur if incompletely resected.
■ What other symptoms are common in patients presenting with this condition?	Because of their slow growth many meningiomas are picked up incidentally after neuroimaging for other reasons. However, large tumors may displace normal brain tissue and cause focal neurologic deficits such as visual disturbances, hearing loss, mental status changes, extremity weakness, obstructive hydrocephalus, and/or seizures.

ORGAN SYSTEMS

NEUROLOGY

► **Case 19**

A 10-year-old boy is brought to his pediatrician because of a painful ear. The pain began 1 week previously concurrent with a runny nose and sinus pressure that progressed to ear pain and dizziness. On otoscopic examination, the child's tympanic membrane is red and bulging. He has a low-grade fever of 37.8°C (100.0°F), but no other physical findings.

■ What is the most likely diagnosis?	Acute otitis media. The bulging, red tympanic membrane is a sign of middle ear infection. The clinical course is suggestive of a viral upper respiratory infection that led to secondary involvement of the middle ear due to inflammation and congestion of the eustachian tube, which connects the middle ear to the nasopharynx.
■ From what embryologic structure is the tympanic membrane derived?	The tympanic membrane is derived from the first pharyngeal membrane. The **pharyngeal membranes** are the tissue between the pharyngeal groove, or cleft, and pharyngeal pouch. Only the first pharyngeal membrane is retained in the adult; the rest are obliterated during development.
■ What three bones are located in the middle ear, and from what embryologic structures do they derive?	The three bones located in the middle ear (auditory ossicles) are the malleus, incus, and stapes (see Figure 10-23). They function to transmit sound from the tympanic membrane to the internal ear. The **malleus**, which articulates with the tympanic membrane, is derived from the first branchial arch. The **incus**, which lies between the malleus and the stapes, is derived from the first branchial arch. The **stapes**, which articulates with the oval window of the inner ear, is derived from the second branchial arch.
■ What two muscles control the movement of the bones of the middle ear, and what is their innervation?	The tensor tympani inserts on the malleus, and dampens the amplitude of the tympanic membrane oscillations, which prevents damage when the inner ear is exposed to loud sounds. Innervation is by the mandibular nerve (cranial nerve [CN] V3). The stapedius inserts onto the neck of the stapes, and dampens movement of this ossicle. It is innervated by the facial nerve (CN VII).
■ What organisms commonly cause pediatric ear infections?	In order of prevalence, common bacteria that cause middle ear infection are: *Streptococcus pneumoniae, Haemophilus influenzae* (although rarely type B since the introduction of the conjugated vaccine), and *Moraxella catarrhalis*. Less common organisms are group A streptococci, *Staphylococcus aureus, Pseudomonas*, and in newborns, gram-negative bacilli. Approximately 15%–20% of middle ear infections are due to viruses, including respiratory syncytial virus, rhinovirus, influenza viruses, and adenovirus.

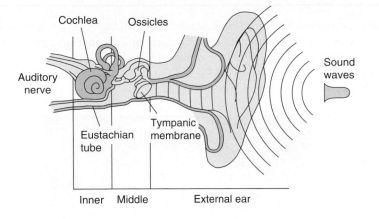

FIGURE 10-23. Anatomy of the ear. (Reproduced, with permission, from Lalwani AK. *Current Diagnosis & Treatment in Otolaryngology—Head & Neck Surgery.* 2nd ed. New York: McGraw-Hill, 2008: 578.)

► **Case 20**

A 54-year-old woman was successfully treated for small cell lung carcinoma 3 years ago. She received chemotherapy and radiation therapy and was declared disease-free via CT scan of the chest 1 year ago. She now comes to her primary care physician with a complaint of nausea, vomiting, and headaches worse on the right side for the past few weeks. A repeat CT scan is shown below in Figure 10-24.

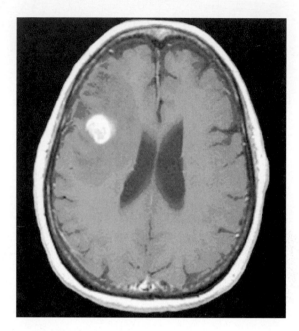

FIGURE 10-24. (Reproduced, with permission, from Kantarjian HM, et al. *MD Anderson Manual of Medical Oncology.* New York: McGraw-Hill, 2006: 797.)

■ **What is the most likely diagnosis?**	Metastatic brain tumor from her small cell lung carcinoma. Brain metastases are more prevalent than primary central nervous system tumors.
■ **What is the differential diagnosis for this condition?**	The differential diagnosis includes a primary brain tumor, metastatic tumor from a second primary, infection, cerebral infarct, or radiation necrosis.
■ **What types of cancer most often metastasize to the brain?**	**L**ung, **B**reast, **S**kin (melanoma), **K**idney (renal cell carcinoma), and **G**astrointestinal, for the mnemonic **L**ots of **B**ad **S**tuff **K**ills **G**lia. Each of these tumors can spread hematogenously to the brain.
■ **Where are these lesions usually located in the brain?**	Metastases are supratentorial, located at the **gray-white matter junction** where the arterial vessels narrow sufficiently for tumor cells to lodge (see Figure 10-24). They are also found at **watershed areas**, or vascular territories situated between two supplying arteries (e.g., middle cerebral artery and anterior cerebral artery).
■ **What are the common symptoms of this condition?**	Symptoms include headaches, seizures, stroke, nausea, vomiting, cognitive dysfunction such as personality changes, and focal neurologic deficits such as aphasia or weakness.
■ **What tests and/or imaging tools could be used to confirm the diagnosis?**	MRI is the imaging modality of choice because of its superior sensitivity for soft tissue. Biopsy of the lesion is often indicated to confirm the diagnosis before a definitive treatment plan is chosen.

An 18-year-old woman goes to her family physician for an evaluation of severe headaches. She describes her headaches as unilateral, beginning with a dull and steady ache and increasing in severity to a throbbing, debilitating pain after several hours. No aura is associated with the headaches, but they are exacerbated by motion and light. Consequently, the patient prefers to remain in a dark room when her headaches occur. She also states this is the second episode she has had; the first episode occurred approximately 4 weeks ago and dissipated within a few days.

■ **What is the most likely diagnosis?**	Migraine headache. Further questioning may reveal that the 4-week interval coincides with menstruation, which is a typical trigger of migraine in young women.
■ **What signs and symptoms are commonly associated with this condition?**	Migraines are unilateral in 60%–70% of cases, while the remaining cases are typically bifrontal or, less frequently, bioccipital. The pain often begins with the gradual onset of a deep, steady ache that crescendos within several hours to a pulsatile, severe pain. Migraines are typically worsened by movement, loud noises, and bright lights. Although **auras** (temporary neurologic symptoms such as light flashes, zigzag lines, or numbness and tingling in the arms and face) are commonly associated with migraine headaches, they are actually seen in only 20% of cases.
■ **How is this condition differentiated from other, more serious pathologic conditions of the head?**	Warning signs that a headache may be serious include: ■ Absence of similar episodes in the past ■ Association with vigorous exercise or trauma (suggestive of carotid dissection) ■ Change in mental status ■ Concurrent infection ■ Sudden onset within seconds to minutes (suggestive of subarachnoid hemorrhage) Physical findings pointing to potentially serious pathology include nuchal rigidity (meningitis), poor general appearance, or papilledema (elevated intracranial pressure).
■ **How can this woman's headache be differentiated from cluster or tension headaches?**	**Tension headaches** are typically bilateral and are often described as a band-like tightness or pressure (as if the patient were wearing a tight hat). They are typically not debilitating, and the pressure waxes and wanes over an unpredictable time course. Tension headaches are closely associated with stress. **Cluster headaches** typically occur in males and are always unilateral. The pain often begins around the eye or temple, is sudden in onset (and could thus be mistaken for subarachnoid hemorrhage), and is described as deep and persistent. The pain often lasts for several hours and can be associated with tearing of the eyes and sweating.
■ **What are the most appropriate treatments for this condition?**	Possible treatments include nonsteroidal anti-inflammatory agents (especially indomethacin), acetaminophen, triptans (i.e., sumatriptan, a serotonin agonist), and less typically ergotamine agents (i.e., dihydroergotamine). For more frequent, chronic migraines, daily treatment with β-blockers such as propranolol or calcium channel blockers such as verapamil can be effective in prevention.

► **Case 22**

A 28-year-old previously healthy woman comes to the physician complaining of weakness in her legs, urinary incontinence, and difficulty speaking. She has also noticed a slight tremor in her hand when she attempts to eat. She says her symptoms have worsened over the previous 4 weeks. She denies any history of fever or vomiting and has no other health problems. Upon questioning, she recalls her mother had similar symptoms when she was young. Physical examination reveals left-sided facial droop, left tongue deviation, and lateral gaze weakness. An MRI is shown in Figure 10-25. Relevant laboratory findings are as follows:

WBC count: 9100/mm³
Hemoglobin: 13.3 g/dL
Hematocrit: 37.1%
Platelet count: 287,000/mm³
Cerebrospinal fluid (CSF) IgG index: 0.89 (normal <0.66)

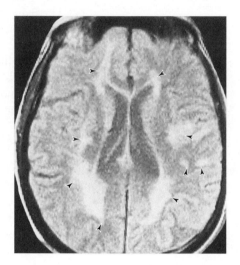

FIGURE 10-25. (Reproduced, with permission, from Waxman SG. *Clinical Neuroanatomy*, 25th ed. New York: McGraw-Hill, 2003: 307.)

▪ **What is the most likely diagnosis?**	Multiple sclerosis (MS). The arrowheads in Figure 10-25 show the lesions of MS.
▪ **What risk factors are associated with this condition?**	▪ Age 20–50 years (mean age of onset is 30 years) ▪ Female gender (female:male ratio 1.77:1.00) ▪ Having been raised in a temperate climate ▪ Having a family history of MS
▪ **What anatomic finding could explain the findings on physical examination?**	A **medial brain stem lesion** involving cranial nerves VI, VII, and XII (see Figure 10-26) would lead to the constellation of facial droop, tongue deviation, and lateral gaze weakness. The intention tremor indicates cerebellar involvement.
▪ **What are the typical CSF findings in this condition?**	**Oligoclonal bands** are seen in 85%–95% of cases. The presence of these immunoglobulins reflects the autoimmune nature of the disease. Similarly, the **IgG index** is elevated in >90% of patients with definite MS. The total CSF WBC count is normal in most patients, so an elevated WBC count is nonspecific.

What is the likely finding on imaging of the brain?

Multiple **demyelinating plaques** are usually present in the brains of patients with MS, especially in the periventricular region, corpus callosum, and centrum semiovale.

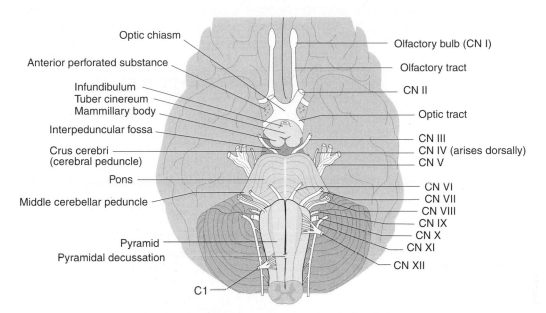

CNs that lie medially at brainstem: III, VI, XII. 3(×2) = 6(×2) = 12.

FIGURE 10-26. Brain stem anatomy. (Reproduced, with permission, from Le T, Bhushan V, Rao DA. *First Aid for the USMLE Step 1: 2008.* New York: McGraw-Hill, 2008: 374.)

▶ **Case 23**

A 12-year-old boy is seen by the dermatologist for numerous skin lesions. Physical examination reveals 10 separate uniformly hyperpigmented macules, 15–25 mm in diameter, scattered over the patient's trunk and limbs. Freckling is present in both armpits and recently dozens of soft, skin-colored, domed nodules on the patient's back have appeared. The dermatologist notes kyphosis and refers the patient for further evaluation by an ophthalmologist.

■ **What is the likely diagnosis?**	Neurofibromatosis type 1 (NF1), or von Recklinghausen's disease, is a common neurocutaneous disorder. NF1 has complete penetrance with variable expression. Diagnosis is made on clinical criteria.
■ **What are the genetics of this condition?**	NF1 is an autosomal dominant disorder caused by mutation in the *NF1* gene found on chromosome **17**. About half of the cases of NF1 are familial and the rest represent new mutations. NF1 codes for the protein neurofibromin, and is thought to be a tumor suppressor gene. **Hint:** "von Recklinghausen" has **17 letters** and is located on chromosome **17**.
■ **What are the typical dermatologic findings of this condition?**	The hallmark is six or more hyperpigmented macules called **café-au-lait** spots. In addition, **neurofibromas**, multiple soft fleshy tumors, usually develop during adolescence. Both can be seen in Figure 10-27. **Freckling** is also present in the axilla and groin.

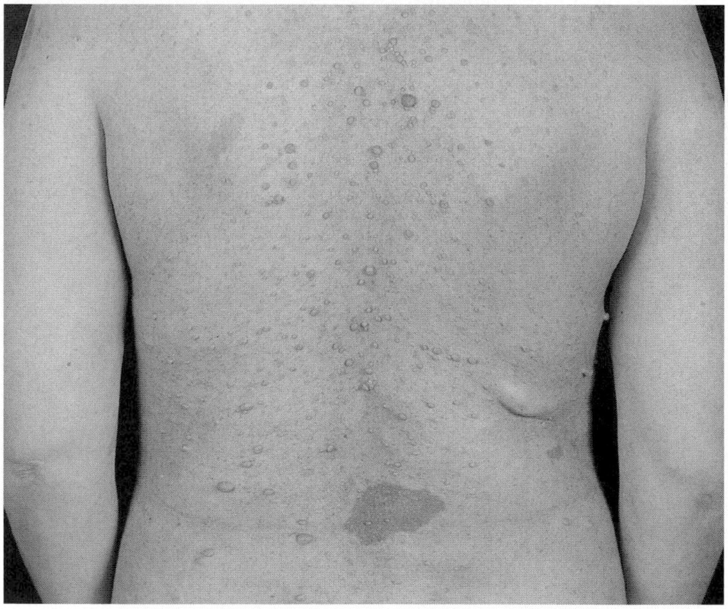

FIGURE 10-27. The multiple small skin-colored papules seen here are neurofibromas. The large hyperpigmented macule is a café-au-lait spot. (Reproduced, with permission, from Wolff K, et al. *Fitzpatrick's Color Atlas & Synopsis of Clinical Dermatology*, 5th ed. New York: McGraw-Hill, 2005: 465.)

▪ What are the typical ophthalmologic findings in this condition?	**Lisch nodules**, which are raised, pigmented, hamartomas, are found on the iris (see Figure 10-28).
▪ Patients with this condition are predisposed to what tumors?	Patients are susceptible to **optic gliomas**, which may arise anywhere along the optic tract, particularly in the optic nerve or chiasm. Patients are also at increased risk for other central nervous system tumors such as astrocytomas and gliomas. Peripheral neurofibromas can undergo malignant transformation into neurofibrosarcomas.

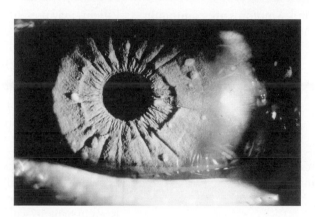

FIGURE 10-28. Multiple hamartomas (Lisch nodules) can be seen on the iris of this patient with neurofibromatosis type 1. (Reproduced, with permission, from Ropper AH, et al. *Adams and Victor's Principles of Neurology*, 8th ed. New York: McGraw-Hill, 2005: 870.)

▶ **Case 24**

A 25-year-old woman presents to her physician with difficulty chewing and swallowing her food. She also complains of occasional double vision. She states her symptoms are often absent in the morning and appear to worsen as the day progresses.

▪ **What is the most likely diagnosis?**	Myasthenia gravis.
▪ **What patient characteristics are typically associated with this diagnosis?**	Myasthenia gravis is more commonly seen in men than in women, and most patients are >50 years old when diagnosed.
▪ **What signs and symptoms are commonly associated with this condition?**	Patients may present with a variety of findings, including ptosis, diplopia, dysarthria, difficulty chewing, and difficulty swallowing. Proximal muscle weakness is usually greater than distal muscle weakness. Weakness increases with use of the muscles.
▪ **What is the pathophysiology of this condition?**	Patients develop antibodies directed toward **acetylcholine** receptors. Because of a higher threshold of activation by acetylcholine, signal transmission across the neuromuscular junction is decreased. This process leads to muscle weakness.
▪ **What tumor is commonly associated with this condition?**	Myasthenia gravis has been associated with an increased frequency of **thymomas.** It is thought that the thymus is the site of production of autoantibodies against acetylcholine receptors. Even in patients with no thymus neoplasm, **thymectomy** has been shown to improve symptoms in 85% of cases.
▪ **How would the clinical presentation differ in a patient with autoantibodies against presynaptic voltage-gated calcium channels?**	**Lambert-Eaton syndrome** presents in a similar manner and is associated with small cell lung cancer. However, symptoms usually **decrease** with muscle use as more calcium is released. This is in contrast to myasthenia gravis, in which weakness **increases** with muscle use.

► **Case 25**

A 66-year-old man presents to his physician with a new-onset tremor in his right hand that worsens when he is watching television. He has also been experiencing some difficulty walking, and his friends complain that he has not been able to keep up with them on the golf course. His wife has noticed he does not seem to get excited about anything.

■ What is the most likely diagnosis?

Parkinson's disease. Parkinson's disease typically presents with symptoms described by the mnemonic **TRAP: T**remor that is worse at rest, **R**igidity, **A**kinesia or bradykinesia, and **P**ostural instability.

■ What neuropathologic findings are associated with this condition?

Parkinson's disease is marked by significant neuronal loss in the **substantia nigra**, which leads to decreased dopaminergic input into the basal ganglia. Characteristic findings include depigmentation of neurons in the substantia nigra and concentric eosinophilic cytoplasmic inclusions called **Lewy bodies** (see Figure 10-29).

■ How does a loss of dopamine release from the substantia nigra lead to a decrease in movement?

Dopamine activates the direct motor pathway in the basal ganglia and inhibits the indirect pathway. Normally, dopamine inhibits the inhibitory motor output from the globus pallidus interna (GPi) via these pathways. Decreased dopamine levels in Parkinson's disease due to substantia nigra compacta (SNc) degeneration result in increased inhibitory output from the GPi and substantia nigra reticulata (SNr) and subsequent bradykinesia.

■ What symptoms are likely to develop over time in this patient?

As the disease progresses, additional symptoms that may develop include shuffling gait, masked facies, and dementia.

■ What are the most appropriate treatments for this condition?

Carbidopa can be used with levodopa in the treatment of Parkinson's disease. Carbidopa, a peripheral dopa decarboxylase inhibitor, reduces peripheral conversion of levodopa. This augments its action in the central nervous system and reduces its action outside the central nervous system (where levodopa can cause arrhythmias and dyskinesias). Pramipexole and bromocriptine, which are direct dopaminergic agonists, can also be used to augment dopamine signaling.

■ What other etiologies might result in a similar presentation?

Typical antipsychotic agents have antidopaminergic activity. Thus, patients taking these medications for schizophrenia can exhibit Parkinson-like symptoms. 1-Methyl-4-phenyl-1,2,3,6-tetrahydropyridine (MPTP) and antiemetic agents can also induce parkinsonian symptoms.

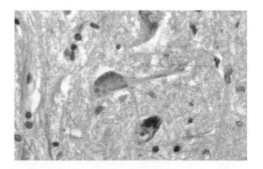

FIGURE 10-29. Lewy bodies in Parkinson's disease. (Reproduced, with permission, of the Pathology Education Instructional Resource Digital Library [http://peir.net] at the University of Alabama, Birmingham.)

► **Case 26**

A 16-year-old boy complains of progressive hearing loss in both ears. His hearing has been deteriorating over the last several months, and this has been accompanied by ringing in his ears (tinnitus). The pediatrician notices hyperpigmented macules on the patient's arms and legs. MRI of the head is shown in Figure 10-30.

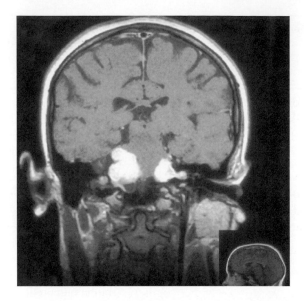

FIGURE 10-30. (Reproduced, with permission, from Riordan-Eva P, et al. *Vaughn & Asbury's General Ophthalmology*, 17th ed. New York: McGraw-Hill, 2008: 301.)

■ What is the likely diagnosis?	**Neurofibromatosis type 2 (NF2)**, an autosomal dominant disorder whose hallmark is bilateral acoustic neuromas.
■ What is the pathogenesis of this condition?	Mutation of the gene *merlin* found on chromosome **22**. Type 2 = 22. *Merlin* codes for a protein involved in cytoskeleton components responsible for contact inhibition of tumor progression.
■ What other signs and symptoms are common in patients with this condition?	Blurry or cloudy vision due to juvenile cataracts is also seen in NF2. Patients may also present with similar skin findings as those seen in neurofibromatosis type 1, such as café-au-lait spots.
■ What are the two forms of hearing loss?	**Conductive hearing loss,** which is hearing loss involving the ear canal, tympanic membrane, middle ear, and ossicles. **Sensorineural hearing loss,** which is hearing loss involving the inner ear (cochlea), vestibulocochlear nerve, or central processing centers in the brain.

■ **How do the Weber and Rinne tests distinguish between the two forms of hearing loss?**

In the **Weber** test, a vibrating tuning fork is placed in the center of the patient's cranium. A patient with **unilateral conductive** hearing loss will have lateralization to the **affected ear** (i.e., the tone will be louder in the affected ear). A patient with unilateral sensorineural hearing loss will have lateralization to the unaffected ear.

In the **Rinne** test, a vibrating tuning fork is placed on the mastoid process behind the ear (bone conduction; BC) and then next to the external auditory canal (air conduction; AC). Normally AC is greater than BC. A patient with **conductive** hearing loss will "hear" the vibration louder when the tuning fork is on the mastoid process, than when placed by the external auditory canal (**BC > AC**). In a patient with sensorineural hearing loss the normal relationship (AC > BC) will be preserved. This patient has **bilateral** sensorineural hearing loss and would test normal in both examinations.

A 36-year-old woman presents to her primary care physician with a 6-month history of occasional milky discharge from her breasts, chronic headaches, and decreased libido. Her past medical history reveals long-standing amenorrhea and infertility. The patient denies any visual disturbances. Laboratory tests reveal a negative urine pregnancy test, a normal thyroid-stimulating hormone level, and a prolactin level of 88 µg/L (normal 5–20 µg/L).

■ What is the most likely diagnosis?	**Hyperprolactinemia** from a prolactin-secreting anterior pituitary adenoma. Classic symptoms in females are amenorrhea, infertility, and galactorrhea.
■ What is the differential diagnosis of a mass in the sella turcica?	The differential diagnosis includes pituitary adenoma, pituitary hyperplasia, craniopharyngioma, meningioma, germ cell tumor, chordoma, primary lymphoma, cyst, abscess, or arteriovenous fistula of the cavernous sinus.
■ What is the pathogenesis of elevated prolactin levels in this condition?	**Dopamine** secreted from the hypothalamus travels to the anterior pituitary where it inhibits prolactin secretion. A mass in the pituitary may compress the infundibulum, causing a "stalk effect," in which dopamine cannot reach its target. Thus, prolactin is continuously secreted. Physiologic hyperprolactinemia may occur during **pregnancy.** You must always rule out pregnancy in any female who presents with amenorrhea!
■ What other hormones are secreted from the anterior pituitary?	Adrenocorticotropic hormone (ACTH), thyroid-stimulating hormone (TSH), growth hormone (GH), luteinizing hormone (LH), and follicle-stimulating hormone (FSH) are also secreted. Although prolactinomas are the most common hyperfunctioning tumor, a pituitary adenoma may secrete any of the above hormones.
■ What is the most appropriate treatment for this condition?	Reduction in tumor size, suppression of prolactin secretion, and return of menses are usually accomplished with a dopamine agonist such as **bromocriptine** or cabergoline. Both are ergot derivatives that act directly on dopamine receptors in the hypothalamus to decrease prolactin secretion. When medical management is no longer effective or the mass is very large, transsphenoidal surgery with resection of a large hyperfunctioning sellar mass is typically undertaken.
■ What visual disturbance is classically seen with this condition?	**Bitemporal hemianopia** results when the growing pituitary tumor impinges on the optic chiasm (see Figure 10-31).

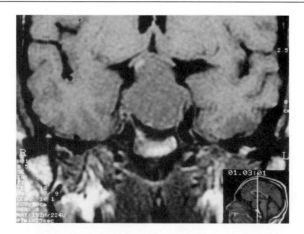

FIGURE 10-31. Pituitary adenoma. MRI showing a pituitary mass elevating the optic chiasm, causing bitemporal hemianopia. (Reproduced, with permission, from Riordan-Eva P, et al. *Vaughn & Asbury's General Ophthalmology*, 17th ed. New York: McGraw-Hill, 2008: 280.)

ORGAN SYSTEMS

NEUROLOGY

► **Case 28**

An emergency medical team is called to help a 30-year-old woman who is unconscious at work. Her coworkers state that before she became unconscious, for the first 10 seconds or so she pointed to her right hand as it began twitching rhythmically, then stiffened every muscle and fell down. After about 15 seconds, she became incontinent and started jerking her arms and legs rhythmically for a few minutes. She then lay still, unresponsive and unconscious, for about 3 minutes. The medical team notes she is now breathing deeply but remains unresponsive.

■ **What is the most likely diagnosis?**	Seizure. Involvement of the left motor cortex is implicated, because the seizure started with a right-handed motor activity.
■ **How is this condition classified?**	This is a simple partial seizure with motor signs secondarily generalizing into a tonic-clonic seizure. During the first 10 seconds, the patient maintained consciousness, pointing to a **"simple" seizure** ("complex" seizures require a loss of consciousness). After the first 10 seconds, her simple partial seizure evolved into a generalized tonic-clonic seizure. The **tonic phase** is characterized by the immobile contraction of all muscles, and the **clonic phase** is characterized by the bilateral rhythmic jerking of the extremities.
■ **Why is the woman breathing deeply after her incident?**	The patient is likely responding to acidosis. A **respiratory acidosis** can develop from the loss of coordinated respirations during the seizure, and a **metabolic acidosis** can develop as muscles contract under anaerobic conditions and produce lactic acid.
■ **What is the most appropriate treatment for this condition?**	Popular antiseizure medications include valproic acid, phenytoin, phenobarbital, primidone, and carbamazepine. Many antiseizure medications work by enhancing γ-aminobutyric acid (GABA) binding on chloride channels. GABA binding allows chloride ions to flow into neurons, thereby inhibiting neuronal firing. Barbiturates act on the same chloride channel as does GABA, and enhances GABA signaling by increasing the **duration** of chloride channel opening. Benzodiazepines act on the same channel and enhance GABA signaling, but they do so by increasing the **frequency** of chloride channel opening.
■ **What are the most common adverse effects of these medications?**	■ Valproate: Hepatotoxicity, neutropenia, thrombocytopenia, teratogenicity (neural tube defects in the fetus). ■ Carbamazepine: Hepatotoxicity (must check liver function), aplastic anemia, agranulocytosis. ■ Phenytoin: Gingival hyperplasia, teratogenicity. ■ Ethosuximide and lamotrigine: Stevens-Johnson syndrome (a bullous form of erythema multiforme that involves mucous membranes and large areas of the body). ■ Carbamazepine and phenobarbital: Induction of cytochrome P450, resulting in drug interactions.

▶ **Case 29**

A 72-year-old woman is at home with her husband when he notices she sounds confused even though she had been speaking clearly just moments before. He brings her into the emergency department, where she is unable to follow commands. Her speech is fluent but does not make any sense. A CT scan of the head is shown in Figure 10-32.

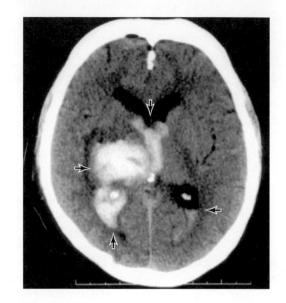

FIGURE 10-32. (Reproduced, with permission, from Aminoff MJ, Greenberg DA, Simon RP. *Clinical Neurology*, 6th ed. New York: McGraw-Hill, 2005: 315.)

▪ **What is the most likely diagnosis?**	Stroke. Figure 10-32 shows extensive hemorrhage in the thalamus (left arrow) and its extension into the third (top arrow), ipsilateral (bottom arrow), and lateral ventricles (right arrow).
▪ **What risk factors are associated with this condition?**	▪ Advanced age ▪ Cardiovascular disease ▪ Carotid disease ▪ Diabetes mellitus ▪ Dyslipidemia ▪ Family or personal history of transient ischemic attack or stroke ▪ Hypertension ▪ Smoking
▪ **What type of aphasia does the patient exhibit?**	The combination of fluent but nonsensical speech with poor comprehension is characteristic of **Wernicke's aphasia** (sensory aphasia). These patients also display poor repetition and naming ability. Other findings commonly associated with Wernicke's aphasia include contralateral visual field cut (due to ischemia of optic radiation) and **anosognosia** (unawareness of one's deficit).
▪ **A lesion in what anatomic area would cause these findings?**	Wernicke's aphasia is usually the result of ischemia in the superior temporal gyrus, which is supplied by the inferior division of the left middle cerebral artery.

- **What speech pattern would result if this condition affected the inferior frontal gyrus?**

The inferior frontal gyrus controls motor aspects of speech. A stroke in this area would cause **Broca's aphasia** (motor aphasia), which is characterized by nonfluent, agrammatic speech. Due to the proximity of the primary motor cortex for the face and arm, **dysarthria** (difficulty in articulating words) and right face and arm weakness are often associated with Broca's aphasia. Comprehension is intact in these patients.

- **If the patient had nail-bed hemorrhages, nodules on her fingers and toes, and retinal hemorrhages, what diagnosis should be considered?**

This constellation of symptoms suggests the diagnosis of **infective endocarditis**, which is characterized by splinter hemorrhages, Osler's nodes on the pads of the fingers and toes, and Roth's spots on the retina. Infective endocarditis can lead to the release of thrombi from the valvular vegetations, resulting in embolic events.

▶ **Case 30**

A 35-year-old woman presents to the emergency department complaining of back pain. Six years ago, she was diagnosed with a 2.5-cm primary breast tumor with metastases to one axillary lymph node. At that time, she underwent a mastectomy and adjuvant chemotherapy. She had been feeling well until 3 months ago, when she began to develop back pain. The pain has become progressively worse, particularly when she lies down. She also notes some weakness in both legs but no leg pain. She denies fever, night sweats, weight loss, or headache. Physical examination reveals no cervical lymphadenopathy; 4/5 muscle strength in the lower extremities bilaterally; normal pain, vibration, and position sensation; 3+ patellar reflexes bilaterally; a positive Babinski's reflex on the right; and normal anal sphincter tone.

▪ What are common causes of back pain?	▪ Musculoskeletal (e.g., muscle strain, osteoarthritis, compression fracture, or ankylosing spondylitis). ▪ Disk herniation. ▪ Metastases. ▪ Osteomyelitis. ▪ Referred pain from visceral disease (e.g., gallstones or kidney stones, pancreatitis, or aortic aneurysm).
▪ What is the likely cause of this patient's back pain?	The patient's history of breast cancer raises concern for the development of metastases resulting in epidural **spinal cord compression.** Her leg weakness, hyperreflexia, and positive Babinski's signs indicate upper motor neuron lesions, which are likely the cause of her weakness as well. Her pain at rest and lack of sciatica argue against disk herniation.
▪ How would signs of upper motor neuron lesions contrast with those of lower motor neuron lesions?	As in this patient, upper motor lesions are characterized by spastic paralysis, hyperreflexia, and a positive Babinski's sign. In contrast, lower motor neuron lesions are associated with flaccid paralysis, muscle atrophy, muscle fasciculations and fibrillations, and hyporeflexia.
▪ What are the most common metastases to bone?	The most common sources of bone metastases are cancers of the breast, prostate, lung, and kidney (renal cell carcinoma).
▪ What are the most appropriate treatments for this condition?	Treatment options include steroids such as dexamethasone, radiation therapy, and surgical decompression. Spinal cord compression is an oncologic emergency because neurologic dysfunction, if present, may become permanent if it is not immediately addressed.

A mother brings a 16-month-old girl to the neurologist for evaluation of new-onset seizures and right-sided hemiparesis. The seizures are tonic-clonic in nature and began at the same time as the hemiparesis. The infant has a port-wine stain on her left face in the distribution of the ophthalmic branch of the trigeminal nerve. The infant has also failed to meet developmental milestones for her age.

■ What is the likely diagnosis?	Sturge-Weber syndrome, a rare congenital disorder with unknown etiology. The disorder is manifested by vascular malformations of the skin (**port-wine stain**) and leptomeninges.
■ What other tests or imaging tools could be used to confirm the diagnosis?	MRI is most useful for identifying a leptomeningeal angioma. Often these tumors are ipsilateral to the port-wine stain. These lesions are responsible for the seizures, hemiparesis, and mental retardation.
■ What ocular features may be present in this condition?	Many patients may also have **glaucoma. Heterochromia** of the iris (the irises are different colors), visual field defects, and vascular malformations of the choroid may also be present.
■ What is the most appropriate treatment for this condition?	Treatment is aimed at alleviating symptoms. Port-wine stains (see Figure 10-33) may be treated with laser therapy. Seizures can be managed with anticonvulsants. Patients with seizures refractory to pharmacotherapy may undergo surgical resection of the lesion, often involving a hemispherectomy of the affected side.

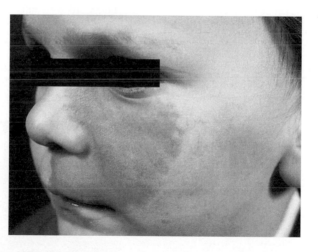

FIGURE 10-33. **This young child has a port-wine stain in the distribution of the second branch of the trigeminal nerve.** Patients with Sturge-Weber syndrome usually have port-wine stains on the forehead in the distribution of the **first** branch of the trigeminal nerve. (Reproduced, with permission, from Wolff K, et al. *Fitzpatrick's Color Atlas & Synopsis of Clinical Dermatology*, 5th ed. New York: McGraw-Hill, 2005: 187.)

▶ **Case 32**

A 43-year-old woman with a history of hypertension presents to her physician with a severe headache. She says this is the most painful headache she has ever experienced. The headache began this morning while she was watching television. She also had two episodes of vomiting earlier in the day. She denies any traumatic events. Cardiac examination reveals a midsystolic click with a late systolic murmur at the apex. A CT scan of the head is shown in Figure 10-34.

■ What is the most likely diagnosis?	Subarachnoid hemorrhage (see arrows in Figure 10-34).
■ What are some common etiologies of this condition?	Most spontaneous subarachnoid hemorrhages occur in the **circle of Willis** (commonly at the bifurcation of the middle cerebral artery) as a result of the rupture of a berry aneurysm (see Figure 10-35; the arrowhead points to a berry aneurysm) or an arteriovenous malformation. The risk is increased by a history of hypertension. The most common location of a **berry aneurysm** is the anterior communicating artery, then the posterior communicating artery, followed by the middle cerebral artery. Trauma causes more subarachnoid hemorrhages than spontaneous ruptures do.
■ Given this patient's symptoms, what is the pathophysiology of this condition?	The murmur on cardiac examination is characteristic of mitral valve prolapse, which is commonly seen in **Marfan's syndrome.** Berry aneurysms have been associated with Marfan's syndrome, Ehlers-Danlos syndrome, adult polycystic kidney disease, and coarctation of the aorta.
■ What are the typical findings on cerebrospinal fluid (CSF) analysis?	The CSF is usually bloody with a xanthochromic or yellow supernatant, reflecting bilirubin release from the breakdown of hemoglobin.
■ Why was the patient vomiting?	Vomiting is a common sign of increased intracerebral pressure, which in this patient would be secondary to the hemorrhage.

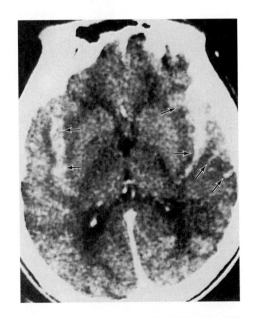

FIGURE 10-34. (Reproduced, with permission, from Waxman SG. *Clinical Neuroanatomy*, 25th ed. New York: McGraw-Hill, 2003: 186.)

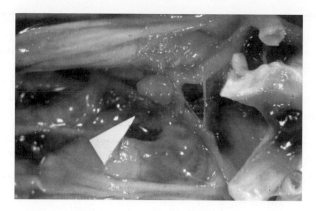

FIGURE 10-35. Berry aneurysm. (Reproduced, with permission, of the Pathology Education Instructional Resource Digital Library [http://peir.net] at the University of Alabama, Birmingham.)

► **Case 33**

A 77-year-old man falls while climbing the stairs to his apartment. He temporarily loses consciousness and awakens with a mild headache. His relatives do not notice any problems until 3 weeks later, when they begin to note a change in his mental status. Typically a personable man, he starts to yell at his family members for no reason and does not recognize people he knows well. He is brought to the emergency department, where a CT scan of the head is obtained (see Figure 10-36).

■ What is the most likely diagnosis?	This is a common history for a chronic subdural hematoma. The diagnosis is confirmed by CT scan (see Figure 10-36), which shows a crescent-shaped area of hemorrhage that crosses cranial suture lines.
■ What is the source of bleeding in this type of injury?	Subdural hematomas result from head trauma that causes venous bleeding, most commonly from bridging veins within the dura, which then bleed into the space between the arachnoid and dura mater.
■ What would explain the delayed onset of symptoms?	Symptoms in chronic subdural hematoma result from an expanding blood accumulation, which slowly and progressively compresses the cerebrum. Deficits in central nervous system functioning may be delayed depending on when specific intracranial areas are affected by the compression.
■ What would one expect to see on CT scan if the patient experienced no loss of consciousness, followed shortly thereafter by mental status changes?	This scenario is more consistent with an **epidural hematoma.** The CT scan of an epidural hematoma (see Figure 10-37) usually shows a biconcave disk formation that does not cross suture lines. The most common source of bleeding in epidural hematoma is lacerations of the middle meningeal artery.

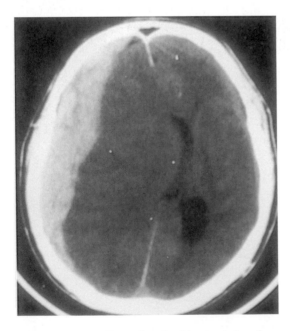

FIGURE 10-36. (Reproduced, with permission, from Aminoff MJ, Greenberg DA, Simon RP. *Clinical Neurology,* 6th ed. New York: McGraw-Hill, 2005: 329.)

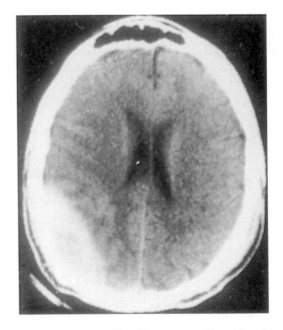

FIGURE 10-37. Epidural hematoma. (Reproduced, with permission, from Aminoff J, Greenberg DA, Simon RP. *Clinical Neurology.* 6th ed. New York: McGraw-Hill, 2005: 329.)

A 61-year-old man with a history of chronic diarrhea presents to the emergency department after fainting. He reports he suddenly collapsed after getting up to go to the bathroom. He did not note any prodromal symptoms or vertigo. The patient has spent the past few days recovering from the flu, during which time he has had a poor appetite. He denies a history of seizures and has no known cardiac or valvular abnormalities. On admission, his blood pressure is 115/80 mm Hg supine and 90/70 mm Hg standing. His pulse is 88/min, and his respiratory rate is 20/min.

▪ What is the most likely diagnosis?	Syncope.
▪ What signs of volume depletion are evident on physical examination?	Orthostatic hypotension, tachycardia, tachypnea, dry mucous membranes, and decreased skin turgor are evident on physical examination.
▪ What are the major causes of this condition?	In order of decreasing frequency: ▪ Vasovagal reflex. ▪ Cardiogenic causes (including arrhythmias, aortic stenosis, tamponade, pulmonary embolism, and aortic dissection). ▪ Neurogenic causes (including transient ischemic attack, migraine, and seizure). ▪ Orthostatic hypotension. ▪ Medications. No cause can be determined in many cases.
▪ What is the most likely cause of this condition in this patient?	The most likely cause of syncope in this patient is orthostatic hypotension secondary to poor food and water intake and chronic diarrhea.
▪ What is the Bezold-Jarisch reflex?	An increase in sympathetic tone induces a vigorous ventricular contraction, leading to a reflex increase in vagal tone. This reflex reaction (the so-called **Bezold-Jarisch reflex**) leads to a decrease in heart rate and/or blood pressure via the vagus nerve.
▪ How does the vascular system compensate for the decrease in venous return following an orthostatic change?	Mechanoreceptors in the heart react to the decrease in blood pressure and compensate by increasing sympathetic tone, which decreases vagal tone and increases release of antidiuretic hormone. This results in increased peripheral vascular resistance (increasing venous return) and an increase in cardiac output, thereby minimizing the drop in blood pressure.

A 57-year-old obese, right-handed man with a history of atrial fibrillation and mitral valve repair is brought to the emergency department by a coworker, who noticed a sudden onset of slurred speech and hand clumsiness. The coworker states the man's speech suddenly became slow, as if he had trouble finding words, as well as slurred. The coworker also notes the patient was generally confused but able to understand and follow commands, and he denied seeing any seizure-like activity or loss of consciousness. The patient denies any recent head trauma. Physical examination reveals an irregularly irregular heartbeat and a left carotid bruit. Neurologic examination reveals the patient's cranial nerves are grossly intact with the exception of mildly decreased facial sensation on the right. He has 4/5 muscle strength in his extremities and diminished sensation in the right arm. A CT scan of the head is negative for bleeding or mass lesion. The patient's symptoms resolve spontaneously within 2 hours of their onset.

■ **What is the most likely diagnosis?**	Transient ischemic attack.
■ **What is the most likely cause of this condition in this patient?**	This is most likely an **embolic stroke**, as the patient has several risk factors for emboli: ■ Carotid stenosis, presumably from atherosclerosis, which can be a source of emboli. ■ History of atrial fibrillation, which can predispose to embolus formation. ■ Mitral valve repair, which can harbor vegetations that may embolize.
■ **What findings on CT scan of the head suggest the presence of cerebral edema?**	Signs of cerebral edema include loss of the gray matter–white matter junction; loss of prominence of sulci; and evidence of a mass effect, such as midline shift, decreased size of the lateral ventricles, and uncal herniation.
■ **What artery supplies the affected area of the brain in this patient?**	The patient experienced right-hand clumsiness, suggesting a left hemisphere event (motor fibers cross at the pyramidal decussation at the level of the midbrain; see Figure 10-38 for a review of the circle of Willis). His speech deficit also suggests a compromise of blood to his left hemisphere, as the verbal center in most right-handed individuals is in the left hemisphere. The left middle cerebral artery, supplying the motor cortex and verbal centers, is the most likely culprit in this patient.
■ **What are the components of a neurologic language examination?**	■ **Comprehension:** This is disrupted in patients with Wernicke's aphasia. ■ **Speech production, or fluency:** This is disrupted in patients with Broca's aphasia. ■ **Repetition.** ■ **Naming.**

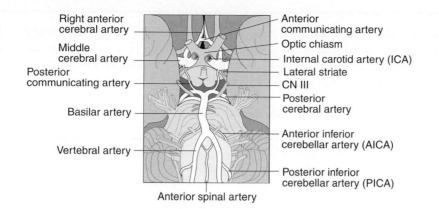

Right anterior cerebral artery

Middle cerebral artery

Posterior communicating artery

Basilar artery

Vertebral artery

Anterior communicating artery

Optic chiasm

Internal carotid artery (ICA)

Lateral striate

CN III

Posterior cerebral artery

Anterior inferior cerebellar artery (AICA)

Posterior inferior cerebellar artery (PICA)

Anterior spinal artery

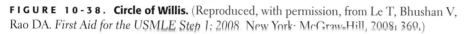

FIGURE 10-38. Circle of Willis. (Reproduced, with permission, from Le T, Bhushan V, Rao DA. *First Aid for the USMLE Step 1; 2008.* New York: McGraw-Hill, 2008; 369.)

▶ **Case 36**

A 6-year-old boy with a history of mental retardation and seizures is brought by his mother to the pediatrician for an evaluation of skin lesions. The pediatrician notes firm, discrete brown papules in the nasolabial folds and on the cheeks. Further examination reveals an elliptical, hypopigmented macule on the patient's abdomen and a pinkish-brown plaque with a cobblestone appearance on his lower back. Funduscopic examination reveals a flat, translucent lesion on the left retina.

■ **What is the most likely diagnosis?**	Tuberous sclerosis, an autosomal dominant syndrome manifested by numerous benign neoplasms of the brain, skin, and kidney, as well as other organs. Tuberous sclerosis demonstrates complete genetic penetrance but highly variable expressivity. Most cases arise from a sporadic mutation, but offspring of an affected individual will inherit the mutation in an autosomal dominant pattern.
■ **What genes are mutated in this condition?**	The tuberous sclerosis complex gene 1 (*TSC1*) and gene 2 (*TSC2*) are mutated. *TSC1* encodes for the protein hamartin, and *TSC2* encodes for the protein tuberin. Both act as tumor suppressor genes, explaining the wide expressivity of the syndrome, as another "hit" is required to produce a tumor.
■ **What dermatologic and ophthalmic abnormalities are common in this condition?**	**Ash-leaf spots**, which are elliptical hypopigmented macules, may develop. In fair-skinned individuals, they can be visualized with a Wood's lamp (see Figure 10-39). **Adenoma sebaceum,** which are small angiofibromas that are typically distributed in a malar fashion on the face are also seen (see Figure 10-40). **Shagreen patches**, which are firm, reddish, raised lesions with a leathery texture are commonly found on the lumbar area of the back. Brown fibrous plaque may be seen on the forehead. Retinal hamartomas, which are seen as gray or yellow lesions on funduscopic examination, may also be present.
■ **What are the cardiac and renal manifestations of the condition?**	Patients classically present with **cardiac rhabdomyomas** that often regress spontaneously over the first few years of life. Renal manifestations include bilateral **angiomyolipomas** as well as cysts.
■ **What are the typical brain lesions in people with this condition?**	Cortical tubers and subependymal nodules are common, and both are considered **hamartomas.** Subependymal nodules can undergo malignant transformation to subependymal giant cell **astrocytomas.** Consequences of cortical hamartomas are seizures and mental retardation.

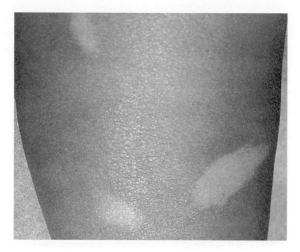

FIGURE 10-39. Hypopigmented macules, or ash-leaf spots. (Reproduced, with permission, from Wolff K, et al. *Fitzpatrick's Color Atlas & Synopsis of Clinical Pathology,* 5th ed. New York: McGraw-Hill, 2005: 461.)

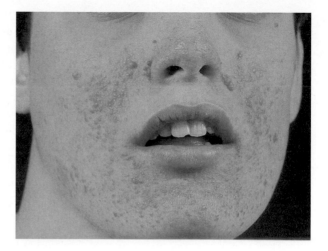

FIGURE 10-40. Small angiofibromas in a malar pattern known as adenoma sebaceum. (Reproduced, with permission, from Wolff K, et al. *Fitzpatrick's Color Atlas & Synopsis of Clinical Pathology,* 5th ed. New York: McGraw-Hill, 2005: 462.)

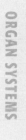

ORGAN SYSTEMS

NEUROLOGY

► **Case 37**

A 14-year-old boy is brought to his family physician complaining of weakness of his left hand and wrist. He is a varsity tennis player and has been having difficulty playing, and over the past week he has developed a burning sensation and numbness of the fourth and fifth fingers of his left hand. He says he woke up with the change in sensation and strength after falling asleep with his left arm over the side of his bed. Physical examination reveals no evidence of fracture, but there is significant edema of his elbow and a generalized weakness of the medial digits.

■ What is the most likely diagnosis?	Injury of the ulnar nerve. Ulnar nerve injuries often present with a partial claw-like deformity.
■ What movements of the hand will be weakened by this injury?	Wrist adduction or ulnar deviation (flexor carpi ulnaris) and adduction and abduction at the MCP joints will be affected. Patients are unable to hold anything between their fingers, and thumb adduction will also be affected. The ulnar nerve regulates sensation in the medial 1.5 fingers and the medial border of the hand.
■ What are the motor and sensory functions of this nerve?	The **ulnar nerve** causes flexion of the medial wrist and flexion of the MCP, proximal interphalangeal (PIP), and distal interphalangeal (DIP) joints of the ring and little fingers (it supplies the flexor carpi ulnaris muscle and the medial part of the flexor digitorum profundus muscles—the extrinsic muscles of the hand). It also innervates all intrinsic muscles of the hand except the thenar muscles and the first two lumbricals. Its functions in the hand, therefore, are adduction at the carpometacarpal joint of the thumb and adduction and abduction at the MCP joints of all fingers. The ulnar nerve also is responsible for flexion at the MCP joint and simultaneous extension of the PIP and DIP joints. It provides sensory information to the medial palm and dorsum of the hand, and the medial half of the ring and little fingers (both palmar and dorsal surfaces).
■ What are the most common causes of this injury?	Injuries include direct trauma and prolonged pressure or compression of the nerve. Ulnar nerve damage is a distal neuropathy. The symptoms occur because the myelin sheath is destroyed, which slows or prevents nerve conduction. The most common site of ulnar nerve injury is at the elbow, because the nerve lies superficially in the groove between the medial epicondyle and the olecranon. A blow to the medial epicondyle often hits the nerve, causing tingling in the territory of the ulnar nerve and the so-called sensation of a "funny bone."
■ What is the most appropriate treatment to reduce the swelling at this patient's elbow?	Corticosteroids are used to treat this disorder.

▶ **Case 38**

A 72-year-old man with a history of coronary artery disease, diabetes, and hypertension is brought to the primary care physician by his wife. She reports a stepwise decline in her husband, beginning with paralysis in one arm, gait disturbance, and now difficulty speaking. Further questioning reveals that the patient frequently misplaces objects, forgets where he is, and repeats the same questions.

▪ **What is the likely diagnosis?**

Vascular dementia, the second most common cause of dementia after Alzheimer's disease. It can be broadly categorized into two groups: multi-infarct dementia and diffuse white matter disease (Binswanger's disease). Vascular dementia can occur simultaneously with other forms of dementia such as Alzheimer's.

▪ **What is the pathophysiology of this condition?**

Recurrent strokes are responsible for the decline seen in patients with vascular dementia. Multiple large cortical infarcts cause multi-infarct dementia, whereas numerous smaller subcortical infarcts (lacunar strokes) cause diffuse white matter disease.

▪ **What features of the clinical history distinguish between the two forms of this condition?**

Multi-infarct dementia is caused primarily by cortical lesions and clinical features are specific to the area affected. Classically, patients will present with a stepwise deterioration in function. Because the lesions in diffuse white matter disease are subcortical, clinical features include focal motor signs, early gait disturbances, urinary frequency, and personality changes. The clinical course is gradual and can help distinguish it from multi-infarct dementia.

▪ **What are the risk factors for development of this condition?**

History of stroke, advanced age, hypertension, vascular disease, diabetes, smoking, and dyslipidemia are all risk factors. Treatment is aimed at any of the above underlying causes. Antiplatelet therapy may be used to prevent further cerebrovascular accidents.

▪ **What imaging tools could be used to confirm the diagnosis?**

MRI is the best imaging choice to determine if vascular dementia is present. The T2-weighted MRI shown in Figure 10-41 of a patient with diffuse white matter disease demonstrates numerous periventricular and corona radiata lesions.

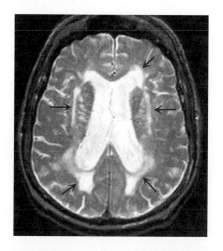

FIGURE 10-41. **T2-weighted MRI of a patient with diffuse white matter disease illustrating multiple lesions in the periventricular white matter and corona radiata.** (Reproduced, with permission, from Kasper DL, et al. *Harrison's Principles of Internal Medicine*, 16th ed. New York: McGraw-Hill, 2005: 2401.)

► **Case 39**

A 45-year-old man visits his primary care physician because he has noticed that his hearing has progressively worsened. Otologic examination reveals the patient's external ear canals are occluded with cerumen. The physician instructs the patient to use a ceruminolytic preparation overnight and to return the next day. On the following day, the physician performs a test that includes placing cold water into the patient's right ear canal. This causes the patient's eyes to move in an unusual way, rhythmically moving slowly toward the right and then jumping quickly back to the midline.

■ **What reflex is being demonstrated here?**

This is the vestibulo-ocular reflex, which is responsible for keeping the eyes stabilized on an object while the head or body is in motion.

■ **What are the patient's eye movements called?**

These rhythmic eye movements are called **nystagmus.** Nystagmus consists of two alternating phases: the slow phase, in which the eyes move slowly and smoothly as if they were following a moving object, and the fast phase, during which the eyes return to midline with rapid, saccadic movements. By convention, nystagmus is labeled according to the direction of the fast phase; this patient thus has a leftward nystagmus.

■ **What is the pathway of this reflex?**

When warm water is introduced to the external ear canal, it induces convection currents that stimulate the semicircular canals. When a patient's head is tilted to about 60°, the horizontal canals are most stimulated. Input from the semicircular canals travels via the vestibular nerve to the vestibular nuclei in the brain stem. From there, projections travel along the medial longitudinal fasciculus to the nuclei of cranial nerves III, IV, and VI (see Figure 10-42). From these nuclei, inhibitory and excitatory motor projections coordinate the eye movements of nystagmus.

■ **How do the semicircular canals sense movement?**

Each semicircular canal has an ampulla at its base that contains hair cells embedded in the crista ampullaris. When the endolymph within the semicircular canals moves as a result of movement of the head, it displaces the hair cells, and this mechanical disruption is translated into **depolarization** if the flow of fluid is one direction, or **hyperpolarization** if the fluid moves in the opposite direction.

■ **If the physician had used warm water to irrigate the ear canal, would the reflex have been elicited?**

Both warm water and cold water can stimulate the vestibulo-ocular reflex. However, because the direction of endolymph flow depends on convection currents set up by the temperature of the water in the external canal, warm water stimulates nystagmus toward the side of stimulation, while cold water stimulates nystagmus away from the side of stimulation. This can be remembered by the mnemonic **COWS** (**C**old = **O**pposite, **W**arm = **S**ame). Note, however, that this maneuver is rarely performed in an awake patient, as it can be associated with nausea. When performed in a comatose patient, the maneuver may elicit only the slow phase.

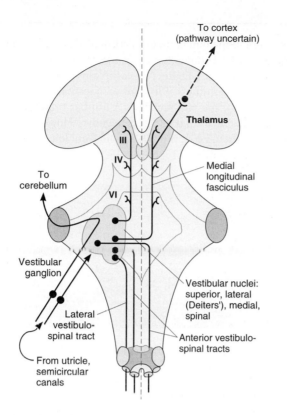

FIGURE 10-42. Principal vestibular pathways superimposed on a dorsal view of the brain stem. (Modified, with permission, from Ganong WF. *Review of Medical Physiology*, 22nd ed. New York, NY: McGraw-Hill, 2005: 174.)

▶ **Case 40**

A 14-year-old boy is sent to the emergency department (ED) by the nurse at his summer camp after he experienced a 1-minute seizure earlier that day. The boy has no previous history of seizure activity. In the ED, the boy complains of lethargy, vomiting, myalgias, severe headache, and neck stiffness. On further questioning, he reveals he has had many of these symptoms for the past few days. A lumbar puncture is performed, and a Gram stain of the cerebrospinal fluid (CSF) is negative. However, polymerase chain reaction (PCR) analysis of the CSF is positive for viral nucleic acid sequences. The cells found in the boy's CSF are shown in Figure 10-43.

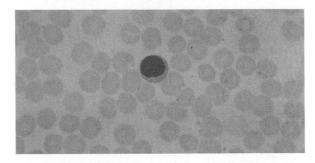

FIGURE 10-43. (Reproduced, with permission, from Berman I. *Color Atlas of Basic Histology*, 3rd ed. New York: McGraw-Hill, 2003: 107.)

▪ **What is the most likely diagnosis?**	This likely represents a viral meningitis.
▪ **What organisms are most likely to cause this condition?**	The most common causative organism of viral meningoencephalitis is **echovirus**, which is part of the Enterovirus subgroup of the picornavirus family. Other causative organisms include coxsackievirus (another enterovirus), adenovirus, human immunodeficiency virus, cytomegalovirus, Epstein-Barr virus, and herpes simplex virus.
▪ **Detection of the most likely viral agent with PCR requires modification of the standard PCR strategy. What type of enzyme is essential to this modification?**	Reverse transcriptase is essential in this type of test. Because enteroviruses are RNA viruses, detection proceeds with reverse transcription-PCR (RT-PCR). Normal transcription is the synthesis of RNA from DNA; this process is the **reverse.** Viral RNA is reverse transcribed into the complementary DNA (cDNA), and that cDNA can then be amplified using the standard PCR DNA amplification strategy.
▪ **What changes in this patient's glucose and protein levels in CSF are most likely to be seen?**	As with most cases of viral meningitis, CSF glucose concentration should be normal and CSF protein concentration should be normal to slightly increased. This is in contrast to CSF findings in bacterial meningitis, in which protein is increased, glucose is decreased, and polymorphonuclear leukocytes are prominent in the CSF. Table 10-1 compares CSF findings in bacterial, viral, and fungal meningitis.
▪ **Some viruses capable of causing this patient's symptoms are sensitive to acyclovir. What is the mechanism of action of this drug?**	Acyclovir targets viral DNA polymerase. Herpesviruses are DNA viruses that are sensitive to acyclovir. Picornaviruses, however, are RNA viruses that do not contain DNA polymerase, and therefore they are not sensitive to acyclovir.

■ What type of cells is shown in Figure 10-43?

The cell in Figure 10-43 is a **lymphocyte**, which is characterized by its small size, with most of the cell volume occupied by the darkly stained and round nucleus. Lymphocytes play a key role in cellular immunity, particularly in combating infection. Lymphocytosis of the CSF is commonly seen in viral meningitis.

TABLE 10-1. CSF Findings in Meningitis

	PRESSURE	CELL TYPE	PROTEIN	SUGAR
Bacterial	↑	↑ PMNs	↑	↓
Fungal/TB	↑	↑ lymphocytes	↑	↓
Viral	Normal/↑	↑ lymphocytes	Normal	Normal

Reproduced, with permission, from Le T, Bhushan V, Rao DA. *First Aid for the USMLE Step 1: 2008.* New York: McGraw-Hill, 2008: 172.

ORGAN SYSTEMS

NEUROLOGY

► **Case 41**

A 26-year-old man is being evaluated by a neurologist for recurrent headaches and changes in vision. A careful ophthalmologic examination reveals multiple hemangiomas of the retina in both eyes, and an MRI of the brain demonstrates three hemangioblastomas of the cerebellum.

▪ **What is the most likely diagnosis?**	von Hippel–Lindau (VHL) disease. This disease is characterized by diffuse hemangioma formation, including cavernous hemangiomas, as well as by an increased incidence of renal cell carcinoma (RCC).
▪ **What is the pattern of inheritance for this condition?**	VHL disease is inherited in an autosomal dominant fashion in 75% of cases. It is associated with deletion of the *VHL* gene, a tumor suppressor gene on the short arm of chromosome 3. Twenty-five percent of cases occur sporadically. In the United States, the incidence of VHL disease is about 1 in 36,000 individuals.
▪ **What is Knudsen's two-hit theory of carcinogenesis?**	Dr. Alfred Knudsen described the recessive nature of target genes involved in the development of retinoblastoma in infancy. The two-hit theory of carcinogenesis describes a gene product whose normal function is to inhibit cell growth (a **tumor suppressor gene**). An individual may inherit one inactive allele (the first "hit"), but expression of the remaining allele can maintain normal cell growth. If, however, a somatic mutation is also acquired, tumor suppressor activity is lost, and there is a tendency toward proliferation and malignant progression. The *VHL* gene on chromosome 3 acts as a classic tumor suppressor gene.
▪ **What is the leading cause of death in patients with this condition?**	RCC, predominantly the clear cell type, is the leading cause of death in patients with VHL, with some case series reporting a prevalence as high as 40%–75% at autopsy. In patients with VHL, RCC develops from malignant degeneration of renal cysts and is usually bilateral. The average age for development of RCC in patients with VHL is 44 years. Because of the high incidence of renal cysts and RCC in patients with VHL, periodic imaging of the kidneys is key in patients and at-risk relatives.
▪ **What other tumors and lesions are patients with this condition at increased risk of developing?**	Patients with VHL disease are at risk for developing multiple cysts in the liver, epididymis, pancreas, and kidneys. Pheochromocytomas, rare pancreatic carcinomas, and endolymphatic sac tumors are also part of the spectrum of VHL. Hemangioblastomas are typically in the cerebellum or medulla, but may also occur in the spinal cord. Hemangiomas of the retina are common and are often bilateral.

A 55-year-old man is brought to the emergency department by a friend who has noticed the patient has had memory lapses and difficulty with walking and balance. The patient has a 26-year history of excessive alcohol use. On further questioning, the patient is unable to relate a consistent history. When asked about his location, the patient states he is at home. Physical examination reveals his left eye does not adduct on rightward gaze, and his gait is ataxic.

■ What is the most likely diagnosis?	These symptoms are suggestive of Wernicke's encephalopathy, which classically presents as the triad of **ophthalmoplegia** (paralysis of one or more eye muscles), ataxia, and encephalopathy. This may progress to Korsakoff's syndrome, which consists of memory lapses, confusion, and confabulation.
■ What type of memory deficit is likely to be seen in this condition?	Patients with Wernicke-Korsakoff syndrome usually suffer from **anterograde amnesia**, which is characterized by an inability to form new memories with general preservation of long-term memories. This is in contrast to **retrograde amnesia**, in which the only memories that are lost are long-term memories that precede the precipitating event.
■ What is the pathophysiology of this condition?	This disease is seen in alcoholics with thiamine deficiency due to poor nutrition and absorption. The thiamine deficiency results in periventricular hemorrhage and degeneration in a symmetric pattern in multiple cerebral areas, including the cerebellum, brain stem, and bilateral mammillary bodies (see Figure 10-44; arrows show abnormal enhancement of the mammillary bodies).
■ What specific cranial nerve pathway is responsible for the abnormality noted on lateral gaze?	Inability to adduct the left eye on rightward gaze suggests a left medial longitudinal fasciculus (MLF) lesion. Normally, the abducens nucleus projects neurons both to the ipsilateral lateral rectus muscle via cranial nerve (CN) VI, and to the contralateral medial rectus muscle via the MLF and CN III. In this case, the contralateral MLF pathway must be damaged, resulting in inability to adduct the contralateral (left) eye during lateral gaze.
■ For which essential biochemical pathways is thiamine required?	Thiamine is needed for the oxidative carboxylation of α-ketoacids and is a cofactor for the transketolase hexose monophosphate shunt.
■ What other disease can result from thiamine deficiency?	**Beriberi** is a deficiency of thiamine (vitamin B$_1$) secondary to malnutrition. It is characterized by peripheral neuropathy and axonal demyelination.

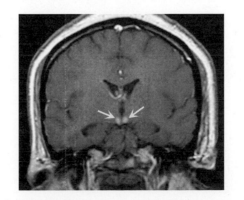

FIGURE 10-44. MRI of mammillary bodies in Wernicke's encephalopathy. (Reproduced, with permission, from Kasper DL, et al. *Harrison's Principles of Internal Medicine*, 16th ed. New York: McGraw-Hill, 2005: 1636.)

Psychiatry

Case 1	382
Case 2	383
Case 3	384
Case 4	385
Case 5	386
Case 6	387
Case 7	388
Case 8	389
Case 9	390
Case 10	391
Case 11	392
Case 12	393
Case 13	394
Case 14	395
Case 15	396

► **Case 1**

A mother brings her 8-year-old daughter to see the pediatrician because of concerns about her behavior. Mother states that her child is unable to finish any activities at home and becomes easily distracted. She is unable to sit still long enough to complete her homework and is constantly "bouncing off the walls." The mother has received complaints from her school about talking back to the teacher and interacting poorly with peers. They are considering making her repeat the third grade.

■ **What is the most likely diagnosis?**	Attention deficit hyperactivity disorder (ADHD). ADHD is estimated to have a prevalence in school-age children as high as 8%. Males are more affected than females.
■ **What are the typical manifestations of this condition?**	ADHD is characterized by **hyperactivity, impulsivity,** and **inattention** that lead to significant impairment. Hyperactivity is manifest as fidgetiness, and an inability to remain seated or play quietly. Impulsivity is displayed as inability to wait for one's turn, talking when inappropriate, and constantly interrupting. Inattention may be seen as forgetfulness, poor concentration, an inability to finish tasks, or a lack of attention to detail. According to the *Diagnostic and Statistical Manual of Mental Disorders, Fourth Edition,* these symptoms have to be present before the age of 7, persist for at least 6 months, and be present in more than one setting (e.g., at home and at school).
■ **What is the appropriate treatment for this condition?**	Treatment may include behavioral interventions, pharmacological therapy, or both. Although it may seem counterintuitive, stimulants have shown great effect in treating patients with ADHD. Stimulants such as methylphenidate and dextroamphetamine act by increasing catecholamine release.
■ **What is the natural course of this condition?**	Many with ADHD find that they "outgrow" it during adolescence. A subset of patients, particularly those with inattentive type, continue to have the disorder as adults and will benefit from pharmacotherapy.

A mother brings her 3-year-old son to the physician because she believes he is not developing normally. She says he does not reach out for her with his arms, show joy, or follow her around like his siblings did. His language development is delayed and he often mechanically repeats other people. He needs to have "everything his way" and has many rituals. "He seems to be in a world of his own," she notes. Tests show a lower-than-average IQ.

■ **What is the most likely diagnosis?**	Autistic disorder. Autism is the most severe of the pervasive developmental disorders which also include Asperger's syndrome, Rett's disorder, and childhood disintegrative disorder.
■ **What is the classic triad of findings in this condition?**	The triad includes: ■ Profound difficulty relating to other people. ■ Severe language disorder: delayed and abnormal speech, poor comprehension, tendency to echo questions. ■ Marked routines and rituals associated with a poverty of imaginative play. Odd motor patterns such as hand flapping and walking on tiptoe are also common.
■ **What is the epidemiology of this condition?**	Autism is rare, with a prevalence of approximately 2 per 1,000 children. More common in boys, it presents in early childhood but is a lifelong condition.
■ **What is the etiology of this condition?**	Autism is a heterogeneous disorder with a significant, though as of yet uncharacterized, genetic component.
■ **What is the differential diagnosis of this condition?**	Differential includes Asperger's syndrome, Rett's disorder and childhood disintegrative disorder. **Asperger's syndrome** is a milder form of autism involving problems with social relationships and repetitive behavior. These children have no cognitive or language delay. They often have stiff, monotonous speech, are clumsy, and express an unusually intense interest in a narrow subject area (like camera models).

▶ **Case 3**

A 22-year-old woman presents to the clinic with an 8-day history of insomnia and increased energy. Her roommate is concerned because the patient has been talking rapidly and loudly. The patient has made several expensive purchases recently and has been exhibiting uncharacteristically seductive behavior, dressing inappropriately for class, and drawing a lot of attention to herself. She denies any substance abuse and urine toxicology screen is negative.

▪ What category of psychiatric disorder does this patient exhibit?	This patient's symptoms are within the spectrum of mood disorders, specifically a manic episode of bipolar disorder. Other disorders in this class include major depressive disorder, dysthymic disorder and bereavement.
▪ How does the epidemiology differ between patients presenting with manic depression and those presenting with depressive disorder?	Manic depression is found in 1% of the population, affects women and men equally, and has a bimodal distribution (early 20's and middle age). Depressive disorder is much more common (15%–25% lifetime prevalence) with women effected 2:1. Depression occurs across the lifespan with particular prevalence in 20's and elderly patients.
▪ What signs and symptoms are commonly associated with this disorder?	▪ Abrupt onset of increased energy ▪ Decreased attention span ▪ Decreased need for sleep ▪ Elevated or expansive mood or irritability ▪ Hyperreligiosity ▪ Pressured speech ▪ Impulsive behavior, including spending, gambling, substance use or sex
▪ How is this disorder classified?	**Mania** presents a significant disability to the patient and usually is associated with psychotic symptoms. Episodes typically last >1 week. In contrast, **hypomania** is associated with a milder variety of similar symptoms as mania, but without gross functional impairment; this diagnosis requires only 4 days of symptoms. ▪ Bipolar I: requires distinct manic and depressive syndromes. ▪ Bipolar II: requires distinct hypomanic and depressive syndromes. ▪ Mixed: presence of both manic and depressive symptoms concurrently over a period of time (often described as dysphoric mania or agitated depression). ▪ Rapid cycling: presence of at least four distinct manic, depressive, or mixed mood episodes over a period of 1 year.
▪ What are the most appropriate treatments for this disorder?	First-line drugs include mood stabilizers (lithium, valproate, or carbamazepine) and antipsychotic agents (olanzapine, haloperidol, or risperidone). Hospitalization can be necessary to ensure patient safety.

► **Case 4**
A 37-year-old pianist visits her physician because of difficulty sleeping over the past 3 weeks. She has been waking up early in the morning, well before her usual waking time. In addition, she does not enjoy playing the piano as much as she used to. She has gained 4.5 kg (10 lb) in the past month. On questioning, she reveals she had a similar episode about 1 year ago.

■ **What is the most likely diagnosis?**	Major depressive disorder.
■ **Which symptoms are most commonly associated with this condition?**	The diagnosis of a major depressive disorder requires two or more episodes consisting of five of the following symptoms, present for at least 2 weeks (**"SIG E CAPS"**): **S**leep disturbances, decreased **I**nterest, **G**uilt, decreased **E**nergy, decreased **C**oncentration, change in **A**ppetite (usually decreased), **P**sychomotor retardation, and **S**uicidal ideations, in addition to depressed mood. A diagnosis cannot be made in this patient without further questioning to elicit additional symptoms.
■ **What other conditions can present with similar symptoms?**	**Bereavement** can present similarly within 1 year of the loss of a loved one. In bereavement, the patient's symptoms are related to the loss of another person. Grief is characterized by shock, denial, guilt, and somatic symptoms. Depressive symptoms also raise the possibility of **dysthymia**, a milder form of depression with less intense symptoms, which lasts >2 years.
■ **What major neurotransmitter disturbances are characteristic of this condition?**	Patients with major depressive disorder commonly have decreased levels of serotonin and norepinephrine. Dopamine may also be decreased in major depression.
■ **What are the most appropriate treatments for this condition?**	Psychotherapy, antidepressants or a combination of both. Cognitive behavioral therapy (CBT) or psychodynamic psychotherapy are effective treatments for depression. Antidepressant therapies, including selective serotonin reuptake inhibitors, monoamine oxidase inhibitors, and tricyclic antidepressants, generally take from 2–6 weeks to take effect. Thus, a change in therapy should not be considered until after the patient has been taking these medications for at least 2 weeks. Electroconvulsive therapy can be used for major depressive disorder that is refractory to other treatments.

ORGAN SYSTEMS

PSYCHIATRY

A 51-year-old woman presents to her primary care physician with complaints of being uncomfortably anxious about "everything." She is unable to identify a precipitating event or particular worry. She worries about her family, about her health, about finances. She has little respite or relief and is frequently irritable, tired and unable to concentrate on her work. She has been a lifelong "worrier" but the symptoms have gotten so intense in the past six months that she is thinking of giving up working.

■ **What type of psychiatric disorder does this patient exhibit?**	Generalized anxiety disorder. This category, anxiety disorders, also includes panic disorder, agoraphobia (fear of open places), obsessive-compulsive disorder, and posttraumatic stress disorder (persistently reexperiencing a past traumatic event).
■ **What signs and symptoms are commonly associated with this disorder?**	■ **Uncontrollable anxiety** ■ Difficulty concentrating ■ Fatigue ■ Insomnia ■ Irritability ■ Restlessness
■ **What are the common sources of anxiety for these patients?**	■ Cleanliness/contamination (washing hands, cleaning house) ■ Doubt/mistrust ■ Sex ■ Symmetry (rituals around doorways, arranging objects) ■ Safety
■ **What other disorders should be considered in this condition?**	"Normal" worry and adjustment disorder. In contrast to normal anxiety, individuals with generalized anxiety disorder have evidence of social dysfunction secondary to the disorder. Adjustment disorder is characterized by emotional symptoms following an identifiable stressor (i.e., divorce, or loss of a job) and lasts <6 months. In contrast, symptoms in generalized anxiety disorder must have been present for >6 months.
■ **What are the most appropriate treatments for this disorder?**	■ Antidepressants (SSRI, chloripramine) ■ Buspirone ■ Benzodiazipines ■ Cognitive behavioral therapy

ORGAN SYSTEMS

PSYCHIATRY

▶ **Case 6**	A 29-year-old well-groomed man, with no prior medical or psychiatric history, consults a psychiatrist for evaluation. The patient has noticed that over the past 6 months he has been preoccupied with counting items, such as bricks in his driveway, raisins in his cereal, and tiles in the ceiling. Moreover, he says he feels compelled to count particularly to the number 30; for example, he must do 30 push-ups in the morning, jog for 30 minutes, and chew his food 30 times. He has not told anyone about his recent habit, and does not believe it is interfering with his work. However, he is troubled by his own behavior and feels unable to stop. During the medical history, the patient reveals his 30th birthday is next week.

▪ **What is the most likely diagnosis?**	Obsessive-compulsive disorder (OCD), as suggested by the patient's obsessions (recurrent thoughts) and compulsions (recurrent acts).
▪ **What is the epidemiology of this condition?**	OCD occurs in about 3% of the general population. Males are much more frequently afflicted than females. The disorder often runs in families, and may be associated with tic disorders (e.g., Tourette's syndrome).
▪ **What are the most appropriate treatments for this condition?**	Pharmacologically SSRIs and clomipramine are common treatments. Cognitive behavioral therapy (CBT) is also used with and without pharmacologic therapy.
▪ **What is cognitive behavioral therapy?**	**Cognitive behavioral therapy** is a manualized, time-limited type of psychotherapy, which seeks to modify a patient's emotions through identification and modification of the patient maladaptive thought patterns and beliefs. So for this patient the thought of turning 30 may mean the beginning of adulthood and end to the impulsiveness of youth. The maladaptive thought may be "if I count to thirty, I am in control and an adult." The cognitive component will challenge his irrational thought about turning 30 and adulthood. The behavioral component will allow him to combat the need to counting or checking. CBT often involves homework (i.e., thought journals) or practice of behavioral techniques between sessions.

► **Case 7**

A 48-year-old man visits his physician for a routine physical examination. During the interview, he mentions he is having some difficulty at work. His boss claims he is unable to finish tasks within a reasonable amount of time. Yet the patient maintains that his coworkers "don't do things the way I tell them to," and he doesn't feel he can delegate tasks because "they don't do things right." He also admits to frequent arguments with his wife, who does not put things away in the places they are supposed to go. He cannot tolerate anything that is not orderly. During the office visit, the patient takes copious notes.

■ **What is the likely diagnosis?**	This patient exhibits traits consistent with obsessive-compulsive personality disorder. Personality **traits** are typical patterns of relating to or thinking about the world that is exhibited in various social and personal contexts. A personality trait becomes a **disorder** when the traits are extreme and lead to the exclusion of other traits, leading to problems with social behavior and functioning and personal distress. A person is often not aware of maladaptive personality traits.
■ **How are these disorders classified?**	The *Diagnostic and Statistical Manual of Mental Disorders, Fourth Edition* (DSM-IV), classifies personality disorders into three clusters: ■ Individuals in cluster A are described as odd or eccentric ("weird"). ■ Individuals in cluster B are described as dramatic or erratic ("wild"). ■ Individuals in cluster C are described as anxious or fearful ("worried"). This patient falls into cluster C, obsessive-compulsive personality disorder (OCPD).
■ **How can this disorder be differentiated from obsessive-compulsive disorder?**	Obsessive-compulsive disorder (**OCD**) is a disease with the presence of obsessions and compulsions, both of which are unable to be resisted and are experienced as unpleasant by patients (**ego-dystonic**). Symptoms are particularly debilitating due to time consumption and interference with daily, social, and occupational functioning. In **OCPD** patients have a rigid preoccupation with order and control. Patients with OCPD their beliefs and way of navigating the world are simply part of who they are (**ego-syntonic**). Their behaviors may bother the people around them, but often do not bother the patient, though they are aware of the consequences (i.e., long days at work due to refusal to delegate, or irritation and distancing of loved ones.)
■ **What is the first-line treatment for OCPD?**	Both cognitive behavioral therapy (CBT) and psychodynamic psychotherapy can be useful in these patients. Medications can be useful in treating comorbid conditions like anxiety and depression.

A 20-year-old woman complains to her physician that she is unable to drive her car because she frequently has overwhelming anxiety while driving. She describes several episodes of palpitations, nausea, sweating, breathlessness, and an intense fear of dying in these situations. These episodes started about 8 months ago, but are increasing in frequency. The episodes begin suddenly at variable times during the car ride and intensify over the course of 5 minutes, so that she must stop the car to calm down. She finds the symptoms confusing and frustrating, stating that she has "never had any problems with cars before" and that she now avoids travel where a car might be involved. Recently, these episodes have become more common, and can occur even while she is at home and have on occasion woken her from sleep.

■ **What is the most likely diagnosis?**	Panic disorder. However, organic causes of her symptoms (including tachycardias, hyperthyroidism, hyperparathyroidism, pheochromocytoma, hypoglycemia, seizures, and drug use) must be ruled out before panic disorder can be diagnosed.
■ **How are panic attacks related to this condition?**	Panic disorder requires repeated **panic attacks** (or episodes), with relevant behaviors or attitudes between attacks, such as worry about not being able to control the panic attacks. They tend to avoid situations where panic attacks occur and modify their lives around fear of having panic attacks. This can lead to agoraphobia.
■ **What type of seizure can mimic panic attacks?**	Medial temporal lobe **seizures** can produce fear and autonomic phenomena. This is thought to occur because the amygdala, located in the temporal lobe, is often associated with responses to fear.
■ **What are the most appropriate treatments for this condition?**	Panic disorder is often treated with selective serotonin reuptake inhibitors (SSRIs), tricyclic antidepressants, and monoamine oxidase (MAO) inhibitors. These drugs influence the central nervous system levels of norepinephrine, serotonin, and α-aminobutyric acid. Benzodiazepines are also useful in the short-term management of patients with panic disorder.
■ **What syndrome can develop when SSRIs are used with MAO inhibitors?**	**Serotonin syndrome** may result from the use of drugs that enhance serotonin signaling. Since MAO inhibitors and SSRIs both enhance serotonin signaling through different mechanisms, the risk of serotonin syndrome is higher when these drugs are taken together. Serotonin syndrome is more likely to occur with this combination of drugs because most MAO inhibitors irreversibly inhibit MAO. Symptoms of serotonin syndrome fit into three main categories: ■ Autonomic dysfunction (e.g., hyperthermia, tachycardia, unstable blood pressure, diarrhea, and sweating). ■ Cognitive and behavioral changes (e.g., agitation, confusion, and coma). ■ Neuromuscular abnormalities (e.g., hyperreflexia, shivering, myoclonus, and ataxia).

► **Case 9**

A 22-year-old man visits his primary care physician with a complaint of difficulty sleeping for the past year. The patient returned home from Iraq a year ago after serving in the Army and states he only gets 4 hours of sleep per night. He describes that when he does fall asleep he has recurring nightmares about the attack he suffered when he was driving a Humvee that was hit by a roadside bomb. The patient states that he has difficulty driving now because he feels like he is "reliving" the experience when he gets in a car. Since coming home he has expressed no interest in returning to college and broke up with his girlfriend because she couldn't deal with his outbursts of anger and "numbness" to her feelings.

■ What is the likely diagnosis?	The patient displays criteria for **posttraumatic stress disorder (PTSD)**. PTSD is a complex and heterogeneous disorder characterized by reexperiencing an extremely traumatic event with symptoms of increased arousal and avoidance. The disturbance must last >1 month and cause significant social and occupational distress.
■ What causes this condition?	Any event that an individual witnesses or experiences that exposes them to real or threatened death and injury. The individual's response to this event must involve intense fear and horror. Common traumas can occur in both childhood and adulthood and include military combat, sexual or physical assault, accidents and natural disasters.
■ How do patients with this condition re-experience the traumatic event?	Recurrent dreams or intrusive thoughts of the event are common. Patients may describe flashbacks in which they feel as if the event were recurring while they are awake. Often flashbacks are triggered by stimuli which are common to the traumatic event such as sights, smells or sounds.
■ What is one of the ways in which patients with this condition cope?	PTSD patients often avoid thoughts, feelings, stimuli, and conversations that are associated with the trauma. Because of this, it is often difficult for patients to talk about their experience. They also display a restricted range of affect often described as feeling "numb" or "detached."
■ What symptoms may be present in this condition?	PTSD is characterized by hyperarousal that may be manifest as insomnia, bouts of rage, hypervigilance, being easily startled, or having poor concentration.

▶ **Case 10**

A mother brings her 3-year-old daughter to see the pediatrician. The mother reports that her daughter has gradually stopped speaking and is doing "weird" things with her hands. The mother states that though she was a normal baby and toddler, but then started to lose interest in her toys and looks at her family less. Now she doesn't speak at all and has screaming spells for hours during the day. Over time she has become unable to feed herself and is constantly wringing her hands. Physical examination reveals decelerated head growth and stereotypic hand wringing.

■ What is the likely diagnosis?	Rett's disorder is a neurodevelopmental disorder characterized by initial normal development during the first few months to years of life followed by a **loss of speech** and purposeful **hand movements.**
■ What are the genetics of this condition?	Rett's disorder is an X-linked disorder affecting only females. Affected males die in utero. The disorder is cause by mutations in the *MECP2* gene which encodes for a methyl binding protein. This protein is most abundant in the brain and is thought to act as a gene suppressor during development.
■ What other symptoms can this patient expect to develop over time?	After the loss of speech and purposeful hand movements, patients usually develop epilepsy, ataxia, and autistic features. After a period of normal growth, patients display decelerated circumferential head growth. Breathing abnormalities are common with periods of apnea and hyperventilation.
■ What is the treatment and prognosis for patients with this condition?	Treatment for Rett's disorder is aimed at alleviating symptoms with careful management of nutrition, pharmacotherapy for seizures, and physical therapy for motor dysfunction. Patients can generally live for decades with successful management of symptoms.

► **Case 11**

The parents of a 22-year-old man bring him to the family physician because they have noticed a distinct change in their son's behavior over the past 4 months. He appears unkempt, does not have any friends at school, and his grades have started to drop. The young man believes that their neighbor has been sent to spy on him, and his parents have heard him carrying on conversations with imaginary partners. The son denies any history of substance use and his urine toxicology is negative.

■ **What is the most likely diagnosis?**	The constellation of symptoms suggests the diagnosis of schizophreniform disorder, which is the presence of psychotic symptoms for >2 weeks, but <6 months. This is in contrast to a diagnosis of schizophrenia, which requires the presence of symptoms for at least 6 months. The majority of patients with schizophreniform disorder ultimately develop schizophrenia.
■ **What symptoms are associated with this condition?**	Positive symptoms include formal thought disorder (disorganized speech and loosening of associations), delusions, hallucinations, and ideas of reference (beliefs or perceptions that irrelevant, unrelated, or innocuous things are referring to a person directly, or have a special significance for that person). Negative symptoms include flat affect, social withdrawal, and avolition (inability to initiate and maintain goal-directed activities).
■ **What is the epidemiology of this condition?**	The lifetime prevalence of schizophrenia is approximately 1%. It occurs equally often in males and females and its incidence does not differ according to race. Males tend to present in late teens to mid 20's; females tend to present about a decade later. Genetic factors are thought to be important in its etiology. Some evidence suggests patients with schizophrenia are more likely to have been born in the winter and early spring. Viral hypotheses are thought to explain these findings.
■ **What neurotransmitter abnormalities are associated with this condition?**	An excess of dopamine and serotonin are thought to contribute to the development of schizophrenia.
■ **What are the most appropriate pharmacologic treatments for this condition?**	Typical antipsychotic agents (such as thioridazine, haloperidol, fluphenazine, and chlorpromazine) block dopamine$_2$ receptors. Atypical antipsychotic agents (clozapine, olanzapine, and risperidone) block serotonin receptors and multiple subtypes of dopamine receptors. With the exception of clozapine, they are equally effective in their treatment of positive symptoms, though differ in their side effect profiles. Clozapine is significantly more effective, though with a much greater side effect profile.
■ **What types of personality disorders are seen in relatives of people with this condition?**	There is a familial association between schizophrenia and cluster A personality disorders (i.e., paranoid, schizoid, and schizotypal personality disorders).

A 28-year-old woman presents to her physician with abdominal pain that has persisted intermittently for the past decade. This pain has been particularly intense for the past several weeks. The patient reports she is unable to sleep at night and has "tried everything for the pain but it won't go away." She reports nausea and diarrhea. She also has longstanding complaints of chronic headaches, muscle spasms, and dysparuenia (painful sexual intercourse.). Review of her chart shows multiple visits over the last several years for similar symptoms with only vague physical exam findings and no laboratory findings. She has had several investigative surgeries and procedures without results. She wonders whether she should have another surgery to find out what is wrong.

■ **What is the most likely diagnosis?**

Somatization disorder. This diagnosis is in the category of somatoform disorders which also include body dysmorphic disorder, conversion disorder, hypochondriasis, and pain disorders.

■ **What are common symptoms of this disorder?**

In order to meet criteria, patients must present with somatic complaints in at least four sites. Complaints in general are longstanding though specific complaints may track different time courses. Complaints must begin before age 40. In order to make the DSM-IV diagnosis, there must be gastrointestinal, neurologic, and sexual symptoms.

■ **How are other disorders in this category differentiated?**

- **Body dysmorphic disorder:** patients are excessively concerned with an imagined or slight physical defect, to the point where social, occupational, or academic functioning is adversely affected.
- **Conversion disorder:** patients unconsciously mimic medical disorders (often neurologic and solitary in nature.)
- **Hypochondriasis:** patients persistently believe they have a particular disease, despite multiple pieces of evidence suggesting absence of that illness.
- **Pain disorder:** patients have complaints of pain, but psychological factors contribute to the onset, severity, maintenance, and exacerbation of these complaints.

These somatoform disorders must be distinguished from factitious disorders in which patients consciously induce or mimic medical disorders (i.e., by contaminating urine specimens or surreptitiously injecting insulin), for the purposes of being sick (i.e., to be taken care of, enjoyment of tricking medical professionals, etc.).

Malingering, in which patients consciously feign medical disorders, provides secondary gain (i.e., getting out of work, collecting disability, shelter).

■ **What are the most appropriate treatments for this condition?**

Continuity of care is very important with these patients. Frequent appointments with the same primary care provider during which the patient can express his/her symptoms and concerns are important. The patient should receive a physical examination to rule out a medical cause, but diagnostic testing should be limited once it is determined that no medical cause underlies the condition. The largest "real" health risks to a patient with somatoform disorders are iatrogenic harm and missed diagnoses due to frustrations of medical professionals. Psychiatric referral are rarely accepted on the basis of their somatoform disorder alone; comorbid depression, anxiety, stress and coping are often grounds upon which a patient can accept psychiatric referral.

ORGAN SYSTEMS

PSYCHIATRY

▶ **Case 13**

A 38-year-old man having a severe asthma attack is brought to the emergency department and given IV steroids, which help to resolve his breathing difficulties. He is sent home on a steroid taper and seen in follow up 2 days later when he reports insomnia and appears agitated with grandiose plans for the future. He has rapid and pressured speech and appears to have a euphoric affect. He is also tachycardic. When asked about his mood, he reports he feels "sunny."

■ What is the most likely diagnosis?	Steroid-induced mania.
■ What drugs are most commonly associated with these symptoms?	Drug-induced mania can be secondary to ingestion of cocaine or amphetamines. Corticosteroids are a common iatrogenic cause of mood symptoms, though depression is more likely than mania.
■ What signs and symptoms are commonly associated with this condition?	■ Dilated pupils ■ ECG arrhythmia or ischemia ■ Hypertension ■ Mood elevation, general activation ■ Tachycardia
■ What laboratory tests are useful in confirming the diagnosis?	Urine or serum toxicology screening can identify specific drugs the patient may have ingested. Medications should be reviewed for possible iatrogenic cause.
■ What are the most appropriate treatments for this condition?	The dose of steroids should be reduced as much as clinically possible. If agitation or psychotic symptoms are present, haloperidol is useful, sometimes also with lorazepam. Calcium channel blockers can be used for the acute autonomic symptoms.
■ These symptoms could also be seen in which other psychiatric disorders?	These symptoms could also be evidence of delirium or a manic phase of bipolar disorder.

A 40-year-old woman is brought to the emergency department (ED) by her brother with the chief complaint of "twitching of lips and tongue." The brother is aware of her diagnosis of schizophrenia about a decade ago, but has not seen his sister in years and is worried about these movements. The patient however is not concerned at all. She has achieved fairly good control of her psychotic symptoms with both oral and intramuscular depot antipsychotic agents. She recalls one prior visit to the ED shortly after she was diagnosed with schizophrenia for evaluation of a neck spasm that was painful and "locked my neck to the left."

▪ **What is the most likely diagnosis?**	Tardive dyskinesia. Extrapyramidal symptoms, such as stereotypic oral, buccal, or lingual movements and choreiform or athetoid movements, can be seen after several months or years of therapy with antipsychotic agents. These symptoms are often irreversible.
▪ **What is the pathophysiology of this condition?**	Dopamine$_2$ receptor supersensitivity after long-term use of antidopaminergic drugs is the likely cause.
▪ **What risk factors are associated with this condition?**	▪ Diabetes mellitus ▪ History of movement disorders ▪ Tobacco use ▪ Typical antipsychotic agents (strong risk factor, especially higher doses for longer periods)
▪ **What other movement abnormalities are associated with the use of antipsychotic agents?**	▪ Acute dystonia (sustained muscular spasms—facial, torticollis, and oculogyric crisis) is the earliest to present (within hours). ▪ Akathisia, characterized by extreme restlessness, is the most common extrapyramidal disorder and is one of the most likely causes of medication nonadherence. ▪ Akinesia, seen after a few days, is the inability to initiate movement.
▪ **What can be done to minimize the future risk of developing these symptoms?**	Lowering the dose of typical antipsychotic agents can result in resolution of symptoms. Paradoxically this may produce a transient worsening of dyskinesia as receptors become desensitized. Switching patients to atypical antipsychotic agents is advised, as they are associated with fewer extrapyramidal symptoms. Clozapine is the least likely of all antipsychotic drugs to cause tardive dyskinesia and is also the only medication to treat it. However, its use is limited by need for routine blood monitoring, high degree of both benign and serious side effects and availability only as an oral preparation. High doses of vitamin E have been used with variable success; its effect is thought to be a result of its antioxidant properties.

▶ **Case 15**

A mother brings her 6-year-old daughter to see the pediatrician because she is concerned about her facial movements. The mother states that her daughter has always "blinked too much" but recently she started jerking her head to the right and sticking out her tongue. These are very quick movements that happen multiple times a day. The mother also reports that the child makes grunting noises. The patient says she doesn't know why she does these things but feels a sense of relief once she does them.

■ What is the likely diagnosis?	This patient displays criteria for Tourette's disorder which is characterized by multiple motor and vocal tics present since childhood. A tic is a sudden, stereotypical, repetitive movement or vocalization. The tics in Tourette's disorder occur many times a day for a period of at least 1 year.
■ What motor abnormalities are seen in this condition?	Motor tics can either be simple or complex and can affect any part of the body. Often patients will initially have simple tics such as blinking, should shrug, head jerking, or grimacing. Complex tics may involve coordinated movement such as jumping, squatting, turning, or obscene gestures (copropraxia).
■ What vocal abnormalities are seen in this condition?	The classic vocal tic is coprolalia, or involuntary vocalization of obscene words. Other vocal tics include echolalia (repetition of others), and sounds such as barking, coughing, sniffing, grunting, or snorting.
■ Are the tics of this condition involuntary?	Yes, but for brief periods patients may be able to consciously suppress the tics. They often describe a sense of relief once the tic is performed. This has been likened to the conscious suppression of the desire to scratch a mosquito bite, with relief once executed.
■ What is the natural history of this condition?	The age of onset is usually during childhood and must occur before the age of 18. The disorder may be lifelong but many patients find that the severity of the tics decreases with age and during adulthood may disappear completely.
■ What is the treatment for this condition?	In many cases, education and reassurance may be sufficient. If the tics significantly interfere with the patient's social interactions or school performance, pharmacotherapy with a dopamine antagonist such as haloperidol or fluphenazine can be effective.

Renal

Case 1	398
Case 2	399
Case 3	400
Case 4	401
Case 5	403
Case 6	405
Case 7	407
Case 8	408
Case 9	410
Case 10	411
Case 11	412
Case 12	414
Case 13	416
Case 14	417
Case 15	418
Case 16	419
Case 17	420
Case 18	422
Case 19	423
Case 20	425
Case 21	426
Case 22	427

▶ **Case 1**

A 29-year-old woman who was involved in a motor vehicle accident is brought to the emergency department, where she is found to be hypotensive with severe internal bleeding. She is given several units of blood by transfusion and is sent to the intensive care unit for monitoring. Within 36 hours, a slight decrease in urine output and an increase in blood urea nitrogen (BUN) are noted, and by 72 hours there is a dramatic drop in urine output. Laboratory studies at 72 hours demonstrate the following:

Serum
    Potassium: 5.1 mEq/L
    BUN: 25 mg/dL
    Creatinine: 2.5 mg/dL
Urinalysis: mild hematuria, mild proteinuria, granular casts, renal tubular epithelial
    cells in sediment
Fractional excretion of sodium (Fe_{Na}): 2.2%

■ **What is the most likely diagnosis?**

The patient is most likely suffering from acute tubular necrosis (ATN) secondary to renal ischemia as a consequence of shock following the accident. ATN is the most common cause of acute kidney injury and is a result of direct injury to the renal tubular epithelia.

■ **What are common causes of this condition?**

Common causes include renal ischemia (shock), crush injury (myoglobin is nephrotoxic), and various toxins, including some chemotherapeutic agents and aminoglycoside antibiotics.

■ **What is the cause of the patient's azotemia?**

ATN involves direct damage to renal tubular epithelial cells (the proximal tubule is particularly vulnerable to ischemic injury because of its high demand for adenosine triphosphate). In addition, the sloughage of intact tubular cells and necrotic cellular debris into the tubular lumen blocks the collecting system. This leads to a back leak of filrate, and consequently, to a decreased glomerular filtration rate (GFR).

■ **How do the laboratory findings assist in establishing the diagnosis?**

Muddy brown epithelial and granular cell casts in the urine are pathognomonic for ATN. Hematuria and proteinuria may also be found, as well as an isotonic urine. Sufficient tubular damage may result in oliguria (<500 mL/24 hr). With ATN, the serum creatinine level rises approximately 0.5 mg/dL/day, but the BUN:creatinine ratio remains nearly normal at 10 to 15:1. Tubular necrosis prevents adequate potassium excretion and sodium reabsorption. The latter is reflected by a urinary sodium concentration that is typically >40 mEq/L and a Fe_{Na} that is >2%. These values are in contrast to the prerenal azotemia, in which urine sodium concentration is usually <20 mEq/L and the Fe_{Na} is <0.7%. These values reflect an adequate renal response to decreased renal perfusion. In ATN the high Fe_{Na} is a sign of sodium wasting due to tubular damage.

■ **What is the prognosis for patients with this condition?**

ATN goes through an initiatory phase within 36 hours of injury with a slight decrease in urine output and an increase in BUN. Within 2–6 days, there is a dramatic fall in urine output that can last for weeks. During this maintenance phase, there is a significant risk of death without proper management. Recovery typically occurs within 2–3 weeks.

► **Case 2**

A 27-year-old man visits his physician because he is concerned about the large amounts of blood he has noticed in his urine over the past week. He denies increased frequency or dysuria but does admit to intermittent aching back pain over the past few months, which he attributes to sitting at his desk for long periods of time each day at work. Ultrasound shows massively enlarged kidneys bilaterally. The surface of the right kidney is studded with several dozen well-circumscribed cysts, and ultrasound of the left kidney demonstrates similar lesions.

■ What is the most likely diagnosis?	Autosomal dominant polycystic kidney disease (ADPKD).
■ What is the mode of inheritance of this condition?	Roughly 85% of cases of ADPKD are due to a mutation in the *PKD1* gene on chromosome 16; the remainder of the cases are caused by mutations in *PKD2*. The disease is inherited in an autosomal dominant fashion.
■ How do patients with this condition typically present?	ADPKD may present at any age but is most frequently diagnosed in the third to fifth decades. Because ADPKD is dominantly inherited, patients may be aware of a family history of the disease. Patients experience chronic flank pain as a result of massively enlarged kidneys, and microscopic or gross hematuria is common. Nocturia may be present if renal concentrating ability is impaired. Hypertension at presentation is not uncommon.
■ What are the extrarenal manifestations of this condition?	Colonic diverticular disease is the most common extrarenal effect of ADPKD. Hepatic cysts (see Figure 12-1) are present in 50%–70% of patients and are generally asymptomatic with little effect on liver function. There is also an association between ADPKD and berry aneurysms of the circle of Willis, which show familial clustering. Rupture of such aneurysms result in subarachnoid hemorrhage and negatively impacts mortality and morbidity. Mitral valve prolapse is found in 25% of patients with this disease.
■ What is the prognosis for patients with this condition?	Progression to chronic renal failure is common, with 50% of patients developing **end-stage renal disease** by age 60 years. There is great variability in the progression of the disease even within families. Early age at diagnosis, male gender, recurrent infection, and hypertension are all associated with an early onset of renal failure. *PKD1* carriers tend to have a more severe course. At present, there is no proven treatment for ADPKD; treatment generally consists of controlling any associated hypertension and/or proteinuria in order to preserve the glomerular filtration rate, but eventually, renal replacement therapies are indicated.

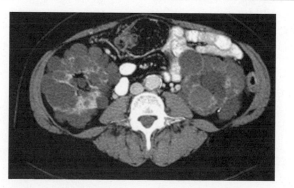

FIGURE 12-1. **Bilateral kidney cysts in polycystic kidney disease.** (Reproduced, with permission, of the Pathology Education Instructional Resource Digital Library [http://peir.net] at the University of Alabama, Birmingham.)

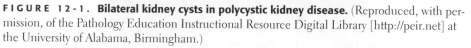

▶ **Case 3**

A 10-year-old boy is brought to his pediatrician for evaluation of bloody urine. A urine sample is positive for hemoglobin and RBC casts. The boy's maternal grandfather suffered from deafness and died of renal failure. The boy also has a 25-year-old male maternal cousin who currently uses a hearing aid and requires dialysis for end-stage renal disease. The family pedigree is shown in Figure 12-2; the boy is indicated by the arrow, his maternal grandfather by the number 1, and his maternal cousin by the number 2. Darkened symbols represent people with known renal disease.

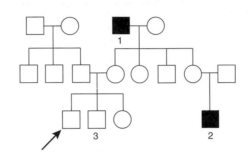

FIGURE 12-2.

■ What is the most likely diagnosis?	The most likely diagnosis is hereditary nephritis, or Alport's syndrome, which consists of glomerular disease, sensorineural deafness, and ocular abnormalities, such as anterior lenticonus, a conical projection of the lens surface. These patients often progress to end-stage renal disease by the second decade of life.
■ This condition is due to a mutation in a gene coding for which protein?	The defective gene codes for the α5 subunit of type IV collagen. Tissue from patients with this mutation fails to stain for this protein.
■ Because of this mutation, the glomerulus loses the ability to selectively filter on the basis of what property?	The glomerulus loses the ability to filter on the basis of size. The glomerular basement membrane is primarily a size-selective (as well as charge-selective) filter, and thus, damage to the basement membrane leads to loss of size selectivity.
■ What is the probability that this patient's brother (person 3 on the pedigree above) has the same disease?	The probability is 50%. The pedigree represents X-linked dominant inheritance. Since the boy's mother is a carrier, each son has a 50% chance (one of two X chromosomes in the mother) of inheriting the mutation. There are also autosomal recessive and autosomal dominant variants of Alport's syndrome.
■ What other screening tests, in addition to urinalysis, could be used to confirm the diagnosis?	Because Alport's syndrome is associated with ocular abnormalities and deafness, an ophthalmological examination and a formal audiogram should be performed, as deficits may be subtle. Skin biopsies can also be useful in diagnosing Alport's syndrome.

► **Case 4**

A 75-year-old woman presents to her physician complaining of a 2-day history of nausea and malaise. She states that she is essentially in good health, although she recently started taking omeprazole for her gastroesophageal reflux disease. The patient denies the use of any other medications, including antibiotics and analgesics. Her physical examination reveals a temperature of 38°C (100.4°F), but it is otherwise unremarkable. Laboratory blood testing demonstrates eosinophilia and an elevated serum creatinine. Urine analysis shows mild proteinuria. Urine microscopy is pending.

■ **What is the most likely diagnosis?**	There is a high clinical suspicion for drug-induced acute interstitial nephritis (AIN) because of the patient's recent initiation of a medication. Drug therapy is responsible for 71% of AIN cases reported, with infections (such as *Legionella*, leptospirosis, cytomegalovirus, and streptococci) and autoimmune disorders responsible for the rest. AIN develops anytime from 1 week to 9 months after drug initiation.
■ **What drugs are associated with this condition?**	Many medications have been associated with AIN, although methicillin remains the classic drug. Antibiotics with a high risk of producing AIN include penicillin, cephalosporins, rifampin, and sulfonamide. Nonsteroidal anti-inflammatory drugs (NSAIDs) are known to lead to AIN, as well as vasoconstriction of the afferent glomerular arterioles by inhibiting prostaglandin production. Proton pump inhibitors have recently been increasingly reported as a cause of AIN.
■ **What other symptoms are common in patients with this condition?**	Other nonspecific complaints, such as weakness, fatigue, and anorexia, are common. Rash can sometimes accompany fever and eosinophilia to complete the classic triad of a drug-induced hypersensitivity reaction. However, only 10% of cases of drug-induced AIN manifest with all three signs. Creatinine concentration can also be acutely elevated.
■ **What are the typical findings on urinalysis?**	Urinalysis often reveals pyuria and hematuria. WBCs, including eosinophils, RBCs, and WBC casts, can also been seen in the urine sediment. Mild proteinuria may be found.
■ **What findings are common on kidney biopsy in this condition?**	A kidney biopsy is the only way to confirm this condition. Renal tissue histopathology often shows interstitial edema along with diffuse cellular infiltration of the interstitium by inflammatory cells including lymphocytes, monocytes, eosinophils, and granulocytes (see Figure 12-3). Tubulitis may also be seen. The presence of granulomas may suggest an autoimmune cause, such as sarcoidosis.
■ **What is the most appropriate treatment for this condition?**	Withdrawal of the offending agent is the primary therapy. The effectiveness of corticosteroid administration has not been proven by a prospective, randomized controlled trial, but prednisone is often tried empirically, especially in cases of failure to induce remission after withdrawal of drug therapy or advanced renal failure.

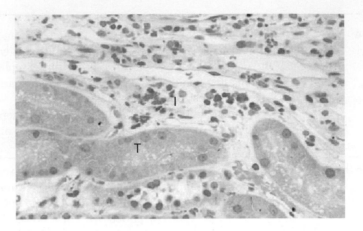

FIGURE 12-3. **Renal biopsy demonstrating interstitial eosinophils. Tubules are indicated by "T," and the interstitium by "I."** (Reproduced, with permission, from Fauci AS et al. *Harrison's Principles of Internal Medicine*, 17th ed. New York: McGraw-Hill, 2008: Figure e9-25.)

A 70-year-old African-American man returns to his physician for his annual follow-up visit for a prior diagnosis of monoclonal gammopathy of undetermined significance (MGUS). He reports he continues to have mild lower back pain and proximal extremity weakness, and notes that he has had polydipsia and polyuria in the past several months. Physical examination is unremarkable. Urinalysis is notable for aminoaciduria, glucosuria, and phosphaturia. Relevant laboratory results are as follows:

Sodium: 133 mEq/L
Potassium: 3.3 mEq/L
Chloride: 110 mEq/L
Bicarbonate: 18 mEq/L

Glucose: 85 mg/dL
Calcium: 8.3 mg/dL
Phosphate: 2.1 mg/dL
Uric acid: 2.0 mg/dL

■ **What is the most likely diagnosis?**

Fanconi's syndrome (FS), which is characterized by a generalized transport defect in the proximal tubules. FS is either acquired or inherited. It can be acquired as a rare complication of plasma cell dyscrasias, including multiple myeloma, MGUS, Waldenström's macroglobulinemia, and primary amyloidosis. FS may also result from Sjögren's syndrome, heavy metal poisoning, and drug reactions. If inherited, FS is mostly transmitted as an autosomal recessive trait.

■ **What are the functions of the proximal convoluted tubules?**

The proximal convoluted tubules are the "workhorses of the nephron," responsible for reabsorbing all glucose and amino acids and the majority of filtered sodium, potassium, phosphate, bicarbonate, and water. Ammonia is also secreted to buffer distally secreted H^+.

■ **What is the pathogenesis of this condition?**

FS is characterized by multiple proximal tubular transport defects. The exact mechanism varies with the etiology of FS. In FS associated with monoclonal gammopathies, kappa-type Bence Jones proteins have been found to be reabsorbed by proximal tubular cells. Subsequent failure to complete proteolysis of these light chains results in cytoplasmic crystalline inclusions, which may eventually compromise tubular function.

■ **What is glomerular filtration rate (GFR)?**

The glomerulus filters plasma predominantly by molecular size and net charge. GFR measures the amount of plasma that is filtered into the Bowman's capsule from the glomerular capillaries within the glomeruli per unit time (milliliters per minute) and is a marker of renal function. Infusion of inulin is necessary for an accurate assessment of GFR because it is fully filtered, but is not reabsorbed, secreted, metabolized, or produced endogenously. GFR, however, is more conveniently approximated by creatinine clearance (C_{Cr}), as represented by: $GFR = U_{Cr} \times V/P_{Cr} = C_{Cr}$, where U_{Cr} and P_{Cr} are the urine and plasma concentration of creatine, respectively, and V is the volume of urine per unit time. Because creatinine, unlike inulin, is secreted, a creatinine-based GFR results in an overestimate of the true GFR. In FS, GFR is normal.

■ **What is the mechanism behind the observed hypokalemia?**

The primary function of the kidneys is to preserve volume though the reabsorption of sodium and free water. In FS, there is an increased distal delivery of sodium due to the incompetent proximal tubules. The principal cells within the collecting ducts will compensate by increasing sodium reabsorption through an exchange for potassium. This results in potassium clearance rates for potassium that may be more than twice the GFR, indicating net tubular secretion. Metabolic acidosis secondary to defective proximal tubule bicarbonate reabsorption may also contribute to potassium loss, as cells tend to remove H^+ from circulation through an exchange for potassium thereby increasing the filtered load of potassium.

A 42-year-old woman presents to her physician after having coughed up blood several times in the past week. She reports she has been coughing more frequently and experiencing difficulty finishing her daily walks in spite of her recent cessation of smoking. She has not noticed any significant changes in her urinary habits. Her physical examination is notable for a blood pressure of 144/82 mm Hg and an absence of fever and dyspnea. An x-ray of the chest demonstrates fluffy infiltrates bilaterally. Urinalysis reveals proteinuria and hematuria, along with RBC casts. A spot protein to creatinine ratio shows significant, but subnephrotic range proteinuria.

■ What conditions should be included in the differential diagnosis?	Acute glomerulonephritis and alveolar hemorrhage suggest Goodpasture's syndrome (GP) or a systemic vasculitis, such as Wegener's granulomatosis, which is more common. Lupus should also be considered, along with other forms of acute glomerulonephritis that are related to pulmonary infection or result in pulmonary edema.
■ Based on the prior differential diagnoses, serologic tests for which antibodies would be most beneficial to identify this patient's condition?	■ Anti–glomerular basement membrane (anti-GBM) antibody ■ Antineutrophil cytoplasmic antibody (vasculitides) ■ Antinuclear antibody and anti-double-stranded DNA (lupus)
■ Only anti-GBM antibodies are subsequently isolated from the patient's serum. What is the epidemiology of the associated condition?	Isolation of anti-GBM antibodies suggests GP, which is a form of anti-GBM disease characterized by rapidly progressive glomerulonephritis, alveolar hemorrhage, and autoantibodies to type IV collagen. GP has a prevalence of 1:1 million. GP occurs with alveolar hemorrhage in 60%–70% of cases. Males are more commonly afflicted in the age range of 5–40 years. Both genders are afflicted equally in older adults. Patients <30 years old are more likely to be severely affected. Untreated, GP has a fatality rate of 50%.
■ What is the pathogenesis of this condition?	IgG (rarely IgA or IgM) autoantibodies against type IV collagen are the distinguishing feature of GP, and they also correlate with the severity of disease. The α3 chains of type IV collagen are present in the basement membranes of glomeruli, alveoli, and several other organs. The antigen targets of GP autoantibodies are normally inaccessible due to the presence of endothelial cells. The exposure of these antigens to circulating antibodies is more likely in the kidneys and lungs because of the fenestrated nature of the endothelial lining of glomerular capillaries and the increased susceptibility of the lungs to injury (due to smoking, toxin inhalation, or infection).
■ What type of hypersensitivity reaction is responsible for this patient's disease process?	A type II hypersensitivity reaction is responsible. Fixation of complement to the anti-GBM antibodies activates the classic complement pathway that results in the recruitment of neutrophils and monocytes.
■ What are the typical findings on kidney biopsy microscopy in this condition?	Light microscopy typically shows crescentic glomerulonephritis (see Figure 12-7 later in the chapter). Immunofluorescence microscopy (see Figure 12-4) demonstrates the nearly pathognomonic finding of a smooth linear deposition of IgG along the glomerular capillaries, occasionally with interruption by C3 deposition.

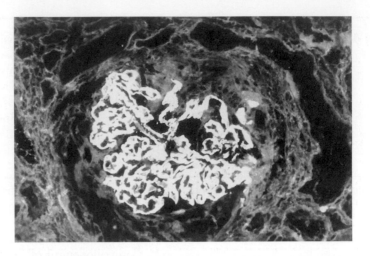

► Case 7

A 4-year-old boy presents with a rash of 2 days' duration that has spread from his legs to his buttocks. He is not febrile and has no sick contacts or other pertinent exposures. The rash consists of nonclustering, nonblanching, raised spots more than 2 mm in size spread over the boy's buttocks and posterior surfaces of his lower extremities. The boy also complains of knee and ankle stiffness and diffuse abdominal pain. His vital signs are stable, and a urinalysis is unremarkable. His laboratory findings are as follows:

Hematocrit: 35%
International Normalized Ratio (INR): 1.0
WBC count: 7000/mm^3
Prothrombin time: 12 sec
Platelet count: 200,000/mm^3
Partial thromboplastin time: 25.2 sec

■ **What is the most likely diagnosis?**

Henoch-Schönlein purpura (HSP). In children, the combination of rash (as described above), arthralgias, abdominal pain, and renal disease is pathognomonic for HSP, although only 63% of patients with HSP actually present with abdominal pain and only 40% with renal disease. An additional 33% of patients also have evidence of gastrointestinal bleeding. Less common symptoms include testicular torsion, intussusception, pancreatitis, cholecystitis, and protein-losing enteropathy. Some 1% of children with HSP progress to end-stage renal disease. HSP is rare in adults.

■ **What are the distinguishing characteristics of this condition?**

Purpura is characterized by nonblanching, flat lesions measuring more than 2 mm in diameter. Related findings are **petechiae**, which are nonblanching, flat lesions measuring <2 mm in diameter. Both are signs of bleeding occurring in the skin. Both purpuric and petechial lesions may be seen in HSP.

■ **What is the pathophysiology of this condition?**

HSP is a small-vessel vasculitis. Although the precipitating factor is unknown, anecdotal evidence points to upper respiratory infection for children. With HSP, IgA deposition in blood vessels causes leaking, which leads to purpura and petechiae. This is pathophysiologically similar to IgA nephropathy.

■ **Which conditions should be considered in the differential diagnosis of this patient's rash?**

The main concerns, in addition to HSP, are clotting disorders and sepsis; as a result, coagulation studies should be performed. A similar rash can be caused by rickettsial infections, although this patient is afebrile. It is very important to distinguish HSP from **hemolytic-uremic syndrome** (HUS), as both present similarly and both can cause extensive renal disease. However, HUS is not likely in this patient, as there are no signs of hemolytic anemia. In adults, HSP must be distinguished from systemic diseases such as hypersensitivity vasculitis and systemic lupus erythematosus.

■ **What are the most appropriate treatments for this condition?**

Treatment is based on the severity of symptoms, as the disease is typically self-limiting. An asymptomatic patient requires no treatment. However, severe symptoms, including signs of renal involvement, may require a renal biopsy and steroids. Regardless of the severity of symptoms, patients with HSP require urinalysis every 3 months for 1 year, as HSP has a high rate of recurrence. Recurrence or flares typically occurs within 4 months after the initial diagnosis, although longer intervals have been observed.

► **Case 8**

A 45-year-old man is brought to the emergency department by his mother after 2 days of worsening confusion, polyuria, polydipsia, and constipation. His past medical history is significant only for chronic osteomyelitis of the right arm secondary to a burn injury sustained in a house fire 5 years ago. Physical examination is unremarkable with the exception of uniformly depressed deep tendon reflexes. The patient is also visibly uncomfortable and disoriented and is uncooperative during much of the examination. ECG reveals a QTc interval of 390 msec. Relevant laboratory findings are as follows:

Serum calcium: 11.88 mEq/L
Serum albumin: 1.45 mEq/L
Ionized calcium: 7.06 mg/dL
Blood urea nitrogen (BUN):creatinine ratio: 29:1.4
Parathyroid hormone (PTH): 12 pg/mL
Alkaline phosphatase: 980 U/L
The patient is immediately started on 1 L of normal saline with a goal of 4–6 L over 24 hours, with furosemide added shortly thereafter.

■ **What other symptoms are common in this condition?**	Symptoms of hypercalcemia include lethargy, hyporeflexia, confusion, depression, headaches, psychosis, bradycardia, a shortened QT interval, nausea, vomiting, constipation, muscle weakness, polyuria, polydipsia, and gastroduodenal ulcer disease (secondary to calcium-induced gastrin release).
■ **What is the importance of ionized calcium and albumin in the diagnosis of this condition?**	Ionized calcium is the primary determinant of cellular and membrane activity. Approximately 45% of calcium circulates in the free or ionized form, while another 40% is bound to albumin. (The remainder is bound to various anions.) Accurate assessment of total calcium levels therefore requires the simultaneous measurement of albumin and ionized calcium levels.
■ **How does hypoalbuminemia affect this condition?**	Hypoalbuminemia can decrease measured serum calcium levels independently of any net change in ionized calcium levels. For each decrease of 1.0 g/dL in serum albumin below the laboratory's reference normal value, 0.8 mg/dL should be added to the total calcium measured. Given the patient's hypoalbuminemia, the actual total serum calcium levels is even greater than the already elevated total calcium observed.
■ **What are pseudohypercalcemia and pseudohypocalcemia?**	**Pseudohypercalcemia** and the converse, **pseudohypocalcemia**, refer to perturbations in net calcium concentration in the setting of a normal ionized fraction. Given a normal ionized fraction, the clinical picture is normal. They are usually caused by alterations in plasma protein concentration.
■ **What is a hypercalcemic crisis?**	This patient presented in a hypercalcemic crisis. Calcium acts as a direct toxin to the renal tubules that blocks antidiuretic activity, as well as causes vasoconstriction and decreases the glomerular filtration rate. This results in polyuria, but increases calcium reabsorption and serum calcium, thereby exacerbating nephrotoxicity.

What are the most appropriate treatments for this condition?

Symptomatic hypercalcemia, as seen in this patient, should first be treated with a saline infusion to expedite renal calcium excretion. Furosemide may be initiated in these patients to promote calciuresis only after the patient is volume repleted. Furosemide serves both to promote natriuresis and to increase calcium excretion. Care must be taken to ensure the patient does not become hypovolemic during calciuresis. Bisphosphonates inhibit osteoclast activity and are efficacious in the treatment of hypercalcemia secondary to this mechanism. Given this patient's past history of chronic osteomyelitis, suppressed PTH, and dramatically elevated alkaline phosphatase levels there is a high clinical suspicion for underlying malignancy.

► **Case 9**

A 57-year-old man with a history of coronary artery disease presents to the emergency department with a 1-week history of progressive weakness, fatigue, and shortness of breath on exertion. On physical examination, the man's heart rate is irregularly irregular, and his lung examination is notable for bilateral crackles that are most pronounced at the bases. An x-ray of the chest demonstrates pulmonary edema, and an ECG reveals he is in atrial fibrillation. The patient is started on digoxin and furosemide. Three days later, he complains of rapid onset of shortness of breath and light-headedness with progressive weakness. His laboratory values are significant for a serum sodium level of 142 mEq/L and a serum potassium level of 2.7 mEq/L. An ECG demonstrates torsades de pointes.

■ What is the most likely diagnosis?	Hypokalemia.
■ What are the two main factors that predisposed the patient to torsades de pointes?	The patient was started on digoxin to increase cardiac output and to treat the atrial fibrillation, and the furosemide was added to treat the pulmonary edema. However, furosemide in the setting of congestive heart failure can lead to severe hypokalemia (serum potassium level <2.5 mEq/L). Digitalis use in the setting of hypokalemia can predispose a patient to possibly fatal arrhythmias.
■ What are the most common causes of this condition?	There are three broad etiologies of hypokalemia: decreased intake, increased losses, and increased translocation into cells. ■ Decreased intake is a very rare cause of hypokalemia. ■ Increased losses can be: 1) Gastrointestinal, from diarrhea, laxative abuse, and/or vomiting. 2) Urinary, as in diuretic use, polyuria and other salt-wasting conditions, hyperaldosteronism, loss of gastric secretions, or metabolic acidosis. ■ Increased translocation into cells occurs with hypothermia, alkalosis, increased insulin availability, β-adrenergic activity.
■ How does alkalosis lead to this condition?	The Na^+-K^+-ATPase pump keeps intracellular potassium levels much higher than the serum/extracellular level. However, in the setting of alkalosis, hydrogen ions leave cells to minimize pH change. In the process, hydrogen ions function in an apparent exchange for potassium that can lead to hypokalemia.
■ How is metabolic acidosis associated with this condition?	**Metabolic acidosis** causes an exchange of hydrogen ions into the cells for potassium ions into the plasma, leading to hyperkalemia. However, in the setting of metabolic acidosis (notably diabetic ketoacidosis), urinary potassium excretion is also increased. This leads to a situation in which potassium is being moved from the cells and then excreted in the urine; so while the serum potassium level is normal or even high in metabolic acidosis, the total body stores are actually low. The hypokalemia will often reveal itself once the acidosis is corrected.
■ What are the most appropriate treatments for this condition?	Potassium can be repleted either directly (i.e., with potassium chloride) or through the use of a potassium-sparing diuretic such as amiloride, spironolactone, or triamterene. Amiloride is often the diuretic of choice, as it lacks the hormonal adverse effects of spironolactone (gynecomastia and amenorrhea).

► **Case 10**

An 86-year-old woman living in a nursing home is brought to the attention of the medical staff due to her lethargy. Relatives note that she has been unable to recognize family members in the past week. Her past medical history is notable for Alzheimer's disease, osteoporosis, and hypertension. Her medications include memantine, donepezil, alendronate, and hydrochlorothiazide, the dose of which was recently increased. Physical examination reveals a blood pressure of 139/80 mm Hg. The patient is sleepy and oriented only to person. CT scan of the head is unremarkable. Laboratory testing is notable for a sodium concentration of 122 mEq/L and normal glucose levels, renal function, and hematocrit.

■ **What is the most likely diagnosis?**	Hyponatremia, which is commonly defined as a serum sodium concentration ≤135 mEq/L. Hyponatremia is more prevalent in the hospital setting or in nursing homes.
■ **What are the common causes of this condition?**	Most cases of hyponatremia can be thought of as arising from two general mechanisms: ■ Too much water, such as in the syndrome of inappropriate secretion of antidiuretic hormone (SIADH), nephrotic syndrome, congestive heart failure, or cirrhosis. ■ Too little salt, such as in salt-wasting conditions (e.g., aldosterone resistance or deficiency), diuretic abuse, dehydration, or vomiting.
■ **What are the typical symptoms associated with this condition?**	The decreased osmolarity causes an osmotic water shift that increases intracellular fluid volume. Clinical manifestations are typically neurologic in nature secondary to cerebral edema within the confines of the cranial vault. Nonspecific symptoms, such as malaise or nausea, are common. Headache, lethargy, confusion, and obtundation may appear as sodium levels fall further. Stupor, seizures, and coma can occur if progression is rapid or concentrations fall below 120 mEq/L.
■ **What is the pathogenesis of this condition in this particular patient?**	This patient is likely suffering from diuretic-induced hyponatremia. Thiazides deplete serum sodium and potassium levels and stimulate ADH-mediated water retention. It should be noted though that loop diuretics are unlikely to cause hyponatremia, as the maximal urine concentrating ability, and thereby water retention, is reduced with the decrease in medullary interstitial tonicity. The brain cells react to hyponatremia by secreting salts, and over time organic osmolytes, to prevent excess water entry and swelling. This may account for the fact that no significant swelling can be seen on CT scan of the head.
■ **What other laboratory test will aid in the identification of the etiology of this condition in this patient?**	Plasma osmolality, urine osmolality, fractional excretion of sodium, urine sodium concentration, and urine potassium concentration would be helpful. If diuretics are responsible as in this case, the plasma osmolality may be slightly low. Urine osmolality would be elevated, as thiazides would stimulate ADH. Urine sodium is elevated due to a thiazide-mediated decrease in reabsorption. However, some of the excess sodium delivered to the collecting duct is reabsorbed at the expense of potassium. Urine potassium therefore would also be elevated.
■ **What is the risk of correcting hyponatremia too quickly?**	This can result in central pontine myelinolysis, a diffuse (not limited to the pons) demyelination syndrome. A rapid increase in serum osmolarity leads to brain cell shrinkage, and this is believed to somehow result in demyelination.

▶ **Case 11**

A 5-year-old boy presents to a physician for a second opinion regarding the bowing of his legs since 2 years of age and short stature. The family history is notable for bowed legs in the maternal grandfather and poor dentition in the mother. Physical examination is remarkable for frontal bossing, dental abnormalities, and tibia vara. Urine electrolyte analysis reveals elevated phosphate levels. Serum calcidiol are within normal limits, but calcitriol levels are low. Other relevant laboratory values are as follows:

Blood urea nitrogen: 16 mg/dL
Creatinine: 0.4 mg/dL (normal for age)
Parathyroid hormone (PTH): 54 pg/mL
 (normal: 10–55 pg/mL)

Serum albumin: 4.5 g/dL
Serum phosphate: 1.3 mg/dL
Alkaline phosphatase: 450 U/L
Total calcium: 8.7 mg/dL

■ **What is the most likely diagnosis?**

Hypophosphatemic (vitamin D–resistant) rickets, as suggested by his slow growth, skeletal findings, and upper normal PTH, normal calcidiol, and calcium levels, but low calcitriol and phosphaturia in the setting of normal renal function. Two inheritable forms exist. X-linked hypophosphatemic rickets (XLH) is more likely in this case, as it generally affects males and presents in childhood. The grandfather likely was similarly affected, while the heterozygous mother is only mildly afflicted with dentition problems. A less common autosomal dominant form also exists, which affects both genders equally, and presents later in life.

■ **What is the pathogenesis of this condition?**

XLH is associated with a loss of function mutation in a gene on the X-chromosome responsible for the clearance of fibroblast growth factor-23. Failure to clear the latter leads to phosphaturia and unchecked 1α-hydroxylase activity in the kidney. Increased excretion of phosphate, decreased calcitriol levels, and ultimately bone deformities result. The previous eponym of vitamin D–resistant rickets derives from the fact that administration of calcidiol (or even calcitriol) by itself is not beneficial in the setting of renal phosphate wasting.

■ **What are the typical radiologic findings in this condition?**

Figure 12-5 shows the typical findings of widened diaphyses, funnel-like beaking of the metaphyses, and increased curvature of the femoral and tibial shafts. Lower extremity deformities develop as the child begins to bear weight with ambulation.

■ **How is phosphate regulated in the body?**

Calcium and phosphate regulation are linked. Phosphate is primarily reabsorbed in the proximal renal tubules. **PTH** release is stimulated by low serum calcium levels, high phosphate levels, and low vitamin D levels. It decreases phosphate levels by inhibiting phosphate reabsorption in the proximal tubules, although this is partially offset by its effect of enhancing resorption of calcium and phosphate from bone.

Calcitriol formation is stimulated by low serum calcium and phosphate levels and high PTH levels. It enhances gut absorption of both calcium and phosphate, induces the osteoclast maturation necessary for bone remodeling, and promotes calcium deposition in the bone. It also decreases PTH secretion.

■ **What is the most appropriate treatment for this condition?**

A combination of phosphorus and calcitriol is required to restore age-appropriate growth velocity. Administration of either alone is insufficient. Phosphorus by itself would decrease ionized calcium levels, which results in PTH release and secondary hyperparathyroidism. Serum phosphorus level normalization also simultaneously decreases calcitriol formation. This removes the inhibitory effect calcitriol has on PTH synthesis and its stimulatory effect on intestinal reabsorption of calcium and calcium deposition in bone. This ultimately causes hypocalcemia, persistent hypophosphatemia, and bone disease.

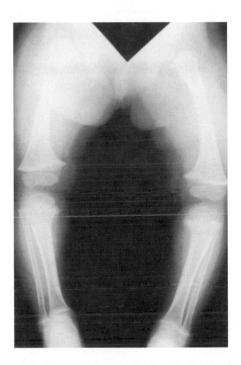

FIGURE 12-5. Bowed long bones and irregular, flared physes. (Reproduced, with permission, from Skinner HB. *Current Diagnosis & Treatment in Orthopedics*, 4th ed. New York: McGraw-Hill, 2006: 603.)

▶ **Case 12**

A 24-year-old woman presents to the emergency department with nausea, vomiting, tachypnea, sweating, and tinnitus. Her mother reports that she found an empty bottle of aspirin in the patient's bedroom. Physical examination reveals a temperature of 38.6°C (101.5°F), a heart rate of 100/min, a respiratory rate of 40/min, and altered mental status. Arterial blood gas is notable for a pH of 7.28, partial carbon dioxide pressure (P_{CO_2}) of 25 mm Hg, and bicarbonate of 17 mEq/L. Her anion gap is 22. Salicylate levels are pending. Intravenous fluids are initiated, and charcoal and sodium bicarbonate are administered orally. The patient is transferred to the intensive care unit for further stabilization.

■ **What is the acid-base disturbance in this patient?**

A mixed metabolic acidosis and respiratory alkalosis. The pH <7.35 indicates an acidemia. Respiratory acidosis is unlikely given the below-normal P_{CO_2} and the anion gap of 22. In this setting the low bicarbonate indicates she has a metabolic acidosis. Applying Winter's formula, the appropriate respiratory compensation is $P_{CO_2} = 1.5(17) + 8 = 33.5 \pm 2$. The "compensation" in this case is therefore excessive, suggesting an independent respiratory alkalotic process.

■ **What are the causes of metabolic acidosis?**

Metabolic acidosis derives from the loss of bicarbonate or the retention of acid. The former results in nonanion gap acidosis and is always the result of conditions that result in hyperchloremia (>109 mEq/L), such as renal tubular acidosis. The excess chloride suppresses bicarbonate reabsorption. Metabolic acidosis that is caused by retention of acid results in an anion gap metabolic acidosis because unmeasured, acidic anions are retained. To recall the major causes of anion gap metabolic acidosis, the mnemonic **MUD PILES** is useful:

Methanol
Uremia
Diabetic ketoacidosis
Paraldehyde or **P**henformin
Iron tablets or **I**soniazid
Lactic acidosis
Ethylene glycol
Salicylates

■ **What are the causes of respiratory alkalosis?**

Anything that stimulates the central respiratory drive and causes hyperventilation, such as cerebrovascular accidents or neurologic disease, can cause respiratory alkalosis. Hypoxia, such as that caused by anemia, high attitudes, and pulmonary disease, can likewise lead to an increased respiratory rate and respiratory alkalosis. It can also be caused by other hyperventilatory states such as mechanical overventilation or voluntary hyperventilation, such as in cases of anxiety.

■ **How is an anion gap calculated?**

The equation $Na^+ - (Cl^- + HCO_3^-)$ is typically used. K^+ is typically not included due to its small contribution as a predominantly intracellular cation. A normal anion gap is 6–12 mEq/L. The presence of unmeasured anions, such as salicylates, displaces and reduces serum bicarbonate, thereby producing an apparently larger gap.

■ **What is the pathogenesis of this patient's condition?**

Aspirin is hydrolyzed to salicylate once ingested. At toxic levels, salicylates cause a primary respiratory alkalosis by stimulating the medullary respiratory center to hyperventilate. Salicylates also stimulate skeletal muscle metabolism, increasing oxygen consumption and carbon dioxide production. This further stimulates hyperventilation. The metabolic acidosis component occurs because salicylates both cause lipolysis and uncoupling of oxidative phosphorylation, thereby resulting in the production of organic acids, pyruvate, and ketones.

► **Case 13**

A 20-year-old man on his first postoperative day after an appendectomy develops nausea and vomiting that is unresponsive to antiemetic therapy. He currently is unable to retain any fluids and has also not consumed anything by mouth. His physical examination is notable for orthostatic hypotension. The patient admits he had discontinued his intravenous (IV) fluids due to discomfort. His arterial blood gas is notable for a pH of 7.48, partial carbon dioxide pressure (P_{CO_2}) of 42 mm Hg, and bicarbonate of 28 mEq/L.

■ What acid-base disturbance is seen in this patient?

Metabolic alkalosis. The pH of the arterial blood is >7.45, which indicates alkalemia. Metabolic versus respiratory alkalosis can be distinguished by examining the P_{CO_2}. A P_{CO_2} >40 mm Hg suggests a metabolic process. A bicarbonate >25 mEq/L is characteristic of a metabolic alkalosis.

■ What does the body do in order to partially compensate for this state?

A patient may hypoventilate to cause a respiratory acidosis that would reduce the pH as a compensatory measure. P_{CO_2} is increased by 0.7 mm Hg for every 1 mEq/L increase in bicarbonate. In this case, the bicarbonate is approximately 3 mEq/L above normal, which translates into an expected P_{CO_2} of 40 + 0.7(3) = 42.1 mm Hg. The metabolic alkalosis here is therefore appropriately compensated.

■ How is this condition classified?

Metabolic alkalosis usually reflects chloride losses. It can be caused by a number of different conditions. Some causes are **saline-responsive**. These are characterized by hypochloremia (<95 mEq/L) and a low urinary chloride (<10 mEq/L). Other conditions are **saline-unresponsive**. These are associated with low serum chloride and a high urinary chloride (>10 mEq/L). Saline-responsive metabolic alkalosis is caused by chloride losses and volume depletion, such as persistent vomiting, cystic fibrosis, hypokalemia secondary to diuretic use, congenital familial chloridorrhea, and post-hypercapnia. Hyperaldosteronism, Cushing's syndrome, alkali administration, and exogenous stimulation of mineralocorticoid production (e.g., licorice) are some disorders responsible for saline-unresponsive metabolic alkalosis.

■ What is the pathogenesis of this patient's condition?

This patient is volume depleted because he stopped his IV fluids. In addition, he has been vomiting, which removes further fluid and chloride (from HCl). His alkalemia is therefore likely saline-responsive. His dehydration stimulates the renin-angiotensin-aldosterone system. Elevated aldosterone causes reabsorption of Na^+ in exchange for K^+ and H^+. This further exacerbates the alkalemia and also leads to hypokalemia. Treatment involves restoration of volume status to prevent further exacerbation of the alkalemia and the complications of hypokalemia.

■ How does aciduria occur in this condition?

Aciduria is paradoxical in the setting of alkalemia. It can occur, however, in the setting of an extended period of volume depletion. The activated renin-angiotensin-aldosterone system exchanges for K^+ and H^+. Over time, the pool of available intracellular K^+ becomes depleted, resulting in the exchange of only H^+. The subsequent aciduria is an indication of a metabolic emergency with severe hypokalemia.

► **Case 14**

A 3-year-old boy is brought to his pediatrician after his mother notices that his limbs seem swollen and his stomach distended. She says the boy received an influenza shot 1 week ago. Physical examination reveals generalized pitting edema and shifting dullness of the abdomen suggestive of ascites. Urinalysis reveals 4+ proteinuria, and laboratory findings show a decreased serum albumin level, hypertriglyceridemia, and a normal serum ionized calcium level. The total Ca may well be low because of the hypoalbuminemia. Blood urea nitrogen (BUN) and serum creatinine values are within normal limits.

■ **What is the most likely diagnosis?**	The boy likely has nephrotic syndrome likely in the form of minimal change disease (lipoid nephrosis). This is the most common manifestation of nephrotic syndrome in children (approximately 90% of cases occur in children younger than 10 years of age).
■ **What are the four classic symptoms of this condition?**	Nephrotic syndrome classically presents with proteinuria, hypoalbuminemia, edema, and hypercholesterolemia.
■ **What pathologic changes at the glomerular level are associated with this condition?**	The glomerular basement membrane contains heparan sulfate, which acts as a negative charge barrier that keeps small and negatively charged proteins such as albumin from crossing the membrane. Minimal change disease is often preceded by a recent infection or vaccination; it is believed that T cells release cytokines that injure glomerular epithelial cells. Consequently, the negative charge barrier is lost, while the size filter provided by the slit diaphragm proteins may remain intact. This leads to renal albumin wasting.
■ **What are the likely findings on histology?**	Glomeruli appear normal on light microscopy; hence, the name "minimal change." However, when the glomeruli are viewed under electron microscopy, effacement or flattening of foot processes can be seen. The electron micrograph in Figure 12-6 shows effacement of the foot processes (arrowhead).
■ **What is the most appropriate treatment for this condition?**	Given the high incidence of minimal change disease in children with nephrotic syndrome, this can be presumed to be the diagnosis until proven otherwise. Corticosteroids are given both as treatment and as a diagnostic tool because the majority with minimal change disease typically promptly responds.

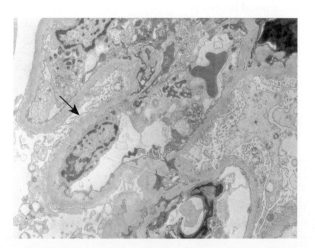

FIGURE 12-6. **Electron micrograph showing effacement of the foot processes in minimal change disease.** (Reproduced, with permission, from Le T, Bhushan V, Rao DA. *First Aid for the USMLE Step 1: 2008.* New York: McGraw-Hill, 2008: Color Image 93.)

▶ **Case 15**

An 11-year-old boy is sent to his school nurse after his gym teacher notes that he was unusually short of breath while playing soccer. After noticing that the boy's socks left deep indentations in his calves and shins bilaterally, the nurse obtains a urine sample that demonstrates proteinuria, but no glucose, no RBCs, and no WBCs. He is then brought to the emergency department for further workup. Relevant laboratory test results are as follows:

Serum
   Sodium: 129 mEq/L
   Potassium: 2.9 mEq/L
   Serum albumin: 2.3 g/dL
Cholesterol levels: elevated

■ What is the most likely diagnosis?	The boy's presentation suggests nephrotic syndrome, which is characterized by the triad of high urine protein losses, hypoalbuminemia, and hypercholesterolemia. Patients often present with periorbital edema, peripheral edema, and/or ascites secondary to decreased plasma protein. This results in decreased plasma oncotic pressure. The latter ultimately leads to sodium and free water retention.
■ What is the most likely mechanism of this patient's proteinuria?	The likely mechanism of action is loss of charge barrier at the glomerular membrane due to effacement of foot processes.
■ What are the typical laboratory findings in this condition?	Serum albumin levels are low, and 24-hour urine protein excretion is high secondary to the massive loss of albumin at the glomerulus. Patients also often demonstrate severe hyperlipidemia.
■ What are the most appropriate treatments for this condition?	It is treated with prednisone. Although the etiology of minimal change disease is unknown, it is thought to be due to an immune system abnormality. Thus, corticosteroids (prednisone) and other immune suppressants are commonly used. Symptomatic treatment should also be initiated for edema, hypercoagulability, infection, decreased intravascular volume, and other clinical manifestations.
■ After 2 months of steroid treatment, the patient shows no decrease in his proteinuria, and a renal biopsy is obtained. What is the most likely diagnosis?	The boy likely has **focal segmental glomerular sclerosis**, which is often resistant to steroid treatment. Light microscopy of the biopsy specimen may demonstrate focal areas of glomeruli with segmental sclerosis. Electron microscopy demonstrates foot process derangement.

► **Case 16**

A 16-year-old previously healthy girl visits her doctor with recent-onset flank pain. She is given ibuprofen and is sent home. Three days later, she develops a fever accompanied by emesis and worsening flank pain. On evaluation, she recalls episodes of urgency as well as decreased urine output. Her physical examination is notable for a temperature of 38.9°C (102.0°F) and costovertebral angle tenderness. Her laboratory findings are as follows:

WBC count: 13,900/mm³   Platelet count: 181,000/mm³
Neutrophils: 74%   Blood urea nitrogen (BUN): 10 mg/dL
Lymphocytes: 10%   Serum creatinine: 1.1 mg/dL
Monocytes: 15%   Hematocrit: 33%
Urinalysis: 2+ protein, small leukocyte esterase, many WBCs, 2–5 RBCs/hpf, few bacteria, and WBC casts

■ **What is the most likely diagnosis?**

Acute pyelonephritis. This diagnosis is suggested by the presence of flank pain, emesis, high fever, and costovertebral angle tenderness on examination. Pyelonephritis is most common in young children and sexually active women. Men are less likely to develop either pyelonephritis (upper urinary tract infection) or acute cystitis (lower urinary tract infection), in part because of their longer urethras. Other predisposing factors include vesicoureteric reflux, flow obstruction, catheterization, gynecologic abnormalities, diabetes, and pregnancy.

■ **What are the most likely pathogens in urinary tract infections (UTIs)?**

Escherichia coli is by far the most common cause of UTI, causing 50%–80% of cases. *Staphylococcus saprophyticus* is the second most common cause of UTI in young, sexually active women. Other common causative organisms include *Proteus mirabilis*, *Klebsiella*, *Serratia*, *Enterobacter*, and *Pseudomonas*. Group B β-hemolytic streptococcal infection can cause UTI in infants as part of the sepsis they develop.

■ **How can this patient's symptoms be distinguished from those associated with cystitis, urethritis, or vaginitis?**

While pyelonephritis classically manifests as flank pain, costovertebral angle tenderness, nausea, and vomiting with high fever, the classic primary complaint in cystitis is dysuria accompanied by frequency, urgency, suprapubic pain, and hematuria. In contrast, urethritis and vaginitis present with dysuria, discharge, pruritus, dyspareunia, and an absence of frequency or urgency.

■ **What are the characteristic laboratory findings in this condition?**

Pyuria is an essential finding for the diagnosis of UTI. Urinalysis typically shows >10 WBCs/mL, whereas significant bacteriuria points toward pyelonephritis rather than cystitis. Hematuria is also common in women with UTI, but not in women with urethritis or vaginitis. Additionally, serum tests will show leukocytosis, an elevated erythrocyte sedimentation rate, and an elevated C-reactive protein level.

■ **What are the most appropriate treatments for this condition?**

The goal of empiric therapy is to use drugs that achieve high concentrations in the renal medulla. Oral medications include the fluoroquinolones (especially ciprofloxacin) and trimethoprim-sulfamethoxazole. Nitrofurantoin, while useful in cystitis because of its activity in urine, poorly concentrates in tissue and is not particularly useful for pyelonephritis. Intravenous options include ceftriaxone, ciprofloxacin, ampicillin and gentamicin, and piperacillin/tazobactam.

▶ **Case 17**

A 37-year-old woman presents to her rheumatologist complaining of increased fatigue, periorbital edema, and swelling of her lower extremities of 3 days duration. One month prior, she had been started on prednisone and hydroxychloroquine for her newly diagnosed lupus. Her previously normal urine analysis now reveals hematuria, proteinuria, dysmorphic RBCs, and RBC casts. Her creatinine is at 2.5 mg/dL. Physical examination at this visit reveals a temperature of 38.3°C (100.9°F), a blood pressure of 150/90 mm Hg, and a weight increase of 5 kg. Moderate ascites and lower extremity pitting edema up to her thighs are present. The next day, a kidney biopsy is performed and is shown in Figure 12-7. The patient is oligo-anuric, and her creatinine rises to 3.2 mg/dL the day of her biopsy.

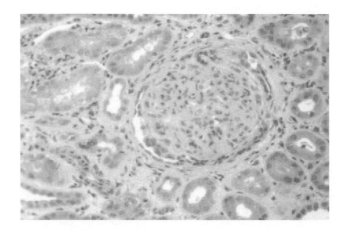

FIGURE 12-7. (Reproduced, with permission, from the Pathology Education Instructional Resource Digital Library [http://peir.net] at the University of Alabama, Birmingham.)

■ **What is the most likely diagnosis?**

Rapidly progressive glomerulonephritis (RPGN) is a clinical diagnosis characterized by a doubling of serum creatinine in a 3-month period and rapid progression to acute renal failure. The latter occurs over weeks to months with associated nephritic urinary sediment, hypervolemia, edema, oliguria, and hypertension. RPGN can result from a primary glomerulopathy or a secondary glomerulopathy mediated by a systemic disease, such as SLE in this case, or a streptococcal infection. Kidney biopsy remains the gold standard for diagnosis.

■ **How does the kidney biopsy aid in the diagnosis of this condition?**

Light microscopy (LM) demonstrates the typical crescent formation of RPGN as seen in Figure 12-7. Immunofluorescence microscopy of a renal specimen distinguishes three major patterns of immunoglobulin deposition, representing three diagnostic categories:

■ Immune-complex glomerulonephritis: Scattered granular deposits of immune complexes. This is the typical "lumpy bumpy" pattern.
■ Anti–glomerular basement membrane disease: Smooth, linear deposition of immunoglobulin as seen in Figure 12-4.
■ Pauci-immune glomerulonephritis: Sparse or absent immunoglobulins.

- **What is the pathogenesis of this condition?**

  RPGN is on the spectrum of immunologically mediated proliferative glomerulonephritides. SLE-associated RPGN is rare, but likely shares a mechanism similar to other types of SLE renal diseases. Mesangial and subendothelial deposition of immune complexes, primarily composed of DNA-anti-DNA, are present. Subsequent activation of complement initiates the immune response.

- **How does the morphology of urine erythrocytes distinguish upper and lower urinary tract disorders?**

  Dysmorphic RBCs suggest upper tract bleeding or inflammatory glomerular or tubulointerstitial disease. RBC casts are also an indication of a glomerular disorder. Normal erythrocytes or eumorphic RBCs support lower urinary tract bleeding.

- **What are the possible clinical presentations of SLE-associated renal disease?**

  Renal involvement occurs in up to 75% of SLE patients. In children with SLE, 90% will have nephritis. Clinical manifestation range from subclinical hematuria or proteinuria to overt nephritic or nephrotic syndrome. The exact underlying type of renal disease is usually identified via kidney biopsy.

► **Case 18**

A 70-year-old man visits his primary care physician after going to a health fair and discovering that his blood pressure is 170/100 mm Hg. The previous year, his blood pressure was 135/85. The man also has a history of hypercholesterolemia. At the physician's office, he has a blood pressure of 150/100 mm Hg and a heart rate of 80/min, and an abdominal bruit is detected in the epigastric region to the right of midline. Laboratory findings are significant for a serum sodium level of 147 mEq/L and a serum potassium level of 3.3 mEq/L.

■ What is the most likely diagnosis?	The man most likely suffers from renal artery stenosis, which is often caused by atherosclerotic plaques in older men (secondary to hypercholesterolemia) and fibromuscular dysplasia in young women. This diagnosis is suggested by the relatively sudden onset of hypertension in addition to hypokalemia.
■ What changes in renin secretion would one expect to see from each kidney?	The kidney ipsilateral to the stenosis will increase renin secretion in response to a perceived decrease in arterial pressure due to decreased flow to the juxtaglomerular apparatus. The contralateral kidney will respond to the patient's resulting hypertension by decreasing its renin secretion (see Figure 12-8).
■ How does an elevated plasma renin level lead to hypertension?	In the plasma, renin converts angiotensinogen to angiotensin I, which is converted to angiotensin II by angiotensin-converting enzyme (ACE). **Angiotensin II** acts on vascular smooth muscle to increase blood pressure. Angiotensin II also acts on the adrenal cortex to stimulate the release of aldosterone, which increases renal absorption of sodium to increase blood volume, thus increasing blood pressure.
■ What electrolyte abnormalities are associated with this condition?	As seen in hyperaldosteronism, the sodium reabsorption is isotonic hence the serum Na is normal but hypertension ensues, and hypokalemia is expected as a consequence of renal potassium losses.
■ What is the diuretic of choice for this condition?	Spironolactone, an aldosterone antagonist, is preferred because of its potassium-sparing properties.
■ Which classes of antihypertensive drugs directly target the effects of renin?	ACE inhibitors (captopril, enalapril, and lisinopril), angiotensin II blockers (losartan), aldosterone-antagonizing diuretics (spironolactone), and renin inhibitors (aliskiren) achieve this goal.

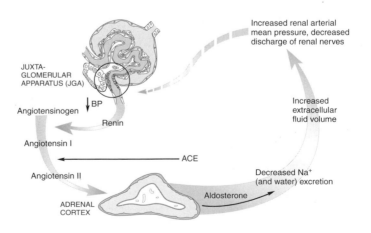

FIGURE 12-8. Renin-angiotensin system. ACE = angiotensin-converting enzyme. (Adapted, with permission, from Ganong WF. *Review of Medical Physiology*, 20th ed. New York: McGraw-Hill, 2001.)

▶ **Case 19**

A 64-year-old woman presents to her physician with sudden onset of nausea and severe back pain on her right side. The patient is in acute distress and is unable to find a comfortable position. She has no prior history of back pain. Her temperature is 36.9°C (98.4°F), her heart rate is 90/min, and her blood pressure is 130/80 mm Hg. Relevant laboratory findings are as follows:

Serum
  Sodium: 140 mEq/L   Chloride: 100 mEq/L
  Potassium: 4 mEq/L   Phosphoric acid: 2.1 mEq/L
  Magnesium: 1.8 mg/dL   Glucose: 100 mg/dL
  Calcium: 13 mg/dL   Blood urea nitrogen (BUN): 15 mg/dL
  Bicarbonate: 25 mEq/L   Creatinine: 1 mg/dL
  Urinary pH: 5.85
  Urinalysis shows RBCs

■ What is the most likely diagnosis?	Nephrolithiasis (kidney stones).
■ How is this condition classified?	Some 85% of renal calculi are **calcium oxalate stones** (see Figure 12-9), which are strongly radiopaque. The second most common kidney stones are **struvite** (ammonium magnesium phosphate), which are radiopaque stones associated with *Proteus vulgaris* and *Staphylococcus aureus* infection. Other, less common stones include **uric acid stones** (radiolucent) and **cystine stones** (moderately radiopaque).
■ What is the pathogenesis of this condition?	Calcium oxalate stones can be caused by hypercalciuria, hyperoxaluria, or hypocitraturia (citrate is a potent inhibitor of calcium precipitation/stone formation).
■ What is the pathogenesis of struvite stones?	Struvite stones form in the presence of alkaline urine, created by urease-splitting organisms. Uric acid stones are associated with hyperuricemia, which is seen in gout and in conditions with high cell turnover, such as leukemia or myeloproliferative disease. Cystine stones are observed in congenital cystinuria.
■ What is the most appropriate treatment for this patient's condition?	Treatment should consist of analgesics, hydration, and if obstructed or infected, antibiotics +/- stenting. Thiazide diuretics are contraindicated in this patient due to her hypercalcemia. Extracorporeal shock wave lithotripsy or surgery may be necessary for stones that do not pass spontaneously.
■ What hormonal imbalance can cause these electrolyte abnormalities?	Hyperparathyrodism may be to blame. The high calcium concentration and low phosphate concentration may be a result of excess parathyroid hormone (PTH). A high PTH level increases renal reabsorption of calcium and decreases renal reabsorption of phosphate. It also stimulates renal activation of vitamin D, which increases calcium and phosphate absorption from the gastrointestinal tract.

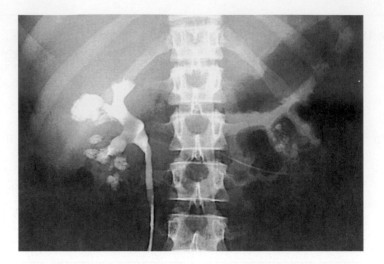

FIGURE 12-9. Kidney stones. (Reproduced, with permission, from Tanagho EA, McAninch JW. *Smith's General Urology*, 16th ed. New York: McGraw-Hill, 2004: 259.)

► **Case 20**

A 60-year-old man with a 30-year smoking history presents to his physician with complaints of cough, fatigue, and a recent 9.1-kg (20-lb) weight loss. An x-ray of the chest reveals a 2-cm hilar mass that is identified on biopsy as small cell lung cancer. On physical examination, the patient has some cachexia but normal skin turgor, no edema or jugular venous distention, and no orthostatic hypotension. Relevant laboratory findings are as follows:

Serum
- Sodium: 128 mEq/L
- Potassium: 4 mEq/L
- Blood urea nitrogen (BUN): 8 mg/dL
- Glucose: 90 mg/dL

Urine
- Sodium: 40 mEq/L
- Osmolality: 610 mOsm/kg H_2O

■ **What is the most likely diagnosis?**

Two possible scenarios exist for his hyponatremia: too much water or too little salt. Too little salt is unlikely here, as the patient has no evidence or any history of renal or extrarenal losses. He is also not hypotensive, orthostatic, or tachycardic. With respect to too much water, he does not have evidence of hypervolemia, distention of jugular veins, or hypertension. His high urinary sodium suggests of at least adequate renal perfusion. The high urine osmolality, which is more than twice the calculated serum osmolality, suggests that antidiuretic hormone (ADH) is present and active in the distal nephron. Since the two physiologic stimuli for ADH secretion, baroreceptor-mediated in hypovolemia and osmoreceptor-mediated in hypernatremia, are absent in this patient, he has the syndrome of inappropriate ADH (SIADH).

■ **What are the major causes of this condition?**

- Ectopic ADH production by a tumor, particularly small cell (oat cell) carcinoma of the lung.
- Intracranial pathology, such as trauma, stroke, tumors, or infection.
- Drugs such as antipsychotic agents, antidepressants, immunosuppressive medications, chemotherapeutic drugs, thiazide diuretics, angiotensin converting enzyme inhibitors, nonsteroidal anti-inflammatory drug, omeprazole, opiates, nicotine, or ecstasy.
- Major surgery, pain.
- Human immunodeficiency virus infection.
- SIADH may also be idiopathic.

■ **How is ADH regulated?**

ADH is the main regulator of serum osmolality. ADH causes water channels (e.g., aquaporin-2) of the principal cells of the kidney's collecting ducts to translocate to the cell membrane, thereby allowing more water to be reabsorbed. Its release from the posterior pituitary is stimulated by hyperosmolarity and by decreased effective circulating volume.

■ **How is this patient's serum osmolality calculated?**

Serum osmolality = $2 Na^+ + glucose/18 + BUN/2.8 = 264$ mOsm/kg

■ **What are the most appropriate treatments for this condition?**

Treatment consists of tumor resection. If evidence of SIADH persists or resection is not possible, treatment involves restriction of free water intake or use of hypertonic saline with loop diuretics. An alternative option is demeclocycline, which poisons the collecting tubule, making it unresponsive to ADH.

▶ **Case 21**

A 5-year-old girl develops a fever of 39°C (102.2°F) 25 days after receiving a well matched deceased donor renal transplant for focal segmental glomerulosclerosis. Her immunosuppression consists of basiliximab, (anti-interleukin 2) prednisone, mycophenolate, and tacrolimus. Blood cultures, and viral titers including cytomegalovirus (CMV), are pending.

▪ What is cross-matching, and what is its benefit?	The process of cross-matching determines whether the recipient has antibodies to the donor's WBCs. This measure prevents hyperacute rejection due to preformed antibodies.
▪ If CMV is present, which fraction of a blood sample will have the highest yield for the virus?	Because CMV invades WBCs, these cells will contain the highest titer of the virus. This portion of the blood separates out as the **"buffy coat"** when blood samples are centrifuged. Figure 12-10 shows a CMV giant cell with multiple hyaline inclusions.
▪ Why is CMV of particular concern in this patient?	The girl is immunosuppressed, and there is a significant probability that she has been exposed to CMV. About 80% of normal adults are infected with CMV yet remain asymptomatic because of their functional immune systems. Thus, there is a high likelihood that the donor may have been CMV-positive. As with other members of the herpesvirus family, CMV is more likely to activate in an immunosuppressed host. In the immunocompromised host CMV can cause a variety of syndromes, including a mild febrile, upper respiratory illness, severe gastrointestinal syndrome with a mild hepatitis, marked pancytopenia, or a pneumonitis. CMV can also directly cause graft dysfunction.
▪ What is the mechanism of action of ganciclovir against CMV?	Ganciclovir is a guanosine derivative that inhibits CMV DNA polymerase.
▪ How does infection lead to fever in a normal individual?	Pyrogenic cytokines released by phagocytic cells of the immune system trigger the release of prostaglandins, including tumor necrosis factor-α and interleukin-1, which causes the hypothalamus to increase the set point of core body temperature. A key factor in the ability to mount a fever is the presence of an intact immune system. Infection is often difficult to detect in patients with poor immune function, as such patients' ability to mount a fever is severely blunted.

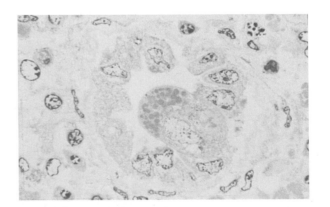

FIGURE 12-10. Photomicrograph of CMV. (Reproduced, with permission, from Le T, Bhushan V, Rao DA. *First Aid for the USMLE Step 1: 2008.* New York: McGraw-Hill, 2008: Color Image 6.)

An 18-month-old boy is brought to the pediatrician with symptoms of his third urinary tract infection since birth. His mother reports the child has malodorous urine, a low-grade fever, and poor appetite. Urinalysis reveals bacteria on Gram stain.

■ Describe the anatomy of the kidney.	If one were to slice a kidney in half, the cortex would be most superficial, with the medulla connecting to calyces, which are connected to the renal pelvis.
■ Explain the anatomic connection between the ureters and the urethra.	There are two ureters that transport urine from each kidney into the bladder. The ureters have three layers of tissue. The most superficial is fibrous tissue, which covers a medial layer of muscle and an inner mucosal layer of epithelial tissue. The urethra exits at the bladder neck at the apex of the trigone. The female urethra is shorter, which predisposes girls and women to urinary tract infections. In infants or young children, frequent urinary tract infections can be a sign of urinary reflux.
■ Where is the bladder located in males versus females?	The bladder sits behind the pubic symphysis and anterior to the rectum in both males and females. The male bladder lies anterior to the seminal vesicles above the prostate gland, and is anterior to the uterus in females.
■ What are the two regions of the bladder?	The lower region is the trigone or the base of the bladder. The entry of the ureters marks the base of the trigone. The apex of the trigone is where the urethral orifice is surrounded by the internal urethral sphincter. The upper region of the bladder holds urine that enters the bladder via the ureteral orifices. The bladder can expand vertically and horizontally to hold up to 300–400 mL (~20-30 mL/kg) of urine before voiding.

■ Describe the innervation of the bladder.	■ Afferent innervation via afferent branches of the visceral nervous system, stretch receptors via parasympathetic nerves, and pain receptors via sympathetic nerves
	■ Efferent innervation:
	  ■ Parasympathetic innervation: The pelvic splanchnic nerves. The preganglionic axons arise from the lateral horn cells at the S2–S4 levels; postganglionic cell bodies are in the bladder wall. These efferent nerves cause detrusor contraction and internal sphincter relaxation during micturition.
	  ■ Sympathetic innervation: The sacral splanchnic nerves. The preganglionic axons arise from lateral horn cell bodies at the T10–T12 and L1–L2 levels. The postganglionic cell bodies are in the inferior mesenteric and hypogastric ganglia. These efferent nerves relax the detrusor and increase the tone of the internal sphincter during bladder filling and prevent reflux of urine into the ureters. In the adult male these efferents also prevent reflux of semen into the bladder at the urethrovesical junction.

ORGAN SYSTEMS

RENAL

Reproductive

Case 1   430

Case 2   432

Case 3   433

Case 4   434

Case 5   435

Case 6   436

Case 7   438

Case 8   440

Case 9   441

Case 10   442

Case 11   443

Case 12   444

Case 13   445

Case 14   446

Case 15   447

Case 16   448

Case 17   449

Case 18   451

Case 19   452

▶ **Case 1**

A 29-year-old woman in week 28 of her third pregnancy is involved in a motor vehicle accident, but does not immediately seek medical attention. Four hours after the accident, she notes lower abdominal pain and vaginal bleeding, and decides to go to the emergency department. Upon presentation, the patient appears quite uncomfortable and says she is experiencing what she believes to be prolonged contractions. Her vital signs are notable for mild hypotension. Relevant laboratory findings are as follows:

Hematocrit: 34%
Platelet count: 80,000/mm^3
Plasma fibrinogen: 180 mg/dL

▪ **What is the most likely diagnosis?**	Abruptio placentae. The presence of painful vaginal bleeding in the second or third trimester is suggestive of abruption, and the presence of contractions is an additional clinical hint. The laboratory values, particularly the mild thrombocytopenia (normal platelet count in pregnancy is >100,000/mm^3) and decreased plasma fibrinogen (should be >400 mg/dL in pregnancy), also suggest placental abruption with developing consumptive coagulopathy.
▪ **What is the differential diagnosis of painful vaginal bleeding in the third trimester?**	Abruption often presents as painful vaginal bleeding, while placenta previa presents as painless vaginal bleeding. Other causes of third-trimester painful bleeding include labor, a genital laceration, and uterine rupture (typically seen in labor in women who are attempting vaginal delivery after cesarean).
▪ **What is the pathophysiology of this condition?**	Abruptio placentae is the premature separation of a normal placenta occurring after 20 weeks' gestation and before delivery. The rupture of maternal blood vessels at the anchoring villi of the placenta causes a separation from the endometrium in which blood can accumulate. The hemorrhage can be either external or concealed, as shown in Figure 13-1 (which also shows placenta previa, another common cause of vaginal bleeding in pregnancy). This in turn disrupts the fetal blood supply, and in severe cases can lead to fetal death.
▪ **What risk factors are associated with an increased incidence of this condition?**	Risk factors typically increase the risk of disruption or weakening of the maternal blood vessels. They include trauma, maternal hypertension, cigarette smoking, cocaine use, thrombophilia, increased parity, direct abdominal trauma, amniocentesis, and multifetal gestation.
▪ **What complication is the patient at greatly increased risk for developing?**	**Disseminated intravascular coagulation** (DIC) occurs in approximately 10%–20% of cases of serious abruption with fetal death. This may be a result of a consumptive coagulopathy. In cases of fetal demise, it is thought that the death of the fetus releases procoagulants into the mother's circulation that provide a trigger for DIC.

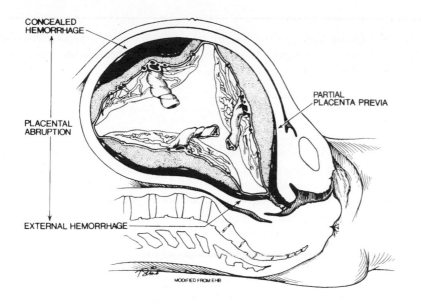

FIGURE 13-1. Layers in abruptio placentae. (Reproduced, with permission, from Cunningham FG, et al. *Williams Obstetrics*, 22nd ed. New York: McGraw-Hill, 2005: 812.)

▶ **Case 2**

A 17-year-old girl presents to clinic for primary amenorrhea. She reports that she has never had a period. On physical examination her breasts are well developed, but she lacks axillary and pubic hair.

■ What is the most likely diagnosis?	Androgen insensitivity syndrome (also known as testicular feminization syndrome).
■ What is the pathophysiology of this condition?	This disorder results from a lack of function of the androgen receptors in a genetically male patient. The testes are present and secrete testosterone and müllerian inhibiting factor (MIF). However, the person cannot use this testosterone because the peripheral receptors are nonfunctional. Instead, the testosterone is converted into estradiol in periperhal tissues (especially adipose tissue), which initiates breast formation. The vagina is often present, but may be short and blind-ending. The MIF secretion inhibits the normal development of ovaries and a uterus.
■ What is the clinical presentation of this condition?	There are two main presentations of this disorder: ■ In newborns it presents as an inguinal mass. ■ In adolescents it presents as primary amenorrhea. The inguinal mass seen in newborns is caused by the aberrant descent of the testes, which usually stay in the abdomen of these patients.
■ What tests and/or imaging tools could be used to confirm the diagnosis?	On karyotype, these patients would be 46,XY. A pelvic ultrasound can be done to look for abdominal testes and the absence of uterus and ovaries. The diagnosis can also be made by analyzing the DNA of the androgen receptor via polymerase chain reaction. Testosterone and dihydrotestosterone (DHT) levels should also be measured. The levels of both should be normal. If the testosterone level is low, this raises concerns about testicular dysgenesis or Leydig cell aplasia/hypoplasia. If testosterone levels are normal but DHT levels are low, one should suspect 5α-reductase deficiency.
■ What is the most appropriate treatment for this condition?	The first treatment is usually removal of the testes, because there is a high risk of cancer development without such a procedure. Thereafter, the treatments are mainly hormone replacement therapy and psychological support. Estrogen is given, but not progesterone because no uterus is present. The estrogen is given to replace the loss of sex hormone production with the removal of the testes. Psychological therapy is also given because of the potential gender confusion. Surgical reconstruction may be needed to create a "functional" vagina.

▶ **Case 3**

A 22-year-old woman presents to the clinic with complaints of itching; burning on urination; and a green, fishy-smelling vaginal discharge. She has had four different sexual partners in the past year, and reports she has used protection in each case. A wet smear of the discharge reveals stippled squamous epithelial cells with smudged borders (see Figure 13-2).

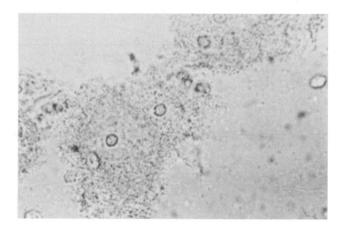

FIGURE 13-2. (Reproduced, with permission, from Kasper DL, et al. *Harrison's Principles of Internal Medicine,* 16th ed. New York: McGraw-Hill, 2005: 767.)

■ **What is the most likely diagnosis?**	Bacterial vaginosis.
■ **What organism causes this condition?**	BV is not generally considered to be a sexually transmitted infection, and can occur in women who have not had intercourse. It is caused by an imbalance of naturally occurring bacterial flora within the vagina, with a decrease in favorable bacteria (lactobacilli) and an overgrowth of existing commensal bacteria (such as *Gardnerella vaginalis*).
■ **What other conditions should be considered in the differential diagnosis?**	*Candida* and *Trichomonas* are other common causes of vaginitis. The presence of **clue cells**, which are squamous epithelial cells with smudged borders (see Figure 13-2), is strong evidence that the infection is bacterial in origin. An elevated pH (>4.5) and a positive **whiff test** (amine release with potassium hydroxide results in a fishy smell) may aid in the diagnosis.
■ **What risk factors are associated with an increased incidence of this condition?**	Risk factors include multiple/new sexual partners, early age at first intercourse, smoking, and use of an intrauterine device. Diabetics, pregnant women, and women with human immunodeficiency virus infection have an increased risk of developing infection with *Candida*. While bacterial vaginosis is commonly thought of as a sexually transmitted disease, it is also seen in women who have not had intercourse.
■ **What is the most appropriate treatment for this condition?**	Metronidazole treats infections with *Gardnerella* and *Trichomonas*. *Candida* (yeast) infections are treated with fluconazole.

► **Case 4**

A 64-year-old man goes to his provider's office complaining of difficulty urinating. He says he has trouble initiating his stream of urine and notes that after it begins, the flow is hard to maintain, and afterwards his bladder still feels full. He says he often finds himself rushing to the bathroom to make it in time and that the need to urinate awakens him several times each night. Besides these complaints, he feels fine, though he has had several urinary tract infections (UTIs) over the past year or so, which is something he never experienced when he was younger.

■ **What is the most likely diagnosis?**	Benign prostatic hyperplasia (BPH).
■ **What are the typical signs and symptoms of this condition?**	The diagnosis is usually based on the history and physical examination, and on occasion, on the results of laboratory studies. The classic signs and symptoms include urinary frequency, urinary urgency, nocturia, difficulty initiating and maintaining a urinary stream, a feeling of postvoid fullness in the bladder, and dribbling. A digital rectal examination can allow one to assess the size of the prostate. A prostate-specific antigen (PSA) test can also be of benefit, since most patients with BPH have mildly elevated levels in the range of 2–10 ng/mL. A markedly elevated PSA (especially values >10 ng/mL) should raise suspicion of prostate cancer.
■ **What is the pathophysiology of this condition?**	In BPH, the central part of the gland, which is the portion that surrounds the urethra, becomes hyperplastic, giving rise to urinary symptoms. In the case of prostate cancer, the peripheral part of the gland is often the hyperplastic part. BPH is a hormonally-mediated disorder, with dihydrotestosterone (DHT) acting as the growth hormone. However, men with BPH do not have higher plasma concentrations of DHT; rather, it is believed that such patients have more DHT receptors on their prostates by virtue of increased estradiol levels, which stimulate the expression of such receptors. By age 80, 90% of men will have BPH.
■ **What are the potential complications associated with this condition?**	One complication is UTI secondary to urine stasis in the bladder. Static urine in the bladder can also result in bladder stone formation. Patients with nocturia often complain of daytime sleepiness and exhaustion due to repeated nighttime awakenings. Rarely, patients can also develop acute urinary retention, which presents with symptoms such as abdominal pain and a suprapubic mass (the filled bladder). This can be a spontaneous occurrence or may be secondary to triggers such as anticholinergics, antihistamines, or α-receptor agonists (e.g., cold medications), all of which decrease bladder contractility.
■ **What is the most appropriate treatment for this condition?**	The principal treatment options are medical and surgical. Medical options include cholinergics (e.g., bethanechol), α-blockers (e.g., prazosin), and 5α-reductase inhibitors (e.g., finasteride). Cholinergics help increase bladder contractility, whereas α-blockers work by relaxing the bladder neck so that urine flows more easily. The 5α-reductase inhibitors prevent the formation of DHT, so that the levels of this growth hormone for the prostate are decreased. Surgery is also an option.

A 24-year-old woman presents to her physician after recently noticing a lump in her left breast that has been associated with some discomfort. The lump moves with touch and she is concerned about cancer, as her mother developed breast cancer at age 62 years. On physical examination, the lump feels firm, has well-defined borders, and is mobile. There are no changes in the skin or nipple and no discharge. No axillary lymph nodes are palpable.

■ **What is the most likely diagnosis and what is its associated prognosis?**	Fibroadenomas are the most common breast tumors seen in young women. They are benign, often arise quickly, and reabsorb within several weeks to months. Fibroadenomas do not carry an increased risk of breast cancer. Note that the risk associated with having a first-degree relative with breast cancer is higher the younger the relative is at diagnosis.
■ **What are Cooper's ligaments?**	The superficial and deep pectoral fascia surrounding the breast are connected by fibrous bands known as **Cooper's suspensory ligaments.**
■ **What is the structure of breast tissue?**	Breast tissue is found between the second and sixth ribs and is made of parenchyma and stroma (see Figure 13-3). The parenchyma has 15–25 lobes, each of which has 20–40 lobules composed of alveoli. Lactiferous ducts offer drainage to the corresponding lobe. The ducts are dilated immediately before the nipple, which forms the lactiferous sinuses.
■ **What are the muscles of the breast tissue, and how are they innervated?**	■ Seratus anterior: Long thoracic nerve ■ Latissimus dorsi: Thoracodorsal nerve ■ Pectoralis minor: Medial pectoral nerve ■ Pectoralis major: Pectoral nerve
■ **What is the most appropriate treatment for this condition?**	Because these growths are benign, no treatment is necessary. The patient should be followed up in 1–2 months to assess for reabsorption. If there is any concern about breast cancer, a needle or excision biopsy is indicated.

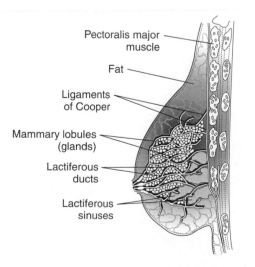

FIGURE 13-3. Normal breast tissue. (Reproduced, with permission, from DeCherney AH, Nathan L. *Current Obstetric & Gynecologic Diagnosis and Treatment*, 10th ed. New York: McGraw-Hill, 2007: 1032.)

▶ **Case 6**

A 17-year-old girl is brought to the emergency department complaining of a 3-day history of nausea and vomiting and intense abdominal pain. Her last menstrual period was 6 weeks ago, but she has a history of irregular cycles. She is not taking oral contraceptives. Her past medical history is significant for an appendectomy at age 13 years. Physical examination reveals a palpable mass in the right lower quadrant. Laboratory tests show her β-human chorionic gonadotropin (β-hCG) level is 1500 mIU/L, and the serum progesterone level is <15 ng/mL. Transvaginal ultrasonography, however, reveals no uterine pregnancy.

▪ **What is the most likely diagnosis?**	Ectopic pregnancy. Ectopic pregnancy occurs at a rate of 17 per 1000 pregnancies. The vast majority (98%) occur in the fallopian tubes, most often (90% of cases) in the ampulla.
▪ **What signs and symptoms are commonly associated with this condition?**	**Nonruptured ectopic pregnancy:** ▪ Abnormal bleeding ▪ Abdominal/pelvic pain ▪ Nausea ▪ Pelvic mass ▪ Vomiting **Ruptured ectopic pregnancy:** ▪ Local or generalized abdominal tenderness. ▪ Orthostatic hypertension. ▪ Shock. ▪ Shoulder pain (due to blood in the abdominal cavity irritating the diaphragm and causing referred pain in the distribution of the phrenic nerve). ▪ Tachycardia.
▪ **What risk factors are associated with an increased incidence of this condition?**	Risk factors include all those conditions that may cause structural or functional damage to the fallopian tubes, including: ▪ Diethylstilbestrol exposure in utero ▪ In vitro fertilization ▪ Pelvic inflammatory disease ▪ Pelvic surgery ▪ Previous ectopic pregnancy ▪ Tubal ligation ▪ Tuboplasty
▪ **What are the typical laboratory findings in this condition?**	The β-hCG level in an ectopic pregnancy is typically <6500 IU/L, which is markedly lower than that in a uterine pregnancy. The serum progesterone level (typically <15 ng/mL) is also much lower than that in a uterine pregnancy.
▪ **What are the likely findings on transvaginal ultrasonography?**	Transvaginal ultrasonography will show no intrauterine gestational sac, a noncystic adnexal mass, or fluid in the cul-de-sac. A gestational sac is visible with a vaginal probe when the β-hCG level is 1500 IU/L, or with abdominal pelvic ultrasonography when the β-hCG level is 6500 IU/L.

■ **What are the most appropriate treatments for this condition?**

The β-hCG levels should be checked every 48 hours. In a normal intrauterine pregnancy, levels of this hormone will double over this time frame; if not, an ectopic pregnancy should be suspected. Methotrexate may be given if the ectopic pregnancy is <3 cm, the β-hCG level is <12,000 IU/L, there is no fetal heart rate, and the mother's liver and renal test results pretreatment are normal. Surgery is indicated if the β-hCG level is higher. Surgery involves removal of part or all of the fallopian tube. Segmental resection might be necessary for an ischemic ectopic pregnancy. Salpingectomy is usually reserved for a ruptured ectopic pregnancy.

ORGAN SYSTEMS

REPRODUCTIVE

▶ **Case 7**

A 26-year-old woman presents to her physician complaining of intense abdominal pain associated with the start of her menstrual periods. She has been trying unsuccessfully to get pregnant for the past 2 years. On questioning, she reports pain with intercourse, especially on deep penetration. Her older sister has a similar history.

▪ What is the most likely diagnosis?	Endometriosis.
▪ What is the pathophysiology of this condition?	In endometriosis, endometrial tissue is found outside the endometrial cavity, usually in the ovary and pelvic peritoneum (see Figure 13-4 for common sites of endometrial implants). It is theorized that this endometrial tissue is either transported via the lymphatic system such that peritoneal tissue undergoes metaplastic transformation into functional endometrial tissue, or that it is transported through the fallopian tubes in retrograde menstruation. Endometrial tissue causes adhesions, fibrosis, and severe inflammation.
▪ What signs and symptoms are commonly associated with this condition?	Cyclic pelvic pain starting 1–2 days prior to the onset of menses and continuing through the first few days of the cycle are characteristic of endometriosis. Dysmenorrhea, dyspareunia, abnormal bleeding, and a history of infertility are also common in these patients. Physical examination typically reveals uterosacral nodularity and a palpable adnexal mass. Laparoscopic evaluation is definitive. Endometrial implants appear as raspberry lesions or **"powder burns"**; these raised, blue or dark brown lesions lead to adhesions. Ovarian cysts can have large collections of old blood called **endometriomas** or **"chocolate cysts."**
▪ What risk factors are associated with an increased incidence of this condition?	Endometriosis occurs in 10%–15% of women overall, but is more common (30%–40%) in women with infertility. The risk of endometriosis is sevenfold higher in women who have a first-degree relative with the condition. Endometriosis has also been linked to autoimmune disorders such as lupus. It is less commonly identified in African-American women.
▪ What are the most appropriate treatments for this condition?	Medical treatment includes treating the symptoms (with nonsteroidal anti-inflammatory drugs) and suppression of menstrual cycles to allow the lesions to involute, such as continuous oral contraceptive pills or medroxyprogesterone (to create a "pseudopregnancy") or androgen derivatives or gonadotropin-releasing hormone agonists (to induce "pseudomenopause"). Surgical treatment may also be necessary in some cases.

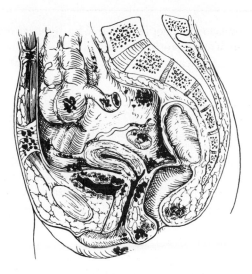

FIGURE 13-4. **Frequent sites of endometriosis deposits (dark areas in image).** (Reproduced, with permission, from Doherty GM. *Current Surgical Diagnosis & Treatment*, 12th ed. New York: McGraw-Hill, 2006: 1075.)

▶ **Case 8**

A 66-year-old man presents to clinic for follow-up of his hypertension. At the end of the visit, he mentions that he has recently had trouble maintaining an erection. He wants to know what the options are for treating this, because he wants to maintain a sexual relationship with his wife.

▪ What is the most likely diagnosis?	Erectile dysfunction (ED), which affects up to 50% of men between the ages 40 and 70.
▪ What are the physiologic steps required to maintain an erection?	Developing and maintaining an erection requires neurologic, vascular, and hormonal factors. Central and peripheral innervation are needed. The main peripheral nerve is the dorsal nerve of the penis, which is a branch of the pudendal nerve, and carries autonomic fibers. From a vascular point of view, there must be significant arterial flow into the penis (specifically into the corpora cavernosa and corpora spongiosum) and prevention of venous outflow. Adequate blood flow is achieved through cGMP-mediated relaxation of the smooth muscle of the corporae, which requires nitric oxide. Adequate production of testosterone is also required.
▪ What risk factors are associated with an increased incidence of this condition?	The main risk factors for developing erectile dysfunction are primarily vascular. There is a strong association with hypertension, cardiovascular disease, and diabetes mellitus. Other risk factors include smoking, obesity, and a sedentary lifestyle. Exercise decreases the risk of ED and has been shown to improve erectile function in some. Other risk factors for ED include injury to the nerve supply for erectile function such as pelvic trauma, pelvic radiation, spinal cord injury, and prostate surgery. Depression, performance anxiety, and fear of sudden death can also result in ED.
▪ What drugs most commonly cause this condition?	Drugs known to be associated with ED include selective serotonin reuptake inhibitors (SSRIs), spironolactone, sympathetic blockers (clonidine, guanethidine, and methyldopa), thiazide diuretics, ketoconazole, cimetidine (but not ranitidine), antipsychotics, cholesterol-lowering drugs, alcohol, and nicotine.
▪ What is the most appropriate treatment for this condition?	The main treatment used for ED is the phosphodiesterase inhibitors. These work by preventing the degradation of cGMP, thereby allowing dilatation of the corpora and adequate blood flow into the penis. Examples of these include sildenafil and vardenafil. Other treatments include the vacuum pump, a prosthesis, and direct injection of α-blockers (i.e., phentolamine) into the penis. If the cause of the ED is depression, treatment of the depression is needed. If the cause is performance anxiety, SSRIs and behavioral therapy are the optimal treatments.

A 22-year-old woman presents to the emergency department with a 3-day history of fever, abdominal pain, pain on inspiration, and vaginal discharge. Her temperature at presentation is 38°C (100.4°F). The patient reports being sexually active and not always using protection. Her last menstrual period ended 5 days ago. She has been with her most recent partner for approximately 1 month. On physical examination, her abdomen is diffusely tender, with more pain in the right upper quadrant, but without rebound or guarding. Cervical motion tenderness is present, as is right-sided adnexal tenderness. Relevant laboratory findings are as follows:

WBC count: 11,000/mm^3
Erythrocyte sedimentation rate (ESR): >15 mm/h
β-Human chorionic gonadotropin: negative
Alanine aminotransferase: 1.5 × normal

■ **What is the most likely diagnosis?**	Fitz-Hugh and Curtis syndrome, a complication of pelvic inflammatory disease (PID), that is characterized by perihepatitis in association with pleuritic right upper quadrant pain and tubal gonococcal or chlamydial infection.
■ **What is the pathophysiology of this condition?**	*Neisseria gonorrhoeae* is responsible for approximately one-third of cases of PID; *Chlamydia trachomatis* is responsible for a slightly higher fraction of cases of PID. Fitz-Hugh and Curtis syndrome is due to a **perihepatitis,** or an inflammation of the underside of the diaphragm and liver capsule. The syndrome is seen in about 5% of patients with PID, and is often mistakenly diagnosed as pneumonia or acute cholecystitis.
■ **What signs and symptoms are commonly associated with this condition?**	Patients with Fitz-Hugh and Curtis syndrome present with PID and pleuritic pain in the upper right quadrant that limits chest expansion. Additionally, patients have an elevated WBC count, fever, pelvic pain, cervical motion tenderness, adnexal tenderness, elevated liver enzyme levels, and an ESR >15 mm/h.
■ **What risk factors are associated with an increased incidence of this condition?**	■ Cigarette smoking ■ High frequency of intercourse ■ Multiple partners ■ New sexual partner within 1 month of symptom onset ■ Recent history of douching ■ Use of an intrauterine device ■ Young age at first intercourse
■ **What are the likely findings on histology?**	If the cause is *N. gonorrhoeae*, Gram staining of the cervical discharge will reveal gram-negative intracellular diplococci. Culture of endocervical samples will reveal *N. gonorrhoeae* and/or *C. trachomatis* infection.
■ **What are the most appropriate treatments for this condition?**	Fitz-Hugh and Curtis syndrome is treated with outpatient antibiotics such as cefoxitin, ceftriaxone, or doxycycline. If the patient is pregnant, has a tubo-ovarian abscess, or cannot tolerate oral medications, she must be hospitalized for administration of intravenous antibiotics. Surgery is indicated only in cases of tubo-ovarian abscess.

▶ **Case 10**

A 36-year-old woman at 24 weeks of gestation presents to the clinic for a routine prenatal visit. Her fetus is large for gestational age, and she is scheduled for an oral glucose tolerance test (OGTT). The mother had one previous pregnancy with no complications and is generally healthy, although obese. Results of the OGGT are as follows:

1-Hour OGGT: Glucose level: 144 mg/dL
3-Hour OGGT: Fasting glucose level: 93 mg/dL
Glucose level at 1 hour: 172 mg/dL
Glucose level at 2 hours: 150 mg/dL
Glucose level at 3 hours: 133 mg/dL

▪ What is the most likely diagnosis?	Gestational diabetes, defined as glucose intolerance first documented in pregnancy.
▪ What is the pathophysiology of this condition?	Gestational diabetes occurs in 3%–5% of all pregnancies. Normal pregnancy is a diabetogenic (pro-diabetic) state characterized by insulin resistance and decreased peripheral uptake of glucose. This is mediated by the production of counterregulatory (anti-insulin) hormones by the placenta, including human placental lactogen, cortisol, and placental growth hormone.
▪ What signs and symptoms are commonly associated with this condition?	This syndrome is most often asymptomatic, and is usually detected between 24 and 28 weeks' gestation by a routine OGTT. Glycosuria, hyperglycemia, and fetus that is large for gestational age raise the suspicion of gestational diabetes.
▪ What risk factors are associated with an increased incidence of this condition?	▪ Age >25 years ▪ Family history of diabetes mellitus ▪ Fetus large for gestational age ▪ Glycosuria at first prenatal visit ▪ Obesity ▪ Past history of gestational diabetes ▪ Polycystic ovarian syndrome ▪ Maternal birthweight of >9 lb ▪ Several previous stillbirths or abortions ▪ Hispanic or African-American ethnicity
▪ What are the common maternal and fetal complications associated with this condition?	**Maternal:** ▪ Cesarean section delivery (due to a large fetus) ▪ Eclampsia/preeclampsia ▪ Glucose intolerance ▪ Increased future risk of diabetes mellitus ▪ Polyhydramnios ▪ Pregnancy-induced hypertension ▪ Preterm delivery **Fetal:** ▪ Congenital defects ▪ Macrosomia ▪ Perinatal mortality (2%–5%) ▪ Shoulder dystocia
▪ What are the most appropriate treatments for this condition?	Affected women should adhere to a diabetic diet. Fasting blood glucose and 2-hour postprandial glucose levels should be routinely monitored. If levels remain high for 2 weeks, insulin therapy should be started. Fetal growth should also be monitored.

▶ **Case 11**

A man and his wife present to a fertility clinic because for a year they have been trying to get pregnant without success. The husband is tall and thin. On physical examination, he has sparse axillary and pubic hair, decreased muscle mass, small testes, and gynecomastia. His urinary gonadotropin levels are elevated and analysis of his sperm reveals azoospermia.

■ What is the most likely diagnosis?	Klinefelter's syndrome.
■ What is the cause and clinical presentation of this condition?	Klinefelter's is estimated to occur in about 1 in 1000 men and is a chromosomal abnormality in which the genotype is **47,XXY.** There is dysgenesis of the seminiferous tubules, which results in primary testicular failure with decreased androgen production. Complications of this include azoospermia and infertility, gynecomastia, small testes and penis, loss of libido, osteoporosis, decreased muscle mass, and sparse axillary and pubic hair. These patients also have a 20 times higher risk of developing **breast cancer** than the typical male. Additional risks include decreased mental capacity and an increased risk of anxiety and depression. All of these complications worsen with an increasing number of X chromosomes.
■ What tests and/or imaging tools could be used to confirm the diagnosis?	Diagnosis should be suspected on the basis of physical examination and laboratory tests. One key laboratory finding is elevated follicle-stimulating hormone (FSH) levels. Because the seminiferous tubules are unformed, there is a lack of Sertoli cells, and hence a lack of the inhibin that these cells usually produce. Without inhibin, there is a loss of negative feedback on FSH, causing FSH levels to be elevated. In addition, testosterone levels will be low, while estradiol levels will be high. The definitive diagnosis requires karyotype.
■ What is the most appropriate treatment for this condition?	The treatment is androgen replacement therapy, which should begin around puberty. This has been shown to help with virilization, psychosocial development, hair growth, muscle mass, libido, testicular size, and precocious osteoporosis.
■ What can be done to increase the fertility of patients with this condition?	Most men with Klinefelter's syndrome produce small amounts of sperm, though usually this sperm cannot be found in the ejaculate. The fact that some sperm are produced allows for extraction of sperm from the testicles to use for in vitro fertilization.

► **Case 12**

A 42-year-old African-American woman visits her physician with a complaint of heavy menstrual periods that last for several days. This has been occurring for the past 3 months, and has been associated with pain and fatigue. Physical examination reveals an enlarged uterus with multiple palpable masses. Laboratory tests show her hemoglobin level is 11.3 g/dL and hematocrit is 33.3%.

■ What is the most likely diagnosis?	Leiomyoma, or uterine fibroids. This diagnosis is suggested by the heavy vaginal bleeding and palpable masses.
■ What is the epidemiology of this condition?	The incidence of leiomyoma is greatly increased in African-American women. It is the most common benign neoplasm in females.
■ Which cells of the uterus are most commonly affected in this condition?	Smooth muscle cells of the myometrium are most commonly affected, although fibroids can also occur in subendometrial or subperitoneal areas (see Figure 13-5). Fibroids within the uterus can be submucosal, subserosal, or intramural. **Submucosal fibroids** are most often associated with abnormal bleeding, while **subserosal fibroids** are most often the cause of pressure due to mass effect.
■ How does the size of this neoplasm change with age?	The estrogen sensitivity of leiomyomas usually results in increased size during the first trimester of pregnancy and shrinkage after menopause.
■ Is this patient at increased risk for uterine malignancy?	Most leiomyosarcomas arise de novo and malignant transformation of leiomyomas into leiomyosarcomas is rare.
■ What uterine abnormality is associated with an increased risk of endometrial cancer?	**Endometrial hyperplasia**, which is characterized by abnormal glandular proliferation, is considered to be a premalignant lesion. This is caused by increased estrogen stimulation, and like uterine fibroids, often presents with abnormal vaginal bleeding. Therefore its presence must be distinguished from abnormal vaginal bleeding secondary to uterine fibroids. This can be accomplished by histological examination of the endometrium obtained by endometrial biopsy.

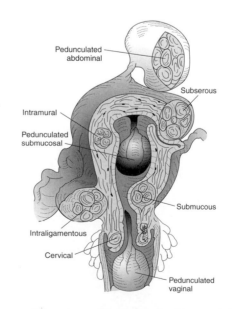

FIGURE 13-5. Myomas of the uterus. (Reproduced, with permission, from DeCherney AH, Nathan L. *Current Obstetric & Gynecologic Diagnosis & Treatment*, 10th ed. New York: McGraw-Hill, 2007: 640.)

▶ **Case 13**

A 51-year-old woman presents to clinic because her periods have become irregular. She says sometimes there are 3 months in between periods, and that the irregularity began about 3 years ago. She complains of hot flashes that occur a few times each day and that sometimes awaken her at night. She says she is less interested in sex because she has begun to find it somewhat painful.

▪ What is the most likely diagnosis?	The start of menopause. Menopause itself is defined as 12 months without a period (amenorrhea).
▪ What is the differential diagnosis for irregular vaginal bleeding and how should it be evaluated?	The differential includes uterine fibroids, uterine polyps, pregnancy complications, menopause, thyroid dysfunction, endometrial hyperplasia (often secondary to anovulatory cycles and chronic estrogen exposure), and endometrial cancer. The gold standard to evaluate these is a uterine biopsy. A transvaginal ultrasound can also be diagnostic.
▪ What are the signs and symptoms of this condition and how might it be reflected in laboratory values?	The first sign of menopause is usually a change in menstrual cycle length. Additionally, a woman might begin to skip periods and experience hot flashes. She may also experience vaginal dryness that results in itching and pain with intercourse (dyspareunia). Her vaginal pH will increase and put her at increased risk for a urinary tract infection (UTI). On laboratory studies, her follicle-stimulating hormone (FSH) level will be elevated. After menopause, the main source of estrogen will be from adipose tissue in the form of estrone. If a woman undergoes menopause before age 40, it is termed premature ovarian failure.
▪ What complications are associated with this condition?	Menopause increases a woman's risk of developing osteoporosis. It is estimated that women can lose up to 20% of their bone density in the years surrounding menopause. This occurs because estrogen, which normally inhibits bone resorption, is decreased. Another risk is coronary artery disease (CAD). Before menopause, women have a lower risk of CAD than men. After menopause, a woman's risk increases until it equals that of a man. Women undergoing menopause are also at risk for depression, though it is unclear whether this is the result of hormonal changes, or the result of other life events that occur around this time (i.e., midlife adjustment, children leaving home, or career disappointments).
▪ What are the most appropriate treatments for this condition and its associated complications?	Hormone replacement therapy (HRT) is usually a combination of estrogen and progesterone. It is commonly given to help with the associated symptoms of menopause and may help prevent CAD and osteoporosis. Contraindications to HRT are severe liver disease, pregnancy, history of venous thrombosis, and history of breast cancer. Topical estrogen can be applied to treat vaginal dryness. Selective serotonin reuptake inhibitors can be given for the depressive symptoms. Other options to prevent osteoporosis include raloxifene, which is a selective estrogen receptor modulator, and the bisphosphonates, which prevent bone resorption.

► **Case 14**

A 17-year-old woman in her second trimester of pregnancy presents to a primary care clinic with painless vaginal bleeding and severe nausea and vomiting. She has not received medical care during her pregnancy. On physical examination, uterine enlargement is noted and grape-like clusters are found on pelvic examination. On ultrasound, a "snowstorm pattern" is seen.

■ **What is the most likely diagnosis?**	Hydatidiform mole or molar pregnancy.
■ **What risk factors are associated with an increased incidence of this condition?**	The main risk factor is extremes of reproductive age (i.e., near menarche or near menopause). The rate of molar pregnancies is 15 times higher in Asian countries and the Far East. A history of molar pregnancy is also predictive.
■ **How does this condition develop?**	A **complete mole** develops when an enucleate egg is fertilized by a haploid sperm that then replicates. This results in 46 chromosomes (all paternal), but no fetal parts. A **partial mole** results from a haploid ovum and two sperm. The karyotpe is typically triploid (69 chromosomes) and fetal parts may be present. There are some cases of recurrent moles that are due to a loss of maternal imprinting.
■ **What are the typical signs and symptoms of this condition?**	The classic triad of symptoms include vaginal bleeding, hyperemesis (due to high levels of β-hCG), and hyperthyroidism. Patients usually present sometime in the second trimester. Most patients do not develop symptoms because of detection of the mole by the patient's obstetrician-gynecologist. In these cases, the presence of a molar pregnancy is detected by an overly large uterus, lack of fetal heartbeat, lack of a fetus on ultrasound, very high levels of β-hCG (levels are often more than 100,000 mIU/mL), and occassinally grape-like clusters exuding from the cervix. The diagnosis is typically made in early pregnancy with evidence of a "snowstorm pattern" on ultrasound.
■ **What are the complications associated with this condition?**	Patients with molar pregnancies are at increased risk for preeclampsia and the development of ovarian theca lutein cysts (which are benign and resolve when the mole is removed). Respiratory distress can result secondary to trophoblastic embolization. Another complication is **choriocarcinoma** (other causes of choriocarcinoma are spontaneous or induced abortion, ectopic pregnancy, and normal pregnancy).
■ **What is the most appropriate treatment for this condition?**	This cancer is highly sensitive to chemotherapy (usually methotrexate or actinomycin D) and has a low rate of recurrence. The most common site of metastasis is the lungs, and the metastases also resolve with chemotherapy. Patients who develop chorocarcinoma are asked not to get pregnant for a year so that they can be monitored for recurrence through serial β-hCG levels.

A 65-year-old woman presents to clinic with several months of abdominal and pelvic pain, vaginal bleeding, and a change in bowel habits. Her physical examination is normal and her CA-125 levels are within normal limits. However, there is a high level of suspicion and a diagnostic laparotomy is recommended.

▪ What is the most likely diagnosis?	Ovarian cancer, which is the second most common and most lethal gynecologic malignancy.
▪ What are the typical signs and symptoms of this condition?	Most patients are asymptomatic or have nonspecific symptoms such as abdominal and pelvic pain, bloating, vaginal bleeding, and changes in bowel habits. In addition, physical findings are rare in early stages of this disease. Because of this, patients usually present when their disease is already advanced. Once the disease is advanced, patients may present with palpable ovarian or pelvic masses, ascites, pleural effusions, or bowel obstruction.
▪ What are the characteristics of this condition?	Most ovarian cancers (90%) are of epithelial origin, of which there are two types: serous and mucinous. The serous type is slightly more common and is often bilateral in its presentation. The mucinous type can progress to pseudomyxoma peritonei. Other types of ovarian cancers include sex cord stromal tumors, germ cell tumors, and metastatic cancer to the ovaries. Germ cell tumors usually present in younger women (before age 20). Sex cord stromal tumors often present with hormonal side effects. Krukenberg tumors are mucin-secreting tumors with signet-ring cells that usually originate in the stomach.
▪ What risk factors are associated with an increased incidence of this disease and what are the protective factors?	Protective factors include multiple pregnancies and oral contraceptive use. It is theorized that the protection results from a decreased number of ovulatory cycles. This theory is consistent with the belief that each ovulatory cycle causes rupture and repair of the ovary that over time can cause cellular changes that lead to cancer. Risk factors include a family history of BRCA1 (a tumor suppressor gene) or HNPCC (a mismatch repair gene) mutations.
▪ What tests and/or imaging tools could be used to confirm the diagnosis?	Initial screening tests include transvaginal ultrasound and CT as well as the tumor marker CA-125. However, the ultrasound and CT often miss cancers and the CA-125 screen is better at detecting recurrences than at establishing an initial diagnosis. As a result, if there is a high level of suspicion based on history, an exploratory laparotomy is usually recommended. This information is then used to stage the disease. Advanced stage disease is present if the cancer is found outside of the pelvis in the peritoneum or lymph nodes (stage III) or outside of the abdominal cavity, such as in the lungs (stage IV).
▪ What is the most appropriate treatment for this condition?	Treatment is usually debulking surgery followed by chemotherapy. The commonly used chemotherapeutic agents are a combination of a platinum (i.e., cisplatin or carboplatin) with paclitaxel. Chemotherapy can be given intraperitoneally or intravenously. Because 50% of women who respond to therapy relapse, some recommend maintenance chemotherapy with paclitaxel.

► **Case 16**

A 57-year-old woman with a history of eczema presents to her primary care physician with a new rash near the nipple of her right breast. She tells her doctor that the rash first appeared 2 months ago, and she had been treating it with the topical corticosteroid prescribed for her eczema. At first the rash improved somewhat, but over the past few weeks it has gotten worse and has expanded in size. Physical examination reveals a raw, scaly lesion around the nipple that is beginning to ulcerate. There is also a palpable mass in the affected breast, a few centimeters deep to the skin lesion.

■ What is the most likely diagnosis?	Paget's disease of the breast, an eczematous skin lesion in the area of the nipple, is associated with underlying invasive or in situ breast carcinoma (see Figure 13-6). In about 50% of cases, Paget's disease is associated with a palpable breast mass. Paget's disease is often mistaken for a benign skin lesion such as eczema.
■ What is the pathophysiology of this condition?	It is thought that the skin lesion develops from underlying ductal carcinoma cells that migrate through the ducts to the epidermis.
■ What are the most likely findings on histology?	The classic histologic findings are large cells with a halo of clear cytoplasm surrounding a prominent nucleolus. The cytoplasm stains positive for mucin.
■ What are the most common sites of metastasis for breast carcinoma?	Bone is the most common site for metastatic disease. Other common organ sites include liver and lung, while less common sites include bone marrow, brain, ovaries, spinal cord, and eye.
■ What is the lymphatic drainage of the breast?	Knowledge of the lymphatic drainage of the breast is important for understanding the metastasis of breast cancer. Approximately 75% of lymphatic drainage of the breast is to the **axillary lymph nodes**, which include the pectoral (majority of drainage), apical, subscapular, lateral, and central node groups. The nipple drains to the pectoral group. The remaining lymph drains to the infraclavicular, supraclavicular, and parasternal (also known as the internal thoracic) nodes.
■ Molecular analysis of a biopsy reveals that the cells express c-erbB-2 (also known as HER-2/neu) in high levels. What is the significance of this, and how does it affect treatment?	The HER-2/neu protein is a transmembrane growth factor receptor kinase (**HER** is an abbreviation for **H**uman **E**pithelial growth factor **R**eceptor). Overexpression of this molecule has been associated with a poorer prognosis. A new medication, trastuzumab (Herceptin™), is a humanized recombinant monoclonal antibody directed against this protein. Clinical trials of adjuvant trastuzumab and chemotherapy have shown a reduction in recurrence risk of up to 50% in HER-2–positive cancers. The binding of trastuzumab to the extracellular portion of the molecule stimulates a cytotoxic immune response, leading to death of the cancer cells.

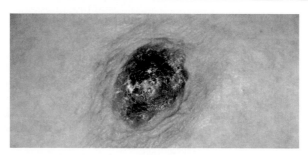

FIGURE 13-6. Paget's disease of the breast. (Reproduced, with permission, from Wolff K, Johnson RA, Suurmond D. *Fitzpatrick's Color Atlas & Synopsis of Clinical Dermatology*, 5th ed. New York: McGraw-Hill, 2005: 495.)

A 36-year-old African-American woman in week 34 of gestation presents to the emergency department with a 2-day history of headache, blurry vision, and sudden right upper quadrant pain. She reports that her husband has noticed increased swelling of her face since yesterday, and her rings are suddenly too tight. She has been healthy except for pregestational diabetes mellitus. Physical examination is notable for hyperactive deep tendon reflexes and jugular venous distention. Her blood pressure at presentation is 165/110 mm Hg; 6 hours later the blood pressure is 170/110 mm Hg. Relevant laboratory findings are as follows:

Serum transaminase: 2 × normal
Creatinine: 1.5 mg/dL
Urinalysis: 3+ protein

■ **What is the most likely diagnosis?**	Preeclampsia and eclampsia are the two most common causes of pregnancy-induced hypertension (PIH). Preeclampsia can occur at 20+ weeks of gestation.
■ **What is the pathophysiology of this condition?**	Systemic endothelial damage is caused by vascular spasm, capillary hyperpermeability, and relatively high levels of thromboxane (vasoconstrictor) relative to prostacyclin (vasodilator). It is a disease of the placenta. Indeed, the primary defect is thought to be abnormal development of the placenta in early pregnancy.
■ **What signs and symptoms are commonly associated with this condition?**	**Mild preeclampsia** is characterized by 1+ proteinuria and a blood pressure >140/90 mm Hg. Common symptoms include headache, rapid weight gain, edema of the face and hands, jugular venous distention, and hyperactive reflexes. **Severe preeclampsia** is characterized by 3+ proteinuria and a blood pressure >160/110 mm Hg. Common symptoms include visual changes, headache, somnolence, right upper quadrant or epigastric pain, oligohydramnios, elevated liver enzyme levels, thrombocytopenia, renal failure, HELLP syndrome, pulmonary edema/cyanosis, and intrauterine growth restriction. **Eclampsia** is characterized by seizures or coma that develop in the setting of preeclampsia.
■ **What risk factors are associated with an increased incidence of this disease?**	■ Abnormal placentation ■ African-American ethnicity ■ Age <20 or >35 years ■ Chronic hypertension ■ Chronic renal disease ■ Cohabitation <1 year ■ Collagen vascular disease (e.g., systemic lupus erythematosus) ■ Diabetes mellitus before pregnancy ■ Family history of preeclampsia ■ Multiple gestation ■ New paternity ■ Nulliparity ■ Previous preeclampsia
■ **What is HELLP syndrome?**	HELLP is a subcategory of preeclampsia that results in a high rate of stillbirth (10%–15%) and neonatal death (~25%). **HELLP** stands for **H**emolysis, **E**levated **L**iver enzymes, and **L**ow **P**latelets.

ORGAN SYSTEMS

REPRODUCTIVE

- **What are the most appropriate treatments for this condition?**

If the baby is term, the fetal lungs are mature, or the case is severe, delivery is the best treatment. Mild preeclampsia is treated with bed rest, close monitoring, and blood pressure control with antihypertensive agents. In severe cases the mother should be hospitalized and magnesium sulfate should be given for seizure prophylaxis (continue for 24 hours postpartum), in addition to antihypertensive agents. In such severe cases, immediate delivery may be indicated to save the life of the mother.

A 17-year-old boy is awakened from his sleep by sudden, sharp scrotal pain. In the emergency department, the patient says he feels nauseous. He reports that the pain is mainly on the left side, and on physical examination, there evidence of swelling and reddening of the scrotum. He has a negative cremasteric reflex.

■ **What is the most likely diagnosis?**	Testicular torsion.
■ **What are the typical signs and symptoms are associated with this condition?**	Testicular torsion is usually seen in adolescent males aged 16–18 years, though it can also occur in infancy. Fifty percent of the time it occurs during sleep, but it can also occur at rest or related to sports and physical activity. Some patients have repeated episodes that spontaneously resolve (presumably the testis is undergoing repeated torsion and untorsion). The main symptoms are sudden, acute onset of pain in the scrotum, often on one side. There can be swelling and reddening of the scrotum, and the affected side may be higher than the other and horizontal in orientation. The cremasteric reflex is often absent. Patients may also complain of abdominal pain, nausea, and vomiting.
■ **What are the complications associated with this condition?**	Testicular torsion results in the twisting of the spermatic cord, which contains the testicular artery, pampiniform plexus, and vas deferens. The main danger is the twisting of the testicular artery, which cuts off the blood supply to the testicle. If this is not reversed rapidly, it will result in **testicular atrophy and necrosis**. This is a true surgical emergency.
■ **What is the most appropriate treatment for this condition?**	One can try to manually untwist the testis, which will result in immediate and dramatic pain relief if successful. The success of this can be confirmed using Doppler ultrasound to look for return of blood flow to the testis. Even if successful, surgery should be performed to suture the testis in place to prevent repeated torsion. If manual detorsion does not work, emergent surgery must be done to untwist the testis and suture it in place. Treatment must be initiated within 6 hours of presentation to assure viability of the testicle. If it is not treated within 24 hours, there is little chance of the testicle's remaining viable.
■ **What conditions should be included in the differential diagnosis?**	Because testicular torsion must be treated emergently, it is the first thing one should rule out. The differential diagnosis for acute scrotal pain with reddening includes orchitis (i.e., secondary to mumps), trauma, hydrocele, varicocele, hernia (suspect bowel entrapment and ischemia if there is pain), tumor, and epididymitis.

ORGAN SYSTEMS

REPRODUCTIVE

► **Case 19**

A 16-year-old girl is brought to her pediatrician because of an absence of menarche. She has short stature, a webbed neck, and a square chest. Physical examination reveals breast buds and female external genitalia. Her blood pressure is normal in both arms. CT scan reveals a small uterus and atretic, fatty ovaries. There is no known history of this condition in her family.

■ **What is the most likely diagnosis?**	Turner's syndrome, characterized by gonadal dysgenesis secondary to the presence of a single X chromosome (XO) (see Figure 13-7). This syndrome is the most common cause of primary amenorrhea.
■ **What other conditions can cause primary amenorrhea?**	Primary amenorrhea refers to the complete absence of menstruation by age 16 (as compared with secondary amenorrhea, which is cessation of menstruation for >6 months after menarche). ■ Absence of uterus, cervix, and/or vagina (**müllerian agenesis**). ■ Hypothalamic hypogonadism (secondary to anorexia, exercise, stress, or gonadotropin-releasing hormone deficiency). ■ Ovarian failure (gonadal dysgenesis, or polycystic ovarian syndrome). ■ Pituitary disease. ■ Transverse vaginal septum or imperforate hymen.
■ **What diagnostic test is indicated based on the patient's clinical features?**	Chromosome analysis should be performed. Typically, 20 cells are analyzed to detect whether mosaicism is present. Additionally, no Barr chromatin body will be seen.
■ **What other conditions are associated with this condition?**	In addition to primary amenorrhea, Turner's syndrome may have a number of other clinical features including: coarctation of the aorta, bicuspid aortic valve, hypothyroidism, sensorineural hearing loss, renal abnormalities, gastrointestinal telangiectasias, and osteoporosis. Mental retardation is not usually present.
■ **What are the most appropriate treatments for this condition?**	Recombinant human growth hormone and hormone replacement therapy can initiate puberty and complete growth.

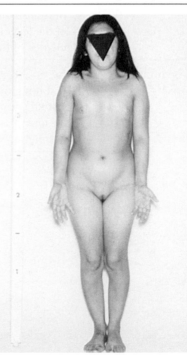

FIGURE 13-7. Turner's syndrome. (Reproduced, with permission, from Le T, Bhushan V, Rao DA. *First Aid for the USMLE Step 1: 2008.* New York: McGraw-Hill, 2008: Color Image 109.)

Respiratory

Case 1	454
Case 2	455
Case 3	456
Case 4	457
Case 5	458
Case 6	459
Case 7	460
Case 8	462
Case 9	463
Case 10	464
Case 11	465
Case 12	467
Case 13	468
Case 14	469
Case 15	470
Case 16	472
Case 17	474
Case 18	475
Case 19	476
Case 20	477

▶ **Case 1**

While working in a laboratory, a medical student accidentally opens a canister containing a highly corrosive gas. Unfortunately, before sealing off the canister, the student inhales a large quantity of the gas. He immediately goes to the emergency department for evaluation and treatment. Physical examination is significant for labored breathing and tachypnea as well as scattered crackles and tachycardia.

■ **What conditions should be included in the differential diagnosis?**	Given this student's history, a differential diagnosis would include conditions such as noncardiogenic pulmonary edema, acute pneumonitis, and diffuse alveolar damage. It should be noted that onset of symptoms may take up to several days depending on the severity of the insult.
■ **If it is found that there is a protein-rich exudate in the patient's alveoli, what diagnosis would be favored and to what condition could it lead?**	The patient is likely to have diffuse alveolar damage, which may lead to acute respiratory distress syndrome.
■ **Describe the process of diffuse alveolar damage?**	There is an increase in alveolar capillary permeability due to the damage caused by an inciting agent, in this case, the corrosive gas and the body's response to it. Initial damage can be attributed to neutrophilic substances that are toxic to tissue, oxygen-derived free radicals, and to activation of the coagulation cascade. This insult leads to protein-rich exudates leaking into the lungs and the formation of an intra-alveolar hyaline membrane.
■ **What further complication can arise if the process of diffuse alveolar damage does not resolve in the first week?**	If the inflammation and hyaline membrane formation do not resolve, the damaged tissue can organize, resulting in fibrosis.
■ **What form of atelectasis will occur if the lung tissue becomes fibrotic?**	Cicatrization atelectasis will occur as a result of the parenchymal fibrosis.

► **Case 2**

A 60-year-old man comes to his primary care physician because of dyspnea on exertion that has been worsening over the past several years. He also reports a nonproductive cough that he has had almost daily over the same period. On questioning, the man says he worked for 30 years as a demolition worker in a shipyard, where he stripped and replaced insulating material. On physical examination, chest expansion appears markedly restricted, and there are fine inspiratory crackles that are most pronounced at the lung bases. Also of note are multiple firm, subcutaneous nodules on the man's hands.

■ What is the most likely diagnosis?	Asbestosis.
■ What conditions should be considered in the differential diagnosis?	One should also consider interstitial lung diseases, especially those caused by occupational exposure, such as silicosis, coal worker's pneumoconiosis, and berylliosis. Conditions not related to occupational exposure including usual interstitial pneumonia and idiopathic pulmonary fibrosis should also be contemplated.
■ What is the pathophysiology of this condition?	The pathophysiologic process involves diffuse pulmonary interstitial fibrosis caused by inhaled asbestos fibers. Asbestos fibers penetrate bronchioles and lung tissue, where they are surrounded by macrophages and coated by a protein-iron complex (ferruginous bodies); Figure 14-1 shows these phagocytosed bodies with Prussian blue iron stain. Diffuse fibrosis around the bronchioles spreads to the alveoli. This causes lung tissue to become rigid and airways to become distorted.
■ What are the most likely findings on x-ray of the chest?	In cases of minor exposure, the only findings may be pleural thickening or calcified pleural plaques. In cases of extensive pulmonary fibrosis, reticular or nodular opacities will be seen throughout the lung fields, most prominently at the bases.
■ What are the most appropriate treatments for this condition?	There is no definitive therapy for asbestosis. As soon as exposure to asbestos is confirmed, the patient should be removed from the exposure and encouraged not to smoke, as the combination of asbestosis and smoking greatly increases the risk of bronchogenic carcinoma. Corticosteroids may have some benefit, although their use is not well established.

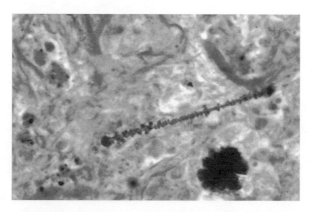

FIGURE 14-1. Asbestos bodies. (Reproduced, with permission, of the Pathology Education Instructional Resource Digital Library [http://peir.net] at the University of Alabama, Birmingham.)

► **Case 3**

A 7-year-old boy is brought to the emergency department (ED) after awakening in the middle of the night with difficulty breathing. He has a 2-day history of worsening productive cough and wheezing. In the ED, the patient is found to be dyspneic and tachypneic and has a decreased inspiratory-to-expiratory ratio. Lung examination reveals diffuse rhonchi and expiratory wheezes in addition to pulsus paradoxus. He is afebrile and has no recent history of fever. This is the patient's second visit to the ED with these symptoms; his first visit was 2 years ago.

■ What is the most likely diagnosis?	Asthma exacerbation. Asthma is a form of obstructive lung disease.
■ What is the pathophysiology of this condition?	Acutely, bronchial hyperresponsiveness leads to episodic, reversible bronchoconstriction. Specifically, smooth muscle contraction in the airways leads to expiratory airflow obstruction. Chronically, airway inflammation leads to histologic changes in the bronchial tree.
■ What histologic findings in the lung are associated with this condition?	Histologic examination reveals smooth muscle hypertrophy, goblet cell hyperplasia, thickening of basement membranes, and increased eosinophil recruitment (see Figure 14-2; arrow points to plate of cartilage, arrowhead points to infiltrate of inflammatory cells). Dilated bronchi are filled with neutrophils and may have mucous plugs.
■ What are some common triggers of this condition?	Viral upper respiratory tract infections, various allergens, stress, cold, and exercise are common triggers of asthma exacerbation.
■ What is the most appropriate treatment for this condition?	Albuterol, a β_2-agonist, helps relax bronchial smooth muscle and decrease airway obstruction. However, for long term control and prevention of acute exacerbations, inhaled corticosteroids are the best treatment.

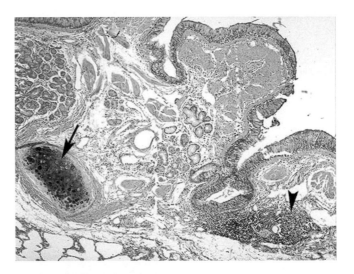

FIGURE 14-2. Histologic findings in asthma. (Reproduced, with permission, from Wilson FJ, et al. *Histology Image Review*. Norwalk, CT: Appleton & Lange, 1997: Figure 19-42.)

A pregnant woman suffering from a markedly elevated blood pressure and thrombocytopenia suddenly starts having seizures. She is rushed to the delivery room where it is determined that she has eclampsia and is immediately taken to the operating room for cesarean section. Her premature baby (<32 weeks) is delivered and is found to have an increased work of breathing and a low heart rate. This baby is intubated and a drug is administered to the neonate for respiratory distress syndrome.

■ What is an example of a drug that is given to the neonate to promote lung expansion?	Surfactant can be given to the neonate directly. Surfactant lowers the surface tension between alveoli, helping the lung to expand. Another important drug that can be used antenatally is dexamethasone. This drug aids in surfactant production and is given to women at risk for a preterm delivery to reduce the chances of RDS.
■ What condition is the neonate suffering from?	The neonate is suffering from neonatal respiratory distress syndrome, which includes progressive and diffuse atelectasis, interstitial edema, and hyaline membrane formation. Atelectasis is defined as the incomplete expansion of the lungs in a neonate or the collapse of a previously inflated lung. Other than in newborns, atelectasis is primarily found in adults.
■ What are the types of adult atelectasis?	There are four subcategories of atelectasis: ■ Adhesive ■ Resorption ■ Cicatricial ■ Passive/Compressive
■ What are the primary types of atelectasis?	Adhesive atelectasis occurs, for example, in patients with insufficient surfactant. In resorption atelectasis, there is an obstruction of an airway, commonly at the level of the smaller bronchi, with collapse of the alveoli distal to the obstruction. A common cause for this type of atelectasis is secretions or exudates. Therefore, this is often seen in people with asthma, bronchitis, aspiration of foreign bodies, and postoperatively. Cicatricial atelectasis occurs in an area of scarred lung tissue. Passive atelectasis occurs due to poor ventilation, for example after surgery. Compressive atelectasis occurs similarly due to a space-occupying mass in the thorax that compresses a region of lung tissue.
■ Does the direction of the mediastinal shift differentiate obstruction from compression atelectasis?	Yes, it does. In obstruction atelectasis the mediastinum shifts towards the atelectasis because there has been loss of lung volume in that area. By contrast the mediastinum will shift away from the atelectasis with compression.
■ During atelectasis, to what is the patient commonly predisposed?	Atelectasis results in a decrease in ventilation and mucus trapping, thereby predisposing the patient to infections.

► **Case 5**

A patient comes to his physician with a hacking cough and purulent sputum. His history is positive for a genetic birth defect called Kartagener's syndrome in which ciliary motion is either abnormal or absent. The patient also claims to have a constantly runny nose, a previous diagnosis of chronic bronchitis, and numerous bouts of pneumonia. Before making a diagnosis, the physician orders a high-resolution CT scan of the patient's lungs seen in Figure 14-3.

■ What is the most likely diagnosis?	This patient clearly has bronchiectasis, which is a permanent dilation of the airways. In the above image, the airways in cross-section have a wide, ring-like appearance. One can clearly note the dilated airways in both lower lobes as well as the lingula.
■ What are the possible etiologies of this condition?	Etiologies include chronic bronchial necrotizing infections, cystic fibrosis, bronchial obstruction from granulomatous disease or neoplasms, α_1-antitrypsin deficiency, an impaired host defense, and inflammation as in bronchiolitis obliterans. Additionally, tuberculosis and primary ciliary dyskinesia should be evaluated.
■ What are the common complications associated with this condition?	Some of the complications include hemoptysis, hypoxemia, cor pulmonale, and amyloidosis.
■ What management is most appropriate for this condition?	If an infection is thought to be the cause, then antibiotics should be given. If the bronchiectasis is very localized, surgery may be an option. For routine management, however, measures include postural drainage and chest percussion.

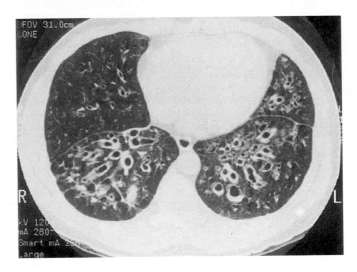

FIGURE 14-3. (Reproduced, with permission, from Weinberger SE. *Principles of Pulmonary Medicine*, 4th ed. Philadelphia, PA: Saunders, 2004.)

A 50-year-old woman visits a community health clinic because of a 1-month history of cough productive of yellow sputum. On questioning, she says she has had several periods of cough lasting 4–6 consecutive months each year for the past 5 years. She has smoked two packs of cigarettes per day for the past 30 years. On examination, the woman's breathing is shallow, and she is exhaling slowly with pursed lips. Her jugular venous pulse is visible to the jaw line when she is reclined at an angle of 45°. Auscultation of the chest demonstrates wheezing and distant heart sounds. A positive hepatojugular reflux is demonstrated, as is 2+ pitting edema up to her knees. A high-resolution CT scan reveals several hyperlucent areas within the lungs.

■ What is the most likely diagnosis?	Chronic obstructive pulmonary disease (COPD) with features of chronic bronchitis. The diagnosis is based on clinical findings of a history of productive cough for at least 3 consecutive months over 2 consecutive years accompanied by emphysema (suggested by pursed-lip breathing).
■ What abnormalities would be expected on pulmonary function testing?	In COPD, the forced expiratory volume in 1 second (FEV_1) is decreased, forced vital capacity (FVC) is normal or decreased, and the FEV_1/FVC ratio is decreased. These findings differ from restrictive lung disease, in which decreased vital capacity and total lung capacity result in a FEV_1/FVC ratio of >80%.
■ How would this condition affect the patient's arterial blood gas levels from normal values for pH, PaO_2, $PaCO_2$, and SaO_2?	pH will decrease as a result of respiratory acidosis. While pH may be normal in a patient with chronic compensated COPD, it will be low in a patient with an acute exacerbation. Arterial oxygen tension (PaO_2) will decrease, arterial carbon dioxide tension ($PaCO_2$) will increase, and oxygen saturation (SaO_2) will decrease secondary to impaired gas exchange (from destruction of alveolar septae and pulmonary capillary bed).
■ Why is breathing with pursed lips adaptive in this condition?	Breathing with pursed lips maintains positive end expiratory pressure. Positive end expiratory pressure prevents alveolar collapse, which is a common occurrence in emphysema. Respiratory therapy often provides supplemental oxygen therapy via a mask or nasal prongs. Positive airway pressure can be provided by using either continuous positive airway pressure, bilevel positive airway pressure, or intubation and ventilatory support.
■ What complication of this condition do the patient's enlarged neck veins, hepatomegaly, and edema suggest?	Cor pulmonale. Right heart failure due to chronic pulmonary hypertension leads to systemic venous congestion, which presents with the symptoms mentioned here. This complication occurs only in patients with severe COPD who develop pulmonary hypertension.

ORGAN SYSTEMS

RESPIRATORY

► **Case 7**

A 67-year-old man comes to the emergency department complaining of a 3-day history of cough and fever and a 1-day history of shaking chills. He has smoked about half a pack of cigarettes per day for the past 45 years. For the past 9 months, the man has had an increasingly severe cough that has been productive of clear sputum. His cough is now productive of rusty sputum. On physical examination, he is found to have a respiratory rate of 24/min and his temperature is 37.8°C (100°F). An x-ray of the chest shows lung consolidation (see Figure 14-4).

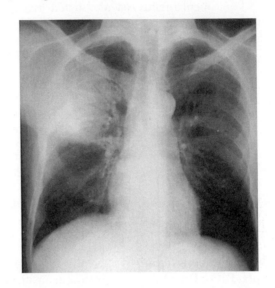

FIGURE 14-4. (Reproduced, with permission, from Le T, Bhushan V, Rao DA. *First Aid for the USMLE Step 1: 2008.* New York: McGraw-Hill, 2008: Color Image 126B.)

■ **What is the most likely diagnosis?**	This patient presents with several of the classic findings of community-acquired pneumonia (CAP): a productive cough, fever, rigors (shaking chills), and tachypnea. His risk factors include an advanced age and a significant smoking history.
■ **What are the likely findings on lung examination?**	Decreased breath sounds, crackles, dullness to percussion, and increased tactile fremitus are probable findings.
■ **What are the most likely causative organisms?**	CAP is most often caused by bacteria, including *Streptococcus pneumoniae* (20%–60%), *Haemophilus influenzae* (3%–10%), *Staphylococcus aureus* (3%–5%), *Legionella* (2%–8%), and *Mycoplasma* (1%–6%), as well as by viruses (2%–15%). Less commonly, they may also be caused by parasites and fungi.
■ **Gram stain of the sputum reveals gram-positive cocci in pairs and short chains. Additional testing reveals that the organism is optochin sensitive, and the Quellung reaction is positive. What is the causative organism?**	*Streptococcus pneumoniae. S. pneumoniae* is a gram-positive, encapsulated organism (see Figure 14-5); hence, the positive Quellung reaction, which is performed by adding anticapsular antisera that cause the capsule to swell. The organism is also catalase negative, α-hemolytic (partial hemolysis; the blood turns greenish), and optochin sensitive (which differentiates it from *S. viridans*, which is also α-hemolytic).
■ **What are the most appropriate treatments for this condition?**	Penicillin V or amoxicillin is rarely used in clinical practice because resistance with these drugs is an increasing problem. The typical treatment is either a macrolide in combination with a cephalosporin, or fluoroquinolone monotherapy.

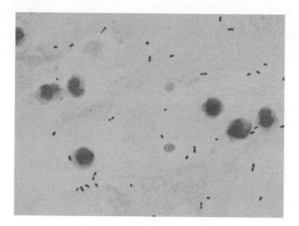

FIGURE 14-5 **Histologic findings of *Streptococcus pneumoniae*.** (Reproduced, with permission, from Le T, Bhushan V, Rao DA. *First Aid for the USMLE Step 1: 2008*. New York: McGraw-Hill, 2008: Color Image 1.)

► **Case 8**

A newborn boy has been diagnosed by prenatal ultrasound with a congenital cystic adenomatoid malformation (CCAM) in the right lower lobe of his lung. CCAMs are hamartomas of terminal bronchioles. In view of the risks of CCAM-associated complications, the boy undergoes a right lower lobe resection.

▪ How many segments of lung will be resected if the entire right lower lobe is removed?	There are five segments in the right lower lobe: superior, medial basal, anterior basal, lateral basal, and posterior basal (see Figure 14-6).
▪ Which vessels supply arterial and venous branches to the lungs, and what paths do the branches follow to supply each lung segment?	The lung alveoli are supplied by branches of the pulmonary artery and vein. The bronchial tree also receives its arterial supply from the bronchial arteries (from the aorta) and venous drainage from bronchial veins that feed into the azygos and accessory hemiazygos veins. Pulmonary and bronchial arteries follow the airways into the periphery. Pulmonary veins course in the septa between adjacent lung segments.
▪ When entering the thoracic cavity through an intercostal space, the surgeon preserves the intercostal nerves and vessels, which lie in what anatomic relationship to the ribs?	The intercostal nerves and vessels lie in the costal groove inferior to each rib. They lie between the innermost intercostal and internal intercostal muscles for the length of those muscles.
▪ During development, the pulmonary arteries arise from which aortic arch?	The sixth aortic arch gives rise to the pulmonary arteries as well as to the ductus arteriosus.
▪ During which week of gestation are the bronchial buds formed from the foregut?	Bronchial buds are formed in the fourth week of gestation. Depending on the histology and other associated anomalies, different types of CCAMs are suspected to result from insults during varying stages of development. For example, **type 2 CCAMs** are associated with anomalies such as esophageal fistulas and bilateral renal agenesis. Thus, type 2 CCAMs are thought to arise early in organogenesis, during the fourth week of gestation.

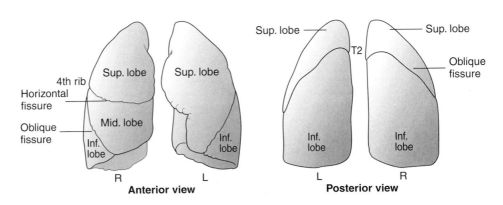

FIGURE 14-6. **Lobes of the lung.** (Reproduced, with permission, from Le T, Bhushan V, Rao DA. *First Aid for the USMLE Step 1: 2008.* New York: McGraw-Hill, 2008: 458.)

▶ **Case 9**

A 15-year-old girl is brought to the emergency department in acute respiratory distress and is stabilized with treatment. On questioning, she reports an increasingly productive cough over the past few days. Her pulse oximetry shows 93% oxygen saturation on 2 L of oxygen, and she often gasps for air midsentence. Examination shows nostril flaring, subcostal retractions, and clubbing of the fingers. A birth history reveals the patient had a meconium ileus.

■ What genetically transmitted disease does this patient likely have?	The patient likely has cystic fibrosis (CF), which is caused by loss-of-function mutations in the CFTR (cystic fibrosis transmembrane conductance regulator) protein, a chloride channel found in all exocrine tissues. As a result of these mutations, secretions in the lung, intestine, pancreas, and reproductive tract are extremely viscous. This can result in obstructions in these organs, leading to disease complications.
■ What test was likely conducted during the patient's infancy to confirm the diagnosis?	A genetic screen was most likely conducted. A sweat chloride test can also confirm the diagnosis, but it may be difficult to collect an adequate amount of sweat in a baby. Patients with CF have elevated chloride levels in their sweat.
■ What is the probable etiology of the patient's current symptoms?	The lungs in patients with CF are colonized at an early age with various bacteria not normally found in the lung. Therefore, patients suffer from repeated pulmonary bacterial infections, leading to increased production of viscous secretions. These increased secretions lead to increased cough and pulmonary obstruction, which can result in acute respiratory distress.
■ What vitamin supplements do patients with this condition usually require?	Patients with CF generally require the fat-soluble vitamins A, D, E, and K. The thick secretions block the release of pancreatic enzymes, resulting in pancreatic insufficiency.
■ What information can be provided if this patient asks for genetic counseling?	CF occurs with a frequency of 1 in 2000 white people; the carrier rate is 1 in 25 white people. CF is an autosomal recessive disease, so all children of a patient with CF will at a minimum become carriers. Some 95% of males with CF are infertile due to defects in the transport of sperm. One or both of the vas deferens are often absent. Infertility affects as many as 20% of women as a result of abnormally thick cervical mucus and amenorrhea from malnutrition.

▶ **Case 10**

A 70-year-old woman with a 65-pack-year smoking history complains to her physician of worsening dyspnea. The dyspnea has now become so severe she is experiencing shortness of breath at rest. She also admits to an occasional cough productive of small amounts of thin sputum. Examination reveals a thin woman with an increased thoracic anteroposterior diameter. The physician notes that his patient breathes through pursed lips, has an increased expiratory phase, and is using her accessory muscles to breathe.

■ **What is the most likely diagnosis?**	Emphysema.
■ **What is the pathophysiology of this condition?**	Destruction of alveolar walls results in enlargement of air spaces. As shown in Figure 14-7, compared with normal lung (A), the lung in emphysema (B) shows destruction of lung parenchyma and marked dilatation of terminal air spaces. Destruction of lung parenchyma also results in decreased elastic recoil, which increases airway collapsibility, causing expiratory obstruction. As a result, patients with emphysema often find it easier to exhale through pursed lips (which maintains a high end expiratory pressure, thereby stenting the alveoli open)—hence the term "pink puffers."
■ **What findings would be expected on lung and heart examination?**	Air trapped in the lungs will cause the chest to sound hyperresonant to percussion. These patients also have decreased breath sounds, wheezing, a prolonged expiratory phase, and diminished heart sounds.
■ **What pattern of lung parenchymal destruction is likely to be found in this patient?**	Smoking results in a destruction pattern termed **centrilobular emphysema,** which affects the respiratory bronchioles and central alveolar ducts. **Panacinar emphysema** is associated with α_1-antitrypsin deficiency and results in destruction throughout the acinus.
■ **What pattern would pulmonary function testing likely reveal?**	One would expect to see values consistent with obstructive lung disease: dramatically reduced forced expiratory volume in 1 second (FEV_1) and reduced forced vital capacity (FVC), resulting in an FEV_1/FVC ratio of <80%.

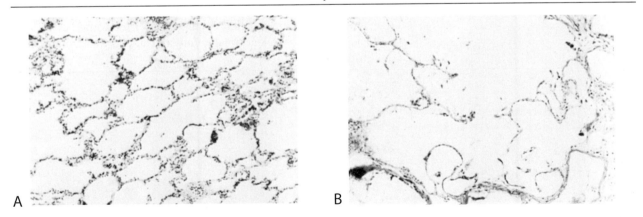

A   B

FIGURE 14-7. (A) Normal lung and (B) lung in emphysema. (Reproduced, with permission, from Chandrasoma P, Taylor CR. *Concise Pathology*, 3rd ed. Norwalk, CT: Appleton & Lange, 1997: Figure 35-6.)

► **Case 11**

A 4-year-old boy is brought to the emergency department (ED) by his mother because he is lethargic and appears to be having difficulty breathing. There is also saliva drooling out of his mouth. Physical examination reveals the patient is febrile, and his lung examination is notable for a high-pitched upper airway wheeze. Further questioning of the patient's mother reveals the child has not received his immunizations.

■ What is the most likely diagnosis?

This is most likely a case of acute epiglottitis, as suggested by the stridor found on lung examination and the drooling saliva—findings consistent with both tracheal and esophageal obstruction. The obstruction is due to swelling of the epiglottis caused by infection. Given the child's unimmunized status, the most likely cause is group b *Haemophilus influenzae* infection.

■ What additional microorganisms can cause this presentation?

Epiglottitis can also be caused by *Pasturella multocida*, which is often transmitted from dog or cat bites, and herpes simplex virus type 1. However, the child's unimmunized status points to *H. influenzae* as the causative agent.

■ What is the main virulence factor of this organism?

The polysaccharide capsule is the major virulence factor of *H. influenzae*. The bacterium has both encapsulated and nonencapsulated strains. The nonencapsulated forms are limited to local infections such as otitis media in children and mild respiratory infection in adults (see Table 14-1). The encapsulated strains are significantly more virulent and can cause disseminated disease such as meningitis, epiglottitis, and septic arthritis. There are six capsular types, designated a through f. The b-type capsule is the subtype that accounts for roughly 95% of serious *H. influenzae* infections in children.

■ How has the vaccine used to prevent this infection been redesigned to improve its efficacy?

The **Hib vaccine** consists of a purified b-type capsule conjugated to diphtheria toxin. The diphtheria toxin activates T lymphocytes, which are required for adequate antibody production against the capsular antigen. The original vaccine consisted only of b capsule and was not effective in eliciting an antibody response.

■ What is the likely source of this infection?

H. influenzae is considered part of the normal flora of the nasopharynx. The organism may thus be spread by direct contact with respiratory secretions and by airborne droplet contamination. Epiglottitis may also represent a primary infection of the epiglottis rather than invasion from the nasopharynx, as is often the case with meningitis and septic arthritis.

ORGAN SYSTEMS

RESPIRATORY

TABLE 14-1. Types of Infection Caused by *Haemophilus*

	H. INFLUENZAE		H. AEGYPTIUS	H. DUCREYI
	TYPE B	NONTYPABLE		
Type of infection	Meningitis Epiglottitis Bacteremia Cellulitis Septic arthritis	Otitis media Sinusitis Tracheobronchitis Pneumonia	Conjunctivitis Purpuric fever (Brazilian)	Chancroid (painful ulcers of genitals, lymphadenitis)
Treatment	Ceftazidime Cefotaxime Ceftriaxone Gentamicin	Cephalosporin Fluoroquinolone Azithromycin	Rifampin	Azithromycin Cephalosporin Ciprofloxacin

ORGAN SYSTEMS

RESPIRATORY

A 60-year-old man visits his doctor complaining of chest pain and difficulty breathing. He states that his symptoms wax and wane but never completely resolve. The patient has an occupational history significant for 30 years as a shipyard worker. Suspecting an occupational exposure to hazardous material, the physician orders a CT scan of the thorax, seen in Figure 14-8.

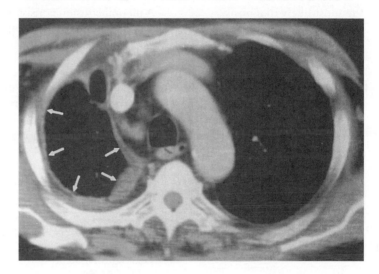

FIGURE 14-8. (Reproduced, with permission, from Chen MYM, Pope Jr. TL, Ott DJ. *Basic Radiology*. New York: McGraw-Hill, 2004: 101.)

■ **What is the most likely diagnosis?**	The pleural thickening indicated by the arrows along with a history significant for exposure to asbestos makes the diagnosis of malignant mesothelioma highly likely. As the disease progresses, the lung is surrounded and compressed by a thick layer of tumor. Common features of the disease include dyspnea, chest pain, and pleural effusions.
■ **What occupations put patients at risk for exposure to the suspected agent?**	Mesotheliomas are rare; however, a history of **asbestos exposure, particularly among smokers,** greatly elevates the risk. Asbestos exposure is commonly seen in pipe fitters, shipyard workers, welders, plumbers, and construction workers. The disease typically manifests itself several decades after asbestos exposure.
■ **What are the typical findings of pulmonary function testing in this condition?**	Pulmonary function testing reveal a **restrictive pattern.** Tumor growth causes decreased lung expansion and total lung capacity. Expect a decrease in both forced expiratory volume in 1 second (FEV_1) and forced vital capacity (FVC), but a preserved FEV_1:FVC ratio.
■ **What is the prognosis for patients with this condition?**	Given strictly supportive care, the median survival for those with malignant mesothelioma ranges from approximately 6 to 8 months. With aggressive therapies such as extrapleural pneumonectomy plus chemotherapy and radiation, the median survival increases to 34 months.

▶ **Case 13**

A 70-year-old man with a history of laryngeal cancer presents to the emergency department with shortness of breath. He complains that for the past 3 days he has been unable to lie flat to sleep and last night he woke up suddenly gasping for air. A decubitus chest film shows layering of fluid.

■ **What is the most likely diagnosis?**

A pleural effusion consists of fluid accumulation in the pleural space (between the visceral pleura and the parietal pleura) of the lung. Normally, the pleural space is only a potential space, with a small amount of fluid.

■ **How is this condition classified?**

There are two types of pleural effusion. **Transudative pleural effusions** are caused by increased hydrostatic pressure of the pleural capillaries (as in congestive heart failure), or by a decrease in plasma oncotic pressure, as seen in disorders with decreased plasma albumin levels (such as renal and hepatic failure). **Exudative pleural effusions** are caused by a change in the permeability of the pleural surface (such as secondary to inflammatory or neoplastic changes). These effusions have a high protein content.

■ **What are the common causes of this condition?**

Transudative pleural effusion:
■ Cirrhosis
■ Congestive heart failure
■ Constrictive pericarditis
■ Nephrotic syndrome
■ Pulmonary embolism

Exudative pleural effusion:
■ Collagen vascular disease
■ Infection (pneumonia, tuberculosis)
■ Malignancy (primary or metastatic lung cancer or mesothelioma)
■ Pulmonary embolism

■ **What are the typical laboratory findings in this condition?**

Analysis of pleural effusion fluid includes measuring pH, total protein, lactate dehydrogenase (LDH), albumin, and cholesterol levels. Cytology (Gram stain, culture) can also be performed to identify infectious causes of effusion. Meeting any one of the three **Light's criteria** qualifies the effusion as an exudate:
■ Protein effusion:serum ratio >0.5
■ LDH effusion:serum ratio >0.6
■ Pleural LDH level greater than two-thirds the upper limit of serum LDH level

■ **What are the most appropriate treatments for this condition?**

Thoracentesis performed by needle insertion into the pleural space is used for diagnostic and therapeutic purposes. The needle is inserted through an intercostal space superior to the rib in order to avoid the intercostal nerve and vessels, which lie in the intercostal groove at the inferior border of the rib. Other treatments include **pleurodesis**, in which the pleura is made adherent and closed by chemical (such as talc or doxycycline) or physical abrasion, and permanent catheter insertion into the pleural space for periodic fluid drainage.

An 18-year-old man comes to the physician complaining of a 3-week history of worsening dry and nonproductive cough. He also has a throbbing headache along with a mild fever and complains of malaise and sore throat. Treatment with penicillin has not relieved his symptoms. Recently, his 16-year-old brother developed similar symptoms.

■ What is the most likely diagnosis?	*Mycoplasma pneumoniae*, which causes primary atypical pneumonia (**"walking pneumonia"**), is the most common cause of pneumonia in teenagers (see Table 14-2). This organism is the smallest free-living bacterium. It has no cell wall and its membrane is the only bacterial membrane containing cholesterol.
■ What diagnostic tests are useful for confirming the diagnosis?	A high titer of cold agglutinins (IgM) and growth on Eaton's agar.
■ What clinical findings are commonly associated with this condition?	Infection with *M. pneumoniae* typically results in mild upper respiratory tract disease including low-grade fever, malaise, headache, and a dry, nonproductive cough. Symptoms gradually worsen over a few days and can last for more than 2 weeks. Fewer than 10% of patients develop more severe disease with lower respiratory tract symptoms.
■ How does this organism cause illness?	*M. pneumoniae* is an extracellular organism that attaches to respiratory epithelium. As the superficial layer of respiratory epithelial cells is destroyed, the normal ability of the upper airways to clear themselves is lost. As a result, the lower respiratory tract becomes contaminated by microbes and is mechanically irritated. Close contact allows for spread of the organism.
■ What are the most appropriate treatments for this condition?	Azithromycin is most commonly prescribed to treat *Mycoplasma* infection. Tetracycline or erythromycin may be prescribed as well.

TABLE 14-2. Most Common Causes of Pneumonia According to Age

6 WEEKS–18 YEARS	18–40 YEARS	40–65 YEARS	>65 YEARS
Viral (respiratory syncytial virus)	*M. pneumoniae*	*S. pneumoniae*	*S. pneumoniae*
Mycoplasma pneumoniae	*C. pneumoniae*	*Haemophilus influenzae*	Viral
Chlamydia pneumoniae	*S. pneumoniae*	Anaerobes	Anaerobes
Streptococcus pneumoniae		*M. pneumoniae*	*H. influenzae*

▶ **Case 15**

A 62-year-old woman presents to the emergency department with acute onset of shortness of breath. She also complains of "stabbing" pleuritic right-sided chest pain. The woman had a stroke 3 months ago but is otherwise healthy. Her temperature is 36.7°C (98.1°F), blood pressure is 90/60 mm Hg, heart rate is 110/min, respiratory rate is 40/min, and oxygen saturation is 77% on room air. Physical examination reveals jugular venous distention, and cardiovascular examination reveals a regular rate and rhythm with no murmurs. The woman's lungs are clear bilaterally with decreased breath sounds in the right middle lobe. She has mild cyanosis in the distal extremities with no clubbing.

■ What is the most likely diagnosis?	This is a case of pulmonary embolism (also known as pulmonary thromboembolism, or PTE).
■ What conditions should be included in the differential diagnosis?	The differential diagnosis includes PTE, myocardial infarction or unstable angina, pneumonia, pneumothorax, exacerbation of chronic obstructive pulmonary disease, pericarditis, and costochondritis or other sources of musculoskeletal pain.
■ What is Virchow's triad?	The three factors increasing a patient's risk for venous thrombosis are local trauma to the vessel wall, hypercoagulability, and stasis. It is believed that patients with PTE have a predisposition toward developing this condition, which is triggered by a stressor such as pregnancy, obesity, or surgery.
■ What is the most likely finding on microscopic examination?	Under low-power magnification, characteristic lines of Zahn will be visible in the thrombus.
■ What test remains the gold standard for diagnosing this condition?	Pulmonary angiography remains the gold standard for diagnosing PTE, as it is the most specific test available for establishing a definitive diagnosis. However, lung scanning remains the most frequently used test. A lung scan showing normal perfusion virtually excludes the possibility of a PTE. Patients who have a physical examination and a lung perfusion scan that cannot exclude PTE should undergo pulmonary angiography. **Plasma D-dimer levels** are elevated in >90% of patients with PTE, but this assay is nonspecific and results may also be elevated in conditions such as myocardial infarction or sepsis. The current strategy for diagnosing PTE and deep venous thrombosis is shown in Figure 14-9.
■ What are the most appropriate treatments for this condition?	PTE should be treated with therapeutic levels of heparin for at least 5 days unless there is a contraindication to anticoagulation (e.g., recent surgery). In most patients, warfarin and heparin may be started together, with oral anticoagulation continued for at least 3 months. If there is a contraindication to anticoagulation or a high risk of recurrence of PTE, an inferior vena cava filter is recommended.

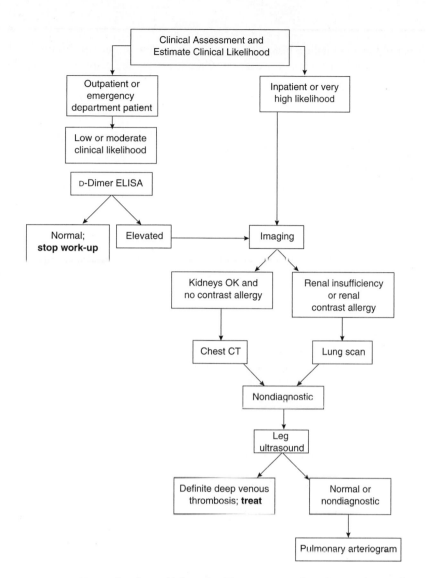

FIGURE 14-9. Diagnosis of PTE. (Adapted, with permission, from Kasper DL, et al. *Harrison's Principles of Internal Medicine*, 16th ed. New York: McGraw-Hill, 2005: 1563.)

▶ **Case 16**

A 40-year-old woman with a history of interstitial lung disease presents to the local hospital complaining of fatigue and weakness. On admission, she is found to have the following laboratory values:

Serum:
    Sodium: 144 mEq/L
    Chloride: 96 mEq/L
    Bicarbonate: 42 mEq/L
    Potassium: 4.2 mEq/L
    Blood urea nitrogen:creatinine
      ratio: 18/1.0 mg/dL

Arterial blood gas values:
    pH: 7.32
    Partial pressure of carbon dioxide (PCO_2):
      91 mm Hg

▪ **What is the most likely cause of these symptoms?**	The patient has respiratory acidosis (pH <7.4, PCO_2 >40 mm Hg) with a compensatory metabolic alkalosis. Respiratory acidosis can be caused by chronic obstructive pulmonary disease, airway obstruction, and hypoventilation. The likely cause of the patient's acidosis is interstitial lung disease, which can chronically impair gas exchange.
▪ **What is the most likely diagnosis?**	The patient has a chronic respiratory acidosis, as indicated by the large compensatory increase in bicarbonate to correct for an elevated PCO_2. Someone with a more acute process would not be able to compensate as robustly.
▪ **In Figure 14-10, label the area that corresponds to chronic respiratory acidosis, and the area that corresponds to acute respiratory acidosis.**	Referring to Figure 14-10, the letter A refers to chronic respiratory acidosis, and the letter B refers to acute respiratory acidosis. Letter C refers to chronic respiratory alkalosis, while letter D refers to acute metabolic alkalosis.
▪ **How is this condition distinguished from metabolic acidosis?**	In respiratory acidosis, the primary disturbance is an increase in PCO_2 to which the body responds by decreasing renal bicarbonate reabsorption. In metabolic acidosis, the primary disturbance is a decrease in bicarbonate, which is compensated for by hyperventilation, resulting in a decreased PCO_2.
▪ **What is the anion gap, and what factors can increase the anion gap in this condition?**	**Anion gap** is defined as $[Na+] - ([HCO_3^-] - [Cl^-])$. Causes of increased anion-gap metabolic acidosis include renal failure, diabetic ketoacidosis, lactic acidosis, and salicylate ingestion. Causes of normal anion-gap metabolic acidosis include diarrhea, renal tubular acidosis, and hyperchloremia.

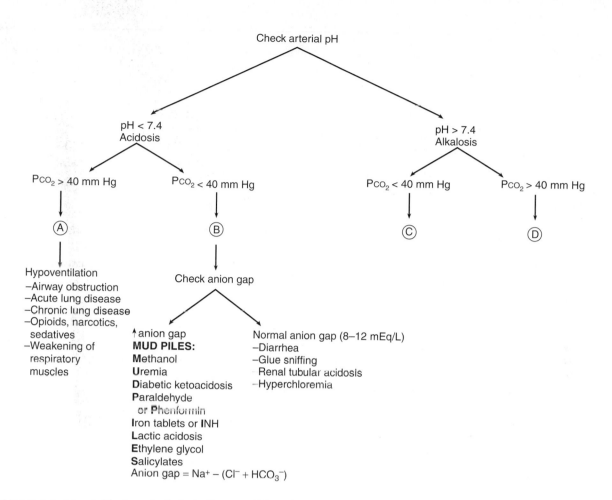

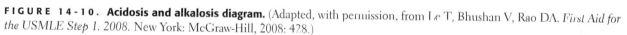

FIGURE 14-10. Acidosis and alkalosis diagram. (Adapted, with permission, from Le T, Bhushan V, Rao DA. *First Aid for the USMLE Step 1. 2008.* New York: McGraw-Hill, 2008: 428.)

▶ **Case 17**

A 35-year-old black man presents to his primary care physician with progressive dyspnea on exertion. He has no history of congestive heart failure or asthma and has had no known contact with any individuals known to have tuberculosis. His laboratory results reveal normal creatinine kinase (CK), CK-MB fraction, and troponin levels. An x-ray of the chest shows bilateral hilar lymphadenopathy and evidence of interstitial lung disease. A thoracoscopic lung biopsy reveals the presence of several small, noncaseating granulomas in both lungs.

■ What are noncaseating granulomas, and what diagnosis does their presence suggest?	Noncaseating granulomas are discrete collections of tissue macrophages, termed *histiocytes*, in the absence of frank necrosis or caseation (as would appear in tuberculosis or histoplasmosis). These granulomas frequently contain multinucleated giant cells and are accompanied by alveolitis. Their presence suggests sarcoidosis.
■ What findings would be expected on pulmonary function testing?	In interstitial lung disease, lung compliance is decreased, reflecting increased stiffness from alveolar wall inflammation and fibrosis. Tidal volume and total lung capacity are typically decreased. Diffusion capacity is also decreased as a result of inflammatory destruction of the air-capillary interface. Unlike most interstitial lung diseases, sarcoidosis has features of both obstruction and restriction.
■ What are common causes of interstitial lung disease, and what is the most likely cause in this patient?	■ Antitumor drugs. ■ Connective tissue disease (e.g., Wegener's granulomatosis, systemic lupus erythematosus, scleroderma, Sjögren's disease). ■ Eosinophilic granuloma. ■ Goodpasture's syndrome. ■ Hypersensitivity pneumonitis; "farmer's lung" or "bird-breeder's lung," in which an immune reaction to a microorganism antigen induces a type III or type IV hypersensitivity reaction. ■ Idiopathic pulmonary fibrosis. ■ Prolonged exposure to occupationally inhaled inorganic agents such as silicone, coal, asbestos, talc, mica, aluminum, and beryllium. ■ Radiation-induced disease. ■ Sarcoidosis (which is the most likely cause of interstitial lung disease in this patient).
■ What are some extrapulmonary manifestations of this patient's interstitial lung disease?	The more common extrapulmonary manifestations of sarcoidosis are in the eye (anterior uveitis) and skin (skin papules and erythema nodosum), but granulomas can also occur in the heart, brain, lung, and peripheral lymph nodes.
■ What is the most appropriate treatment for this condition?	Corticosteroids.

► **Case 18**

A 56-year-old man presents to his physician complaining of fatigue, cough, and a 9.1-kg (20-lb) weight loss over the past 8 weeks. His voice is hoarse and he is unable to keep up with his work as a construction worker. The patient has a 30-pack-year cigarette smoking history. The physician orders posteroanterior and lateral chest radiographs shown in Figure 14-11.

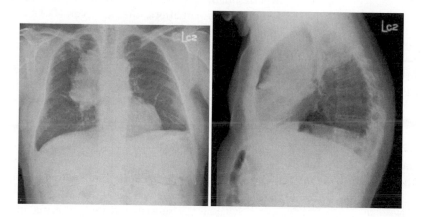

FIGURE 14-11. (Reproduced, with permission, from Kantarjian HM, Wolff RA, Koller CA. *MD Anderson Manual of Medical Oncology*. New York: McGraw-Hill, 2006: 239.)

▪ What is this most likely diagnosis?	The central, hilar nature of the lung mass along with a history significant for a 9.1-kg weight loss is strongly suggestive of small cell lung carcinoma.
▪ What additional symptoms can arise from an intrathoracic cancer?	Due to limited space within the thoracic cavity, cancer masses may cause superior vena cava obstruction, hoarseness of the voice due to recurrent laryngeal nerve compression, phrenic nerve palsy resulting in dyspnea, dysphagia from esophageal compression, and stridor due to tracheal compression.
	Symptoms can also arise due to metastasis to sites such as the brain, bone, and liver.
▪ Which paraneoplastic processes are associated with this condition?	Small cell lung carcinoma is known to cause hormonally mediated Cushing's syndrome due to ectopic secretion of ACTH as well as the syndrome of inappropriate antidiuretic hormone secretion (SIADH). In addition, up to 3% of patients with small cell lung carcinoma develop Eaton-Lambert myasthenic syndrome.
▪ To which areas does this condition commonly metastasize?	Small cell lung carcinoma is notable for its metastasis to the central nervous system, liver, and bone. As a result, patients may present with bone pain, neurologic symptoms such as seizures or focal deficits, and pain in the right upper quadrant.
▪ What is the prognosis for patients with this condition?	Untreated patients with this disease have a median survival of only 6–17 weeks. However, with combination chemotherapy, this median survival may increase to up 70 weeks. The prognosis largely depends on the tumor's reaction to chemotherapy with drugs including etoposide and cisplatin. Surgery is not an option in small cell carcinoma due to early and highly aggressive metastasis.

► **Case 19**

A 55-year-old man comes to the emergency department after he suddenly experienced severe right-sided chest pain followed by profound difficulty breathing. The man informs the physician that he has severe emphysema due to an extensive history of tobacco use. On physical examination, the patient is markedly tachypneic and tachycardic. His breath sounds are diminished at the right apex, and his chest wall is hyperresonant to percussion. No tactile fremitus is noted. Arterial blood gas analyses demonstrate a partial pressure of oxygen (PO_2) of 60 mm Hg and a partial pressure of carbon dioxide (PCO_2) of 50 mm Hg.

■ **What is the most likely diagnosis?**	Pneumothorax—or, more specifically, secondary spontaneous pneumothorax. Whereas primary spontaneous pneumothorax occurs in the absence of underlying lung disease, secondary spontaneous pneumothorax occurs in the setting of chronic lung parenchymal disruption.
■ **What is the pathophysiology of this condition?**	Spontaneous pneumothorax is most likely caused by rupture of a **subpleural bleb,** which allows air to escape into the pleural cavity. A tension pneumothorax ensues when a one-way valve is essentially created, allowing air to gradually accumulate with each inspiration. This air cannot be expelled during exhalation.
■ **What diseases most likely underlie this condition?**	The most common underlying condition is chronic obstructive pulmonary disease. Additionally, patients with acquired immunodeficiency syndrome, *Pneumocystis jiroveci* (formerly *carinii*) pneumonia, cystic fibrosis, and tuberculosis are at higher risk for spontaneous pneumothorax.
■ **What is the most common clinical presentation of this condition?**	Dyspnea with pleuritic chest pain on the same side of the pneumothorax is a common presentation. Typical physical examination findings include diminished breath sounds, hyperresonance, and absent fremitus over the pneumothorax. Arterial blood gas testing typically shows hypoxia and hypercapnia.
■ **What are the typical radiologic findings in this condition?**	Partial collapse of the lung on the side of the pneumothorax with a thin line parallel to the chest wall is occasionally visible. In a **tension pneumothorax,** tracheal and mediastinal deviation can be present away from the pneumothorax. In a **nontension pneumothorax,** however, the trachea and mediastinum will shift toward the side of the collapsed lung.
■ **What is the most appropriate treatment for this condition?**	Chest tube (thoracotomy) with parenchymal sclerosing agents.

After a difficult labor, a baby is delivered breech, with her arms above her head. Physical examination reveals the newborn's right hand is slightly contracted, with the fingers curled towards the palm. The infant seems unable to extend the fingers on the right hand.

■ What is the most likely diagnosis?	Klumpke's palsy. This palsy results from birth injury to the lower trunk of the brachial plexus (C8 and T1 nerve roots). It is a proximal brachial plexus neuropathy.
■ What motor deficits are likely to result from this condition?	The C8 and T1 nerve roots contribute to the ulnar and median nerves. The muscles affected are the medial part of the flexor digitorum profundus and the flexor carpi ulnaris (these two are the only extrinsic muscles of the forearm supplied by the ulnar nerve), and all intrinsic muscles of the hand, including those innervated by the ulnar nerve (interosseous muscles, the second and third lumbrical muscles, and the adductor pollicis brevis muscles) and those innervated by the median nerve (thenar muscles and the first two lumbrical muscles). Over time, wasting of the thenar and hypothenar eminences occurs. Marked wasting between the metatarsals on both palmar and dorsal surfaces of the hand results from paralysis of the lumbricals and interossei.
■ What sensory deficits are involved in this condition?	The lower trunk from C8 and T1 contributes to the medial cutaneous nerves of the arm, forearm, and the ulnar and median nerves. Thus, in this case there will be loss of sensation on the medial side of the arm; the forearm; the dorsal and palmar surface of the fifth finger and half of the fourth finger; the palmar surface of the first, second, and third fingers and lateral half of the fourth finger extending onto the nail beds on the dorsal surface as far as the distal interphalangeal joints; and the palmar surface of the hand.
■ What other injuries can cause this condition?	■ **Thoracic outlet syndrome:** This is a congenital defect in which a cervical rib or a scalenus minimus muscle compresses the lower trunk at C8 and T1. ■ **Trauma:** Injuries to the inferior brachial plexus are much less common than injuries to the superior brachial plexus; traumatic injury can occur when a person grabs something to break a fall, or a baby's upper limb is pulled too hard during delivery. ■ **Tumor infiltration:** Tumor infiltration from the apex of the lung (**Pancoast's tumor**) can be associated with compression of the stellate ganglion, resulting in **Horner's syndrome.**
■ What is another nerve lesion that can cause claw hand?	An ulnar nerve injury will also present with claw hand. However, with ulnar nerve injury only the little finger and the ring finger are clawed because the median nerve is spared (resulting in normal thenar muscles). Also, the sensory deficit involves only the ulnar nerve distribution: the palm and dorsal surfaces of the medial part of the hand and the dorsal and palmar surfaces of the fifth finger and half of the fourth finger.

ORGAN SYSTEMS

RESPIRATORY

APPENDIX

CASE INDEX

Case Title	Chapter	Page
11β-Hydroxylase Deficiency	Endocrine	178
21β-Hydroxylase Deficiency	Endocrine	180
Abdominal Aortic Aneurysm	Cardiovascular	138
Abruptio Placentae	Reproductive	430
Acanthamoeba Infection	Microbiology and Immunology	45
Acetaminophen Overdose	Pharmacology	118
Achalasia	Gastrointestinal	208
Actinomyces vs *Nocardia*	Microbiology and Immunology	46
Acute Intermittent Porphyria	Hematology and Oncology	247
Acute Lymphoblastic Leukemia	Hematology and Oncology	248
Acute Myelogenous Leukemia	Hematology and Oncology	250
Acute Pancreatitis	Gastrointestinal	209
Acute Respiratory Distress Syndrome/Diffuse Alveolar Damage	Respiratory	454
Acute Tubular Necrosis	Renal	398
Addison's Disease	Endocrine	181
Agranulocytosis Secondary to Drug Toxicity	Pharmacology	119
Alcohol Withdrawal	Behavioral Science	4
Alcoholic Cirrhosis	Gastrointestinal	210
Alkaptonuria	Biochemistry	22
Alport's Syndrome	Renal	400
Alzheimer's Disease	Neurology	321
Amyotrophic Lateral Sclerosis	Neurology	324
Androgen Insensitivity Syndrome	Reproductive	432
Anorexia Nervosa	Behavioral Science	6
Anthrax	Microbiology and Immunology	47
Aortic Stenosis	Cardiovascular	139
Aplastic Anemia	Hematology and Oncology	251
Appendicitis	Gastrointestinal	212
Asbestosis	Respiratory	455
Ascariasis	Microbiology and Immunology	48
Aspergillosis	Microbiology and Immunology	49
Asthma	Respiratory	456
Atelectasis	Respiratory	457
Atherosclerosis	Cardiovascular	140
Atrial Fibrillation	Cardiovascular	141
Atrial Myxoma	Cardiovascular	142
Atrioventricular Block	Cardiovascular	144
Attention Deficit Hyperactivity Disorder	Psychiatry	382

CASE TITLE	CHAPTER	PAGE
Autism	Psychiatry	383
Autoimmune Hemolytic Anemia	Hematology and Oncology	254
Autosomal Dominant Polycystic Kidney Disease	Renal	399
Bacterial Vaginosis	Reproductive	433
Barbiturate vs. Benzodiazepine	Pharmacology	120
Barrett's Esophagus	Gastrointestinal	213
Benign Prostatic Hyperplasia	Reproductive	434
Benzodiazepine Overdose	Behavioral Science	5
Benzodiazepine Overdose	Pharmacology	121
β-Adrenergic Second Messenger Systems	Pharmacology	122
β-Thalassemia	Hematology and Oncology	252
Bias	Behavioral Science	8
Bipolar Disorder	Psychiatry	384
Botulism	Microbiology and Immunology	50
Breast Cancer	Hematology and Oncology	255
Breast Mass	Reproductive	435
Bronchiectasis	Respiratory	458
Brown-Séquard Syndrome	Neurology	322
Burkitt's Lymphoma	Hematology and Oncology	258
Candidiasis	Microbiology and Immunology	51
Carcinoid Syndrome	Hematology and Oncology	256
Central Cord Syndrome	Neurology	326
Chagas' Disease	Microbiology and Immunology	52
Cholangitis	Gastrointestinal	220
Choledocholithiasis	Gastrointestinal	214
Cholera	Microbiology and Immunology	53
Cholinergic Drugs	Pharmacology	123
Chronic Granulomatous Disease	Microbiology and Immunology	54
Chronic Myelogenous Leukemia	Hematology and Oncology	259
Chronic Obstructive Pulmonary Disease	Respiratory	459
Clostridium difficile Infection	Microbiology and Immunology	55
Coarctation of the Aorta	Cardiovascular	145
Colorectal Cancer	Hematology and Oncology	260
Community-Acquired Pneumonia	Respiratory	460
Confidentiality and Its Exceptions	Behavioral Science	9
Congenital Cystic Adenomatoid Malformation of the Lung	Respiratory	462
Congenital Rubella	Cardiovascular	146
Congenital Syphilis	Microbiology and Immunology	56
Congestive Heart Failure	Cardiovascular	150
Conn's Sydrome	Endocrine	183
Core Ethical Principles	Behavioral Science	10
Corneal Abrasion/Eye Injury	Neurology	325
Coronary Artery Disease	Cardiovascular	148
Costochondritis	Musculoskeletal	296
Craniopharyngioma	Neurology	328
Creutzfeldt-Jakob Disease	Microbiology and Immunology	57
Crigler-Najjar Syndrome	Gastrointestinal	216
Cryptococcal Meningitis	Microbiology and Immunology	58
Cushing's Syndrome	Endocrine	184
Cutaneous Squamous Cell Carcinoma	Musculoskeletal	297
Cyanide Poisoning	Biochemistry	23
Cystic Fibrosis	Respiratory	463
Cysticercosis	Microbiology and Immunology	59
Cytomegalovirus Infection	Microbiology and Immunology	60

Case Title	Chapter	Page
Damage to Recurrent Laryngeal Nerve	Neurology	329
Deep Venous Thrombosis	Cardiovascular	151
Delirium	Behavioral Science	11
Dengue Fever	Microbiology and Immunology	62
Depression	Psychiatry	385
Diabetes Mellitus	Endocrine	185
DiGeorge Syndrome	Biochemistry	24
Dilated Cardiomyopathy	Cardiovascular	152
Diphtheria	Microbiology and Immunology	63
Disseminated Intravascular Coagulation	Hematology and Oncology	261
Diverticulitis	Gastrointestinal	218
Down Syndrome	Biochemistry	26
Drug Development	Pharmacology	124
Drug Intoxication	Behavioral Science	12
Drug-Induced Acute Interstitial Nephritis	Renal	401
Drug-Induced Lupus	Pharmacology	126
Ectopic Pregnancy	Reproductive	436
Ehlers-Danlos Syndrome	Biochemistry	28
Elephantiasis	Microbiology and Immunology	64
Emphysema	Respiratory	464
Endocarditis	Cardiovascular	154
Endometriosis	Reproductive	438
Epiglottitis Due to *Haemophilus influenzae* Infection	Respiratory	465
Erectile Dysfunction	Reproductive	440
Esophageal Atresia/Fistula	Gastrointestinal	221
Ethylene Glycol Poisoning	Pharmacology	128
Evaluation of Diagnostic Tests	Behavioral Science	13
Ewing's Sarcoma	Musculoskeletal	300
Familial Hypercholesterolemia	Biochemistry	25
Fanconi's Syndrome	Renal	403
Femoral Neuropathy	Neurology	330
Fitz-Hugh-Curtis Syndrome	Reproductive	441
Fragile X Syndrome	Biochemistry	30
Fructose Intolerance	Biochemistry	31
Gastric Cancer	Hematology and Oncology	262
Gastrinoma	Gastrointestinal	222
Generalized Anxiety Disorder	Psychiatry	386
Gestational Diabetes	Reproductive	442
Giardiasis	Microbiology and Immunology	65
Gigantism	Endocrine	186
Glaucoma	Neurology	331
Glioblastoma Multiforme	Hematology and Oncology	263
Glioblastoma Multiforme	Neurology	332
Glucose-6-Phospate Dehydrogenase Deficiency	Hematology and Oncology	264
Gonorrhea with Septic Arthritis	Microbiology and Immunology	66
Goodpasture's Syndrome	Renal	405
Gout	Endocrine	188
Graves' Disease	Endocrine	189
Group B *Streptococcus* in Infant	Microbiology and Immunology	68
Guillain-Barré Syndrome	Neurology	334
Gunshot Wound to Left Flank	Musculoskeletal	298

CASE TITLE	CHAPTER	PAGE
Hand, Foot, and Mouth Disease	Microbiology and Immunology	69
Head and Neck Cancer	Hematology and Oncology	265
Hemochromatosis	Gastrointestinal	223
Hemochromatosis	Hematology and Oncology	266
Hemophilia	Hematology and Oncology	270
Henoch-Schönlein Purpura	Renal	407
Hepatitis B Virus Infection	Gastrointestinal	224
Hepatitis C Virus Infection	Gastrointestinal	225
Hepatocellular Carcinoma	Gastrointestinal	226
Herpes Simplex Virus Type 2	Microbiology and Immunology	70
Hip Fracture	Musculoskeletal	301
Hodgkin's Lymphoma	Hematology and Oncology	268
Homocystinuria	Biochemistry	32
Homonymous Hemianopia	Neurology	342
Hookworm	Microbiology and Immunology	72
Horner's Syndrome	Neurology	336
Huntington's Disease	Neurology	340
Hurler's Syndrome	Biochemistry	33
Hydrocephalus	Neurology	338
Hyperbilirubinemia	Gastrointestinal	227
Hypercalcemia	Renal	408
Hyperparathyroidism	Endocrine	190
Hypertension	Cardiovascular	158
Hypertrophic Cardiomyopathy	Cardiovascular	156
Hypokalemia	Renal	410
Hyponatremia	Renal	411
Hypophosphatemic (Vitamin D–Resistant) Rickets	Renal	412
Hypothyroidism	Endocrine	191
I-cell Disease	Biochemistry	34
Idiopathic Thrombocytopenic Purpura	Hematology and Oncology	272
Infant Development	Behavioral Science	14
Inflammatory Bowel Disease	Gastrointestinal	228
Influenza	Microbiology and Immunology	73
Inguinal Hernia	Musculoskeletal	302
Isolated IgA deficiency	Microbiology and Immunology	74
Kaposi's Sarcoma	Microbiology and Immunology	76
Kartagener's Syndrome	Biochemistry	35
Kawasaki's Disease	Cardiovascular	159
Klinefelter's Syndrome	Reproductive	443
Knee Pain	Musculoskeletal	303
Lead Poisoning	Pharmacology	129
Lead Poisoning	Hematology and Oncology	274
Legionella Infection	Microbiology and Immunology	78
Leiomyoma	Reproductive	444
Leishmaniasis	Microbiology and Immunology	77
Leprosy	Microbiology and Immunology	80
Lesch-Nyhan Syndrome	Biochemistry	36
Listeria Meningitis	Microbiology and Immunology	82
Liver Cysts/Echinococcus	Microbiology and Immunology	83

CASE TITLE	CHAPTER	PAGE
Lower Gastrointestinal Bleeding	Gastrointestinal	229
Lung Cancer (Pancoast's Syndrome)	Hematology and Oncology	275
Lyme Disease	Microbiology and Immunology	86
Macrocytic Anemia	Hematology and Oncology	276
Macular Degeneration	Neurology	341
Malaria	Microbiology and Immunology	84
Malignant Mesothelioma	Respiratory	467
Malignant Pleural Effusion	Respiratory	468
Malpractice	Behavioral Science	15
McArdle's Disease	Biochemistry	37
Measles	Microbiology and Immunology	87
Meckel's Diverticulum	Gastrointestinal	230
Medulloblastoma	Neurology	344
Melanoma	Musculoskeletal	304
Meningioma	Neurology	345
Menopause	Reproductive	445
Metabolic Acidosis with Respiratory Alkalosis	Renal	414
Metabolic Alkalosis	Renal	416
Metabolic Syndrome	Endocrine	192
Metastatic Brain Tumor	Neurology	348
Microcytic Anemia	Hematology and Oncology	277
Middle Ear Infection/Ear Anatomy	Neurology	346
Migraine	Neurology	349
Minimal Change Disease	Renal	417
Mitral Valve Prolapse	Cardiovascular	160
Molar Pregnancy and Choriocarcinoma	Reproductive	446
"Monday Disease"	Cardiovascular	161
Mononucleosis	Microbiology and Immunology	88
Mucormycosis	Microbiology and Immunology	89
Multiple Endocrine Neoplasia Type IIA	Endocrine	194
Multiple Myeloma	Hematology and Oncology	280
Multiple Sclerosis	Neurology	350
Mumps	Microbiology and Immunology	90
Muscular Dystrophy	Musculoskeletal	305
Myasthenia Gravis	Neurology	354
Mycoplasma Pneumonaie Pneumonia	Respiratory	469
Myocardial Infarction	Cardiovascular	162
Neisseria meningitidis Meningitis	Microbiology and Immunology	91
Nephrotic Syndrome	Renal	418
Neuroblastoma	Hematology and Oncology	278
Neurofibromatosis	Musculoskeletal	308
Neurofibromatosis Type 1	Neurology	352
Neurofibromatosis Type 2	Neurology	356
Neuromuscular Blocking Agents	Pharmacology	132
Non-Insulin-Dependent (Type 2) Diabetes	Endocrine	196
Obsessive-Compulsive Disorder	Psychiatry	387
Obsessive-Compulsive Personality Disorder	Psychiatry	388
Obstruction of Superior Mesenteric Artery/ Inferior Mesenteric Artery	Cardiovascular	164
Oligodendroglioma	Hematology and Oncology	281

CASE TITLE	CHAPTER	PAGE
Onchocerciasis	Microbiology and Immunology	92
Operant Conditioning	Behavioral Science	16
Opioid Withdrawal	Behavioral Science	17
Osteoarthritis	Musculoskeletal	306
Osteogenesis Imperfecta	Musculoskeletal	309
Osteomyelitis	Microbiology and Immunology	93
Osteoporosis	Musculoskeletal	312
Ovarian Cancer	Reproductive	447
Ovarian Cancer (Sertoli-Leydig Tumor)	Hematology and Oncology	282
Paget's Disease of the Breast	Reproductive	448
Painless Jaundice	Gastrointestinal	232
Pancreatic Cancer	Hematology and Oncology	283
Panic Disorder	Psychiatry	389
Parkinson's Disease	Neurology	355
Patent Ductus Arteriosus	Cardiovascular	166
Pellagra	Gastrointestinal	233
Pericarditis	Cardiovascular	163
Pharmacodynamics	Pharmacology	130
Pharmacokinetics	Pharmacology	133
Phenylketonuria	Biochemistry	38
Pheochromocytoma	Endocrine	198
Pinworm	Microbiology and Immunology	94
Pituitary Adenoma	Neurology	358
Pneumocystis jiroveci Pneumonia	Microbiology and Immunology	95
Poison Ivy	Microbiology and Immunology	96
Polio	Microbiology and Immunology	97
Polyarteritis Nodosa	Cardiovascular	168
Polycythemia	Hematology and Oncology	284
Post-traumatic Stress Disorder	Psychiatry	390
Preeclampsia	Reproductive	449
Primary Biliary Cirrhosis	Gastrointestinal	234
Pseudohypoparathyroidism	Endocrine	199
Pseudomembranous Colitis/*Clostridium difficile* Infection	Gastrointestinal	236
Pseudomonas aeruginosa Infection	Microbiology and Immunology	98
Pulmonary Embolism	Respiratory	470
Pyelonephritis	Renal	419
Pyloric Stenosis	Gastrointestinal	237
Pyruvate Dehydrogenase Deficiency	Biochemistry	39
Rabies	Microbiology and Immunology	99
Rapidly Progressive Glomerulonephritis	Renal	420
Renal Artery Stenosis/Hypertension/Renin-Angiotensin-Aldosterone Axis	Renal	422
Renal Calculi	Renal	423
Respiratory Acidosis	Respiratory	472
Retinoblastoma	Hematology and Oncology	285
Rett's Disorder	Psychiatry	391
Reye's Syndrome	Gastrointestinal	238
Rheumatic Heart Disease	Cardiovascular	169
Rheumatoid Arthritis	Musculoskeletal	310

CASE TITLE	CHAPTER	PAGE
Ringworm	Microbiology and Immunology	100
Rocky Mountain Spotted Fever	Microbiology and Immunology	101
Rotator Cuff Tear	Musculoskeletal	314
Rotavirus Infection	Microbiology and Immunology	102
Sarcoidosis	Respiratory	474
Schistosomiasis	Microbiology and Immunology	103
Schizophrenia	Psychiatry	392
Seizures/Status Epilepticus	Neurology	359
Sheehan's Syndrome	Endocrine	200
Shigella and Hemolytic-Uremic Syndrome	Microbiology and Immunology	104
Shingles	Microbiology and Immunology	105
Short Bowel Syndrome/Malabsorption	Gastrointestinal	239
Sickle Cell Anemia	Hematology and Oncology	286
Sleep Physiology	Behavioral Science	18
Sleep Stages	Behavioral Science	19
Small Cell Carcinoma	Respiratory	475
Small Cell Lung Carcinoma	Hematology and Oncology	288
Somatoform Disorder	Psychiatry	393
Spherocytosis	Hematology and Oncology	289
Spinal Cord Compression	Neurology	362
Splenic Injury	Hematology and Oncology	290
Spontaneous Pneumothorax	Respiratory	476
Steroid-Induced Mania	Psychiatry	394
Stomach Cancer	Gastrointestinal	240
Stroke	Neurology	360
Strongyloidiasis	Microbiology and Immunology	107
Sturge-Weber Syndrome	Neurology	363
Subarachnoid Hemorrhage	Neurology	364
Subclavian Stab Wound	Musculoskeletal	313
Subdural Hematoma	Neurology	366
Syncope	Neurology	367
Syndrome of Inappropriate Secretion of ADH	Renal	425
Systemic Lupus Erythematosus	Musculoskeletal	316
Systemic Mycoses	Microbiology and Immunology	108
Systemic Sclerosis (Scleroderma)	Musculoskeletal	317
Tardive Dyskinesia	Psychiatry	395
Tay-Sachs Disease	Biochemistry	40
Temporal Arteritis	Cardiovascular	170
Teratoma	Hematology and Oncology	271
Testicular Cancer	Hematology and Oncology	291
Testicular Torsion	Reproductive	451
Tetralogy of Fallot	Cardiovascular	171
Thoracic Outlet Obstruction (Klumpke's Palsy)	Respiratory	477
Thrombotic Thrombocytopenic Purpura/ Hemolytic-Uremic Syndrome	Hematology and Oncology	292
Thyroglossal Duct Cyst	Endocrine	201
Thyroid Cancer	Endocrine	202
Thyroidectomy	Endocrine	203
Tourette's Disorder	Psychiatry	396
Toxic Multinodular Goiter	Endocrine	204
Toxic Shock Syndrome	Microbiology and Immunology	109
Toxoplasmosis	Microbiology and Immunology	111
Transient Ischemic Attack	Neurology	368

CASE TITLE	CHAPTER	PAGE
Transplant Immunology	Renal	426
Transplant Reaction	Microbiology and Immunology	112
Truncus Arteriosus	Cardiovascular	172
Tuberculosis	Microbiology and Immunology	114
Tuberous Sclerosis	Neurology	370
Turner's Syndrome	Reproductive	452
Ulnar Nerve Damage	Neurology	372
Upper Gastrointestinal Tract Bleeding	Gastrointestinal	241
Urinary Reflux	Renal	427
Vascular Dementia	Neurology	373
Vestibulo-Ocular Reflexes	Neurology	374
Viral Meningitis	Neurology	376
Vitamin B_1 (Thiamine) Deficiency	Biochemistry	41
Vitamin B_{12} Deficiency	Gastrointestinal	242
von Gierke's Disease	Biochemistry	42
von Hippel-Lindau Disease	Neurology	378
von Willebrand's Disease	Hematology and Oncology	293
Wegener's Granulomatosis	Cardiovascular	176
Wernicke-Korsakoff Syndrome	Neurology	379
Wolff-Parkinson-White Syndrome	Cardiovascular	174
Yellow Fever	Microbiology and Immunology	113
Zollinger-Ellison Syndrome	Gastrointestinal	244

Index

A

Abdominal aortic aneurysm, 138
Abruptio placentae, 430–431
Absidia, 89
Acanthamoeba infection, 45
Acanthosis nigricans, 192–193
Acetaminophen overdose, 118
Acetylcholine, 19, 132
Achalasia, 208
Acidosis and alkalosis diagram, 473
Aciduria, 416
Acquired immunodeficiency
    syndrome (AIDS), 58, 60,
    209, 476
Acromegaly, 186–187
Actinic keratosis, 297
Actinomyces, 46
Actinomyces israelii, 46
Actinomycin D, 446
Acute chest syndrome, 286
Acute dystonia, 395
Acute inflammatory demyelinating
    polyradiculoneuropathy,
    334
Acute intermittent porphyria (AIP),
    247
Acute interstitial nephritis (AIN),
    drug-induced, 401–402
Acute respiratory distress
    syndrome, 454
Acute tubular necrosis (ATN), 398
Acyclovir, 376
Addison's disease, 181–182
Adenohypophysis, 328
Adenoma sebaceum, 370, 371
Adenosine triphosphate (ATP), 122
Adenovirus, 346, 376
Adrenal insufficiency
    primary, 181–182
    secondary, 182
    tertiary, 182
Adrenal steroid synthesis, 179
Adrenalectomy, 183

Adrenergic agonists, 331
β-Adrenergic antagonists, 157
β-Adrenergic second messenger
    systems, 122
Adrenocorticotropic hormone
    (ACTH), 184, 200, 358
Adult polycystic kidney disease,
    364
Aedes aegypti mosquito, 62
Aflatoxin, 226
African sleeping sickness, 77
Age-related macular degeneration
    (ARMD), 341
Agoraphobia, 386
Agranulocytosis, secondary to drug
    toxicity, 119
Akathisia, 395
Akinesia, 395
Alanine, 39
Albendazole, 72, 83, 94
Albinism, 297
Albuminocytologic dissociation,
    334
Albuterol, 456
Alcohol
    intoxication, 12
    withdrawal, 4, 12, 120, 121
Alcohol dehydrogenase, 128
Aldolase B deficiency, 31
Alkalemia, 416
Alkali syndrome, 190
Alkaptonuria (ochronosis), 22
All-*trans* retinoic acid (ATRA), 250
α-Fetoprotein (AFP), 226
Alport's syndrome, 400
Alveolar damage, diffuse, 454
Alzheimer's disease, 321, 373
Amastigote, 77
Amenorrhea, 358, 452
American trypanosomiasis, 52
Amnesia
    anterograde, 379
    retrograde, 379
Amsler grid, 341

Amyloid plaques, 321
Amyloidosis, 458
Amyotrophic lateral sclerosis
    (ALS), 324
Anaplasma phagocytophila, 101
Ancylostoma duodenale, 72, 107
Androgen insensitivity syndrome,
    432
Androgen replacement therapy,
    443
Anemia
    aplastic, 251, 272, 276
    Cooley's, 252
    hemolytic, 252, 289
        autoimmune, 254
        cold agglutinin, 254
    iron deficiency, 72, 277
    macrocytic, 6, 264, 276
    megaloblastic, 242, 276
    microcytic, 6, 252, 264, 274,
        277
    normocytic, 264
    pernicious, 242
    sickle cell, 286–287
    sideroblastic, 129, 277
Angina, 139, 140
    Prinzmetal's, 140
    stable, 140
    unstable, 140
Angiodysplasia, 229
Angiomyolipomas, 370
Angiotensin-converting enzyme
    (ACE) inhibitors, 158, 422,
    425
Angiotensin II, 422
    receptor blockers, 158, 422
Anion gap, 472–473
Anitschkow myocytes, 169
Ankylosing spondylitis, 228, 362
Anopheles mosquito, 62
Anorexia nervosa, 6–7
Anosognosia, 360
Anterior cruciate ligament, 303
Anthrax, 47

Antibody-dependent enhancement, 62
Anticholinesterases, 123
Antidepressant therapies, 385, 386
Antigenic drift, 73
Antigenic shift, 73
Anti–glomerular basement membrane disease, 420
Antimitochondrial antibodies (AMA), 234
Antipsychotic agents, 384, 392, 395, 425, 440
α_1-Antitrypsin deficiency, 226, 458
Aortic aneurysm, 362
Aortic dissection, 367
Aortic stenosis, 139, 367
Apgar score, 14
Appendicitis, 212
Arthritis, 86, 228
    osteoarthritis, 306
    rheumatoid (RA), 163, 234, 310–311
        radiographic changes in, 311
    septic, 66
        Haemophilus influenzae, 466
Arthrocentesis, 306
Asbestosis, 455
Ascaris lumbricoides, 48
Ascariasis, 48
Aschoff bodies, 169
Ascites, 210, 232, 418
Ash-leaf spots, 370, 371
Asperger's syndrome, 383
Aspergilloma, 49
Aspergillosis, 49
Aspergillus, 49
Aspergillus flavus, 226
Asthma, 456
Astrocytomas, 370
Atelectasis, 457
    cicatrization, 454
Atherosclerosis, 25, 140
Athlete's foot, 100
Atrial fibrillation, 141
Atrial myxoma, 142–143
Atrial septal defect, uncorrected, 284
Atrioventricular block, 144
Atropine, 123
Attention deficit hyperactivity disorder (ADHD), 382
Auer rods, 250
Autistic disorder, 383

Autonomy, 10
Autosomal dominant polycystic kidney disease (ADPKD), 399
Avascular necrosis, 301
Azoospermia, 443
Azotemia, 398

B

B-cell development, stages in, 75
B-cell lymphoma, body-cavity, 76
Babinski reflex, 14
Bacillus anthracis, 47
Bacteremia, 98
    Haemophilus influenzae, 466
Bacteroides fragilis, 212
Bacterial vaginosis (BV), 433
Balloon valvotomy, 139
Barbiturates, 4, 12
    vs. benzodiazepines, 120
    overdose, 120
Barrett's esophagus, 213
Bartonella henselae, 101
Behavioral science, 3–19
Bell's palsy, 86
Bence Jones proteins, 280, 403
Beneficence, 10
Benign prostatic hyperplasia (BPH), 434
Benzodiazepines, 4, 12, 19, 359, 386, 389
    vs. barbiturates, 120
    overdose, 5, 120, 121
Bereavement, 385
Beriberi, 41, 379
Berry aneurysm, 364, 365, 399
β-Adrenergic second messenger systems, 122
β-blockers, 158, 204, 331, 349
Bezold-Jarisch reflex, 367
Bias
    late-look, 8
    recall, 8
    sampling, 8
    selection, 8
Bicuspid aortic valve, 452
Bile salts, malabsorption of, 239
Biliary tree, anatomy of, 220
Binswanger's disease, 373
Biochemistry, 21–42
Bipolar disorder, 384, 394
"Bird-breeder's lung," 474
Bisphosphonates, 312

Bitemporal hemianopia, 358
Blastomycosis, 108
Blumer's shelf, 240
Body dysmorphic disorder, 393
Bone marrow biopsy, 251
Bone marrow transplant, 54, 112
Borrelia burgdorferi, 86
Botulism, 50
Boutonniere deformity, 310
"Bow-string" sign, 310
Bowel wall, layers of, 231
Brain stem anatomy, 351
Brain tumor, metastatic, 348
Breakbone fever, 62
Breast cancer, 255, 443
Breast mass, 435
Brittle bone disease, 309
Broca's aphasia, 361, 368
Bromocriptine, 358
Bronchiectasis, 458
Bronchiolitis obliterans, 458
Brown-Séquard syndrome, 322–323
Bruton's agammaglobulinemia, 75
Bulimia nervosa, 5
Burkitt's lymphoma, 88, 258
Burton's lines, 274
Buspirone, 386

C

Café-au-lait spots, 352, 356
Calcinosis, 317
Calcitonin, 190, 195, 312
Calcitriol, 312, 412, 413
Calcium channel blockers, 157, 349, 394
Calcium deficiency, 6
Campylobacter jejuni, 334
Candida, 49, 154, 433
Candida albicans, 51
    KOH mount of, 51
Candidiasis, 51
    oral, 119
Caput medusae, 226
Carbachol, 331
Carbamazepine, 359, 384
Carbidopa, 355
Carcinoembryonic antigen (CEA), 195
Carcinoid syndrome, 256–257
    clinical characteristics in patients with, 256
Cardiac rhabdomyomas, 370

Cardiac tamponade, 162, 163, 367
Cardiomyopathies, 150
    dilated (DCM), 152–153
    hypertrophic (HCM), 156–157
Cardiovascular system, 137–176
Castleman's disease, 76
Cat scratch fever, 101
Catecholamines, 195, 198
Celiac sprue, 242, 276
Cellulitis, 250
    Haemophilus influenzae, 466
Central cord syndrome, 326–327
Central pontine myelinolysis, 411
Chagas' disease, 52, 77, 208
Chancroid, 466
Charcot's triad, 220
Chédiak-Higashi syndrome, 35
Chickenpox, 106
Childhood disintegrative disorder,
    383
Chlamydia, 78
Chlamydia pneumoniae, 469
Chlamydia trachomatis, 66, 441
Chloridorrhea, congenital familial,
    416
Chloripramine, 386
Cholangitis, 214, 220
Cholecystitis, 214, 407
Choledocholithiasis, 214–215
Cholelithiasis, 214
Cholera, 53
Cholinergic drugs, 123
Choriocarcinoma, 446
Christmas disease (hemophilia B),
    270
Chronic granulomatous disease
    (CGD), 54
Chronic inflammatory
    demyelinating
    polyradiculopathy, 334
Chronic obstructive pulmonary
    disease (COPD), 241, 459
Churg-Strauss syndrome, 168
Chvostek's sign, 199
Circle of Willis, 364, 368, 369,
    399
Cirrhosis, 210–211, 223, 226, 234,
    241, 266
    alcoholic, 210–211
    micronodular pigment, 223
    primary biliary (PBC), 234
Citrate, 39
Clindamycin, 236
Clomipramine, 387

Clostridium botulinum, 50
Clostridium difficile infection, 55,
    236
Clozapine, 119
Coarctation of the aorta, 145, 364,
    452
Coccidioidomycosis, 108
Cognitive behavioral therapy
    (CBT), 385, 386, 387,
    388
Collagen, 29, 138, 309, 405
    synthesis, 29, 309
    types, 29, 309
Colorectal cancer, 260
Common pathway, 261
Community-acquired pneumonia
    (CAP), 460–461
Confidentiality and its exceptions,
    9
Congenital adrenal hyperplasias,
    179, 180
Congenital rubella syndrome
    (CRS), 146–147
Congestive heart failure, 150, 152
Conjunctivitis, 466
Conn's syndrome, 183
Conversion disorder, 393
Coombs' test, 254, 272, 289
Cooper's suspensory ligaments, 435
Coprolalia, 396
Copropraxia, 396
Cor pulmonale, 150, 458, 459
Coracoacromial arch, 315
Corneal abrasion, 325
Coronary artery disease (CAD),
    148–149, 445
Cortisol, 182, 200
    deficiency, 182, 200
Corynebacterium diphtheriae, 63
Costochondritis, 296
Councilman bodies, 113
Coxiella burnetii, 101
Coxsackie viruses, 69, 90, 97, 101,
    159, 376
Cranial nerves
    III, 374, 379
    IV, 374
    V, 325
    VI, 350, 374, 379
    VII, 325, 350
    VIII, 308
    X, 329
    XII, 350
Craniopharyngioma, 328

CREST syndrome, 317
Creutzfeldt-Jakob disease (CJD),
    57
Crigler-Najjar syndrome, 216–217
    principal differential
    characteristics of, 216
Crohn's disease (CD), 228, 242
Cryptococcosis, 111
Cryptococcus neoformans, 58
Cryptosporidium, 209
Cushing's disease, 184
Cushing's syndrome, 184, 275,
    416, 475
Cutaneous squamous cell
    carcinoma, 297
Cyanide poisoning, 23
Cyanosis
    central, 172
    peripheral, 172
Cyclic adenosine monophosphate
    (cAMP), 122
Cyclic guanosine monophosphate
    (cGMP), 161
Cystic adenomatoid malformation
    of the lung, congenital
    (CCAM), 462
Cystic fibrosis, 98, 416, 458, 463,
    476
Cystic hygroma, 201
Cysticercosis, 59, 263
Cystitis, 419
Cytomegalovirus (CMV) infection,
    60–61, 70, 111, 146, 209,
    376, 401, 426

D

D-dimer, 151, 470
de Quervain's thyroiditis, 204
Deafness, sensironeural, 400
Deep venous thrombosis, 151, 470,
    471
Delirium, 11
Delirium tremens, 4, 120
Delusions, 392
Dementia
    Alzheimer's, 373
    multi-infarct, 373
    vascular, 373
Dengue fever, 62, 113
Depression, 18, 385
Dermacentor tick, 101
Dexamethasone suppression test,
    184

Dextroamphetamine, 382
Diabetes insipidus, 328
Diabetes mellitus, 185, 196–197,
    223, 266, 360, 440
  pharmacologic agents for
      treatment of, 197
  Type 1, 185
  Type 2 (non-insulin-dependent),
      185, 196–197
Diabetic ketoacidosis (DKA), 185,
    410
DiGeorge syndrome, 24, 172
Dilated cardiomyopathy, 152–153
Dimercaprol, 129
Diphtheria, 63
Diphyllobothrium latum, 242
Disk herniation, 362
Displacement, 16
Disseminated intravascular
    coagulation (DIC), 181,
    250, 261, 430
  pathophysiology of, 261
Diuretics, thiazide, 158, 440
Diverticulitis, 218–219
Diverticulosis, 229
Donovan bodies, 77
Dopamine, 355, 358, 385, 392
Dose-response curves, 130, 131
Double-blind study, 124
Down syndrome, 26–27, 221, 321
DPT vaccine, 63
Dressler's syndrome, 163
Drug development, 124–125
Drug elimination, 133
  first-order kinetics, 133
  zero-order kinetics, 133
Drug intoxication, 12
Drug metabolism, phase I and II
    reactions of, 127
Drusen, 341
Dual-energy x-ray absorptiometry
    (DEXA) scans, 312
Duchenne's muscular dystrophy
    (DMD), 305
Dukes' classification, 260
Duodenal atresia, 221
Dysarthria, 361
Dysentery, amebic, 65
Dysgerminoma, 291
Dyskeratosis congenita, 251
Dysmetabolic syndrome, 192–193
Dyspareunia, 445
Dysthymia, 385
Dystonia, acute, 395

E

Ear anatomy, 346–347
Eaton-Lambert syndrome, 275, 475
Echinococcus, 83
Echolalia, 396
Echovirus, 69, 90, 376
Eclampsia/preeclampsia, 442,
    449–450
Ectopic pregnancy, 436–437
Ehlers-Danlos syndrome, 28–29,
    138, 160, 364
Ehrlichia chaffeensis, 101
Eisenmenger's syndrome, 284
Electrical alternans, 163
Electroconvulsive therapy, 385
Elephantiasis, 64
Emphysema, 464
Encephalitis, 86, 99
  granulomatous amebic (GAE),
      45
  hepatic, 118
  from HSV-1, 71
  from HSV-2, 71
Encephalopathy, postinfectious,
    263
End-stage renal disease, 399, 400,
    407
Endocarditis, 98, 154–155, 361
  acute, 154
  infective, 361
  Libman-Sacks, 154
  subacute, 154
Endocrine system, 177–205
Endolymphatic sac tumors, 378
Endometrial hyperplasia, 444
Endometriosis, 438–439
Endometritis, 67
Endoscopic retrograde
    cholangiopancreatography
    (ERCP), 220
Entamoeba histolytica, 65
Enterobacter, 419
Enterobacter cloacae, 214
Enterobius vermicularis, 94
Enterococcus, 214
Enterovirus, 97
Enuresis, 19
Enzyme-linked immunosorbent
    assay (ELISA), 86, 102, 113
Eosinophilic granuloma, 474
Epidermophyton, 100
Epidural hematoma, 366
Epiglottitis, 465–466

Haemophilus influenzae,
    465–466
Epinephrine catabolism, 198
Epstein-Barr virus (EBV), 70, 88,
    251, 269, 376
Erectile dysfunction (ED), 440
Erythema chronicum migrans, 86
Erythema nodosum, 474
Erythropoietin, 284
Escherichia coli, 68, 82, 212, 214,
    419
  enterohemorrhagic (EHEC)
      serotype O157:H7, 104, 292
Esophageal adenocarcinoma, 213
Esophageal atresia, 221, 237
Esophagitis, 241
Estrogen deficiency, 312
Ethical principles, core, 10
Ethylene glycol poisoning, 128
Ethylenediaminetetraacetic acid
    (EDTA), 129
Ewing's sarcoma, 278, 300
Exotoxin A, 63
Extinction, 16
Extracorporeal shock wave
    lithotripsy, 423
Extrinsic pathway, 261
Eye injury, 325

F

Fabry's disease, 40
Familial adenomatous polyposis
    (FAP), 344
Fanconi's syndrome, 403–404
"Farmer's lung," 474
Favism, 264
FDA review process, phases of, 125
Femoral neuropathy, 330
Femoral triangle, 330
Ferruginous bodies, 455
Fibrillin, 138
Fibroadenomas, 435
Fibromas, 282
Fitz-Hugh and Curtis syndrome,
    441
Flexor carpi ulnaris, 372
Floppy baby syndrome, 50
Flumazenil, 120, 121
Focal segmental glomerular
    sclerosis, 418
Folate
  deficiency, 6, 226, 242, 252, 264,
      276

role of in nucleic acid and
myelin metabolism, 243
Follicle-stimulating hormone
(FSH), 200, 358, 443, 445
Fovea, 341
Fragile X syndrome, 30, 340
Friedreich's ataxia, 30
Fructose intolerance, 31

G

G protein–linked receptors, 122
Galactorrhea, 358
Gallstones, 214, 220, 362
Gametocytes, 81
Gardnerella vaginalis, 433
Gastric acid secretion, regulation
of, 211
Gastric cancer, 262
Gastric lymphoma, 240
Gastrinoma, 222, 244
Gastritis, acute hemorrhagic, 241
Gastroenteritis, 102
Gastroesophageal reflux disease
(GERD), 213, 222, 237
Gastrointestinal bleeding
lower, 229
upper, 241
Gastrointestinal system, 207–244
Gaucher's disease, 40
Generalized anxiety disorder, 386
Gestational diabetes, 442
Giardia lamblia, 65
Giardiasis, 65
Gigantism, 186–187
Glaucoma, 363
open-angle, 331
Gleevec (imatinib), 259
Glioblastoma multiforme (GBM),
263, 332–333
Glomerulonephritis, rapidly
progressive (RPGN),
420–421
anti–glomerular basement
membrane disease, 420
immune-complex, 420
pauci-immune, 420
Glucose-6-phosphatase deficiency,
42
Glucose-6-phosphate
dehydrogenase (G6PD)
deficiency, 264
Glucose tolerance test, oral, 186
Glucuronyl transferase, 216

Goiter
retrosternal, 329
toxic multinodular 189, 204–205
Golgi apparatus, 34
Gonorrhea
with septic arthritis, 66–67
Goodpasture's syndrome, 176,
405–406, 474
Gout, 42, 188, 423
Gower's sign, 305
Graft-versus-host disease, 112
Gram-positive bacteria, algorithm
for differentiating, 109
Granulomatous amebic
encephalitis (GAE), 45
Granulosa cell tumors, 282
Graves' disease, 189, 204
Grief, 385
Group B *Streptococcus*, 68, 82
in infant, 68, 82
Growth hormone, 186, 187, 200,
358
deficiency, 328
feedback control of secretion, 187
Guillain-Barré syndrome (GBS),
247, 334–335
Gunshot wound to left flank, 298
Gynecomastia, 443

H

Haemophilus, types of infection
caused by, 466
Haemophilus aegyptius, 466
Haemophilus ducreyi, 466
Haemophilus influenzae, 82, 346,
460, 465–466, 469
Half-life ($t_{1/2}$), 133
Hallucinations, 392
hypnagogic, 18
hypnopompic, 18
Hamartomas, 370
Hand, foot, and mouth disease, 69
Hapten, 96
Hartnup's disease, 233
Hashimoto's thyroiditis, 191, 203
Head and neck cancer, 265
Headache
cluster, 349
migraine, 349
tension, 349
Health Insurance Portability and
Accountability Act
(HIPAA), 9

Hearing loss
conductive, 356–357
sensorineural, 356–357
Heart murmur, 139, 146, 157
crescendo-decrescendo, 157
mitral valve (MV) regurgitation,
157
systolic ejection, 139
Helicobacter pylori, 65, 240, 241
HELLP syndrome, 449
Hemangioblastomas, 378
Hematology and oncology,
245–293
Hemianopia, homonymous,
342–343
Hemochromatosis, 223, 226, 307
hereditary (HH), 266–267
iron deposits in the liver in, 267
Hemolytic-uremic syndrome, 104,
272, 292, 407
Hemophilia, 270
Henoch-Schönlein purpura (HSP),
407
Heparin, 141, 293, 470
Hepatitis, 115, 224, 251
A virus, 69, 97
B virus, 168, 224, 226, 232
serologic responses to, 224
C virus, 62, 113, 225, 226, 232
serologic pattern of acute, 225
Hepatocellular carcinoma (HCC),
226, 232, 284
Hereditary nonpolyposis colorectal
cancer (HNPCC), 344
Hermaphroditism, true, 180
Hernia, inguinal, 302
Herpangina, 69
Herpes simplex virus, 60, 105, 111,
146, 376
type 1 (HSV-1), 70, 71
type 2 (HSV-2), 70–71
Herpes zoster, 105–106
Hesselbach's triangle, 302
Heterochromia of the iris, 363
Hexose monophosphate (HMP)
shunt, 41
Hexosaminidase A deficiency, 40
Hiatal hernia, 237
Hib vaccine, 465
Hip fracture, 301, 312
Histiocytes, 474
Histoplasmosis, 108
Hodgkin's lymphoma, 268–269
variants of, 269

Homer-Wright pseudorosettes, 278, 344

Homocystinuria, 32

Homogentisate oxidase, absence of, 22

Hookworm, 72, 277

Hormone replacement therapy (HRT), 445

Horner's syndrome, 275, 322, 336–337, 477
  nerve pathways disrupted in, 337

Human granulocytic anaplasmosis, 101

Human herpesvirus-6, 70

Human herpesvirus-8, 70, 76

Human immunodeficiency virus (HIV), 98, 181, 209, 376, 425, 433

Hunter's syndrome, 33

Huntington's disease, 30, 340

Hurler's syndrome, 33

Hyaluronidase, 155

Hydatidiform mole, 446

Hydralazine, 126

Hydrocele, 302

Hydrocephalus, 338–339
  obstructive, 344

11β-Hydroxylase deficiency, 178–179

21β-Hydroxylase deficiency, 180

Hyper-IgM syndrome, 75

Hyperaldosteronism, 416, 422
  primary, 183
  secondary, 183

Hyperbilirubinemia, 220, 227

Hypercalcemia, 408–409

Hypercalciuria, 423

Hypercitraturia, 423

Hypercoagulability, 151

Hypercholesterolemia, 417, 418, 422
  familial, 25

Hyperinfection syndrome, 107

Hyperkalemia, 180, 181, 200, 258

Hyperlipidemia, 42, 140

Hyperoxaluria, 423

Hyperparathyroidism, 190, 244, 389, 423
  primary, 190
  secondary, 190
  tertiary, 190

Hyperparesis, 263

Hyperphosphatemia, 258

Hyperplasia, 239

Hyperprolactinemia, 358

Hypersensitivity
  type II, 405
  type III, 474
  type IV, 96, 474

Hypersensitivity pneumonitis, 474

Hypertension, 140, 150, 158, 178, 360, 422
  pregnancy-induced (PIH), 442, 449

Hyperthyroidism, 389
  autoimmune-induced, 189

Hypertrophic cardiomyopathy (HCM), 156–157

Hypertrophic osteoarthropathy, 275

Hypertrophy, 239

Hyperuricemia, 188, 258, 423

Hypoalbuminemia, 408, 418

Hypocalcemia, 199, 258, 413

Hypochondriasis, 393

Hypocortisolism, 200

Hypoglycemia, 389

Hypokalemia, 178, 183, 403–404, 410, 416, 422
  ECG in, 183
  secondary to diuretic use, 416

Hypomania, 384

Hyponatremia, 78, 180, 181, 200, 411

Hypoparathyroidism, 24

Hypophosphatemia, 413

Hypopituitarism, 191

Hypotension, 180
  orthostatic, 200, 367

Hypothyroidism, 191, 200, 276, 328, 452
  primary, 191
  secondary, 191

I

I-cell disease, 34

Idiopathic thrombocytopenic purpura (ITP), 272–273

Imatinib (Gleevec), 259

Immunoglobulin A (IgA) deficiency, isolated, 74–75

Incus, 346

Infant development, 14

Inferior mesenteric artery (IMA), obstruction of, 164–165

Infertility, 358, 443

Inflammatory bowel disease, 228

Influenza, 73, 346

Insulin-like growth factor-1 (IGF-1), 186

Insulin, 196, 197
  actions of on human tissues, 197
  structure of, 196

Insulin resistance syndrome, 192–193

Insulinoma, 222

Intrinsic factor, 242

Intrinsic pathway, 261

Intussusception, 230, 407

Irish node, 240

Ixodes tick, 86

J

Japanese encephalitis virus, 72, 113

JC virus, 57

Jock itch, 100

Justice, 10

K

Kala azar, 77

Kaposi's sarcoma, 76

Kartagener's syndrome, 35, 458

Kasabach-Merritt syndrome, 261

Katayama fever, 103

Kawasaki's disease, 159

Keratitis, 45

Kernicterus, 216, 217

Kidney
  anatomy of, 427
  blood supply to, 298

Kidney disease, autosomal dominant polycystic (ADPKD), 399

Kidney stones (nephrolithiasis), 362, 423–424

Klebsiella, 214, 419

Klinefelter's syndrome, 443

Klumpke's palsy, 477

Knee
  anatomy of, 303
  pain, 303

Knudsen's two-hit hypothesis, 285, 378

Koplik's spots, 87

Korsakoff's syndrome, 379

Krebs cycle, 22

Krukenberg's tumor, 240, 447

Kuru, 57

Kussmaul's hyperpnea, 185

Kussmaul's sign, 163

L

Lambert-Eaton myasthenic
        syndrome, 288, 354
Lead poisoning, 129, 264, 274, 277
Leishmania donovani, 77
Legionella infection, 78, 401, 460
Leiomyoma, 444
Leishmaniasis, 77
Leprosy, 80–81
Leptomeninges, 363
Leptospirosis, 401
Lesch-Nyhan syndrome, 36, 188
Leukemia
        acute lymphoblastic (ALL),
                248–249
        acute myelogenous (AML), 250,
                261
                acute promyelocytic, 250
        chronic myelogenous (CML),
                259
Levodopa, 355
Lewy bodies, 355
Light's criteria, 468
Lines of Zahn, 470
Lingual thyroid, 201
Lisch nodules, 353
Listeria monocytogenes, 68, 82
Lithium, 384
Liver cysts, 83
Liver transplantation, 42
Lou Gehrig's disease, 324
Low-density lipoprotein (LDL), 25
Lowenstein-Jensen agar, 114
Lumirubin, 227
Lung abscess, 46
Lung cancer (Pancoast's
                syndrome), 275
        non–small cell, 275
                adenocarcinoma, 275
                bronchoalveolar carcinoma,
                        275
                large cell carcinoma, 275
                squamous cell carcinoma, 275
        small cell carcinoma (SCLC),
                275, 288, 425, 475
Lung, congenital cystic
        adenomatoid malformation
        (CCAM) of, 462
Lung infection, 98
Lung, lobes of, 462
Lupus, drug-induced, 126, 316
Luteinizing hormone (LH), 200
Lyme disease, 86

Lysergic acid diethylamide (LSD)
        intoxication, 12
        withdrawal, 12

M

Macular degeneration, 341
Major depressive disorder, 385
Malaria, 84
Malignant melanoma, 285, 304
Malingering, 393
Malleus, 346
Mallory-Weiss tears, 241
Malpractice, 15
Mania, 384
        steroid-induced, 394
Marfan's syndrome, 28, 138, 160,
                364
McArdle's disease, 37
McBurney's point, 212
McCune-Albright syndrome,
                186
McCune-Albright's hereditary
                osteodystrophy, 199
Measles, 87
        virus, 57, 87
Mebendazole, 72, 83, 94
Meckel's diverticulum, 230–231
Medial brain stem lesion, 350
Medial collateral ligament, 303
Medulloblastoma, 278, 344
Melanoma, malignant, 285, 304
Melanotropin, 200
Meningioma, 345
Meningitis
        aseptic, 90
        bacterial, 82
        cryptococcal, 58
        CSF findings in, 82, 377
        Haemophilus influenzae, 466
        Listeria, 82
        and migraine, 349
        Neisseria meningitidis, 91
        neonatal, 68
        viral, 376–377
Meningococcemia, 159, 181
Meningoencephalitis, 89, 376
Meniscus, 303
Menopause, 445
Merlin gene, 356
Merozoites, 84
Mesenteric ischemia, 164–165
Mesothelioma, 278, 345, 467
        malignant, 345, 467

Metabolic acidosis, 359, 410,
                414–415
        with respiratory alkalosis,
                414–415
Metabolic alkalosis, 416
Metabolic syndrome (MS),
                192–193
Metamorphopsia, 341
Methotrexate, 446
Methylphenidate, 382
Metronidazole, 65, 433
Meyer's loop, 342
Microbiology and immunology,
                43–115
Microsporum, 100
Migraine headache, 349
Minimal change disease, 417
Mitral stenosis, 169
Mitral valve prolapse (MVP), 160,
                309, 364, 399
Monday disease, 161
Monoamine oxidase (MAO)
                inhibitors, 385, 389
Monoclonal gammopathy of
                undetermined significance
                (MGUS), 280, 403
Mononucleosis, 88, 254
Monospot test, 88
Mood stabilizers, 384
Moraxella catarrhalis, 346
Moro reflex, 14
Mucocutaneous lymph node
                syndrome, 159
Mucopolysaccharidoses, 33
Mucor, 89
Mucormycosis, 89
Müllerian agenesis, 452
Multiple endocrine neoplasia
                (MEN)
        type I (Wermer's syndrome),
                186, 244
        type IIA, 194–195
        type IIB, 194
Multiple myeloma, 280, 403
Multiple sclerosis, 263, 336,
                350–351
Mumps, 90
Murphy's sign, 214
Muscular dystrophy, 305
Musculoskeletal system, 295–317
Myasthenia gravis, 123, 354
Mycobacterium avium complex,
                209
Mycobacterium leprae, 80–81

Mycoplasma, 78, 254, 460
Mycoplasma pneumoniae, 469
Mycoplasma tuberculosis, 114
Mycosis, systemic, 108
Myelodysplastic syndrome, 276
Myocardial infarction, 150, 152, 163
  acute (AMI), 162
Myocarditis, 86, 150
Myotonic dystrophy, 30, 340

N

Naegleria fowleri, 89
Narcolepsy, 18
Nasopharyngeal carcinoma, 88
Necator americanus, 107
Necrotizing enterocolitis, 166
Negative predictive value (NPV), 13
Negative reinforcement, 16
Negri bodies, 99
Neisseria gonorrhoeae, 66, 154, 441
Neisseria meningitidis, 66, 82, 91
Neonatal abstinence syndrome, 17
Neonatal respiratory distress syndrome, 457
Nephritis
  acute interstitial (AIN), drug-induced, 401–402
  hereditary, 400
Nephrolithiasis (kidney stones), 423–424
Nephropathy, 42
Nephrotic syndrome, 417, 418
Neural crest cells, 308
Neuroblastoma, 278–279
Neurofibrillary tangles, 321
Neurofibromatosis, 308
  type 1 (von Reckinghausen's disease), 352–353
  type 2, 356–357
Neurology, 319–379
Neuromuscular blockade, 123
  agents, 132
    depolarizing, 132
    nondepolarizing, 132
Neutrophils, autoimmune destruction of, 119
Niacin (vitamin B$_3$)
  deficiency, 233
  overdose, 233

Nicotinamide adenine dinucleotide phosphate (NADPH) oxidase deficiency, 54
Niemann-Pick disease, 40
Night terrors, 19, 120
Nitroglycerin, 161
Nocardia, 46
Non-Hodgkin's lymphoma, 258
Nonmaleficence, 10
Norepinephrine, 385, 389
Nystagmus, 374

O

Obesity, 140
Obsessive-compulsive disorder (OCD), 386, 387
Obsessive-compulsive personality disorder (OCPD), 388
Ochronosis (alkaptonuria), 22
Octreotide, 222, 239, 257
Oligoclonal bands, 350
Oligodendroglioma, 281
Onchocerca volvulus, 92
Onchocerciasis, 92
Oophoritis, 67
Operant conditioning, 16
Opioids
  intoxication, 12
  withdrawal, 12, 17
Optic gliomas, 353
Orchitis, 90
Organophosphates, 123
Osler's nodes, 361
Osteoarthritis, 306, 362
Osteogenesis imperfecta, 309
Osteogenic sarcoma, 285
Osteomyelitis, 93, 98, 362
  Salmonella, 286
Osteoporosis, 312, 443, 452
Otitis externa, 98
Otitis media, acute, 346
  Haemophilus influenzae, 466
Ovarian cancer, 282, 447
  serous papillary cystadenocarcinoma, 345
Ovarian failure, 452
  premature, 445
Oxytocin, 200

P

P-ANCA (perinuclear pattern of antineutrophil cytoplasmic antibodies), 168

Paget's disease
  of bone, 190
  of breast, 255, 448
Pain disorder, 393
Palmar reflex, 14
Pancoast's syndrome (lung cancer), 275, 336, 477
Pancreatic cancer, 283, 378
Pancreatitis, 362, 407
  acute, 209
Panic disorder, 5, 121, 386, 389
Papilledema, 263, 334, 349
  of the optic nerve, 335
Paracoccidioidomycosis, 108
Parathyroid hormone (PTH), 190, 195, 199, 412, 423
  recombinant, 312
Parathyroidectomy, 190
Parkinson's disease, 355
Parvovirus B19, 251, 286
Pasteurella multocida, 465
Patent ductus arteriosus (PDA), 166–167
  uncorrected, 284
Pellagra, 233, 256, 276
Pelvic inflammatory disease (PID), 67, 441
Pemberton's sign, 204
Pentadecacatechol, 96
Peptic ulcer disease, 222, 241
Pericarditis, 163
  fibrinous, 162
  hemorrhagic, 163
  serous, 163
Perihepatitis, 441
Peripheral neuropathy, 86, 115, 274
Petechiae, 407
Pharmacodynamics, 130–131
  antagonists, 130, 131
  efficacy, 130
  potency, 130
Pharmacokinetics, 133
Pharmacology, 117–133
Pharyngeal membranes
Phencyclidine
  intoxication, 12
  withdrawal, 12
Phenobarbital, 359
Phenylalanine, metabolism of, 38
Phenylketonuria (PKU), 38
Phenytoin, 359
Pheochromocytoma, 194, 195, 198, 378, 389

Philadelphia chromosome, 259
Phlebotomy, 284
Picornavirus, 69, 97, 376
Pilocarpine, 331
Pinocytosis, 338
Pinworm infection, 94
Pituitary adenoma, 184, 358
Placenta previa, 430, 431
Plasmodium falciparum, 84, 85
Pleural effusion, malignant, 468
Pleurodesis, 468
Plummer-Vinson syndrome, 204, 277
Plummer's disease, 189, 204–205
Pneumococcus, 286
Pneumocystis jiroveci (carinii), 82, 476
Pneumonia, 98, 476
    atypical, 469
    community-acquired (CAP), 78, 460–461
    Haemophilus influenzae, 466
    most common causes of by age, 469
    Mycoplasma pneumoniae, 469
    neonatal, 68
    Pneumocystis jiroveci, 82
Pneumothorax, spontaneous, 476
Podagra, 188
Poison ivy, 96
Poliomyelitis, 97
Poliovirus, 69, 97
Polyarteritis nodosa, 168
Polycystic ovarian syndrome (PCOS), 192, 442, 452
Polycythemia rubra vera, 284
Polyhydramnios, 221, 442
Polymerase chain reaction (PCR), 30, 105, 376, 432
    reverse transcription (RT-PCR), 376
Polymyalgia rheumatica, 170
Porphyria, 274
Port-wine stain, 363
Portal-systemic anastomoses, 165
Positive predictive value (PPV), 13
Positive reinforcement, 16
Posterior cruciate ligament, 303
Posttraumatic stress disorder (PTSD), 386, 390
Pouch of Douglas, 240
Pralidoxime (2-PAM), 123
Preeclampsia/eclampsia, 442, 449–450

Pregnancy
    ectopic, 436–437
    molar, 446
Prevalence, 13
Priapism, 286
Primary sclerosing cholangitis (PSC), 228, 234
Primidone, 359
Prions, 57
Progressive multifocal leukoencephalopathy, 263
Prolactin, 200
Promastigote, 77
Protein-losing enteropathy, 407
Proteus mirabilis, 419
Proteus vulgaris, 423
Proton pump inhibitors, 222, 244, 401
Psammoma bodies, 345
Pseudohermaphroditism, 180
Pseudohypercalcemia, 408
Pseudohypocalcemia, 408
Pseudohypoparathyroidism, 199
Pseudomembranous colitis, 65, 236
Pseudomonas, 93, 346, 419
Pseudomonas aeruginosa infection, 98
Psychiatry, 381–396
Psychotherapy, psychodynamic, 385, 388
Pulmonary embolism, 367, 470–471
Pulmonary hypertension, 252
Pulmonary stenosis, 171
Pulsus paradoxus, 163
Punishment, 16
Purified protein derivative (PPD) test, 114
Purine salvage pathway, 36
Purpura, 407
Purpuric fever (Brazilian), 466
Pyelonephritis, 419
Pyloric stenosis, hypertrophic, 237
Pyoderma gangrenosum, 228
Pyrantel pamoate, 72, 94
Pyruvate dehydrogenase deficiency, 39
Pyruvate metabolism, 39
Pyuria, 419

Q

Q fever, 101
Quellung reaction, 460

R

Rabies, 99
Radius fractures, 312
Rapidly progressive glomerulonephritis (RPGN), 420–421
    anti–glomerular basement membrane disease, 420
    immune-complex, 420
    pauci-immune, 420
Rathke's pouch, 328
Raynaud's phenomenon, 317
Recurrent laryngeal nerve, damage to, 329
Reduviid bug, 52, 77
Reed-Sternberg cells, 268, 269
Reiter's syndrome, 228
Renal artery stenosis/hypertension, 422
Renal calculi, 423–424
Renal cell carcinoma (RCC), 284, 362, 378
Renal failure, chronic, 399
Renal system, 397–427
Renin-angiotensin system, 152, 153, 180, 422
Renin-angiotensin-aldosterone axis, 422
Reproductive system, 429–452
Respiratory acidosis, 359, 472–473
Respiratory alkalosis, 414–415
Respiratory syncytial virus, 346
Respiratory system, 454–477
Retina, 325
    hemangiomas of, 378
Retinoblastoma, 278, 285
Rett's disorder, 383, 391
Reye's syndrome, 238
Reynolds' pentad, 220
Rhabdomyosarcoma, 278
Rheumatic fever, 154, 163, 340
Rheumatic heart disease, 169
Rheumatoid arthritis (RA), 163, 234, 310–311
    radiographic changes in, 311
Rhinovirus, 69, 97, 346
Rhizopus, 89
Rickets, hypophosphatemic (vitamin D–resistant), 412–413
Rickettsia akari, 101
Rickettsia rickettsii, 101
Rickettsia typhi, 101

Rickettsial pox, 101
Riedel's thyroiditis, 191
Ringworm, 100
Rinne test, 357
River blindness, 92
Rocky Mountain spotted fever
        (RMSF), 101, 159
Rooting reflex, 14
Rotator cuff tear, 314–315
Rotavirus infection, 102
Roth's spots, 361
Rouleaux formation, 280
Rubella, 60, 111
    congenital, 146–147

S

Sabin vaccine, 97
Salk vaccine, 97
Salmonella, 82, 93, 286
Salpingitis, 67
Sarcoidosis, 80, 190, 474
Schilling test, 276
Schistosoma haematobium, 103
Schistosoma japonicum, 103
Schistosoma mansoni, 103
Schistosomiasis, 103
Schizonts, 84
Schizophrenia, 392
Schizophreniform disorder, 392
Sclerodactyly, 317
Scleroderma (systemic sclerosis),
        234, 317, 474
Scotch tape test, 94
Scurvy, 309
Seizures, 359, 389
    medial temporal lobe, 389
Selective estrogen receptor
        modulator (SERM), 312
Selective serotonin reuptake
        inhibitors (SSRIs), 385,
        386, 387, 389, 440, 445
Seminoma, 291
Sensitivity, 13
Sepsis
    burn, 98
    neonatal, 68, 82, 98
Serotonin, 19, 257, 385, 389, 392
Serotonin syndrome, 389
Serratia, 419
Sertoli-Leydig cell tumor, 282
Shagreen patches, 370
Sheehan's syndrome, 200
Shigella, 104

Shingles, 105–106
Short bowel syndrome, 239
Sicca syndrome, 234
Sickle cell disease, 93, 286–287
Signet-ring cells, 240
Sildenafil, 440
Sinusitis, *Haemophilus influenzae*,
        466
Sipple's syndrome, 194–195
Sister Mary Joseph's node, 240
Situs inversus, 35
Sjögren's syndrome, 234, 403, 474
Skin, layers of, 299
Sleep
    apnea, 18
    disorders, 121
        insomnia, 121
    night terrors, 19, 120
    non–rapid eye movement (non-
        REM), 19
    physiology, 18
    rapid eye movement (REM), 18
        physiologic changes in, 19
    sleepwalking, 19, 120
    stages, 19
Slow viruses, 57
Soft tissue sarcoma, 285
Somatization disorder, 393
Somatoform disorders, 393
Somatostatin, 222
Specificity, 13
Spherocytosis, hereditary, 289
Sphingolipidoses, 40
Spinal cord and associated tracts,
        323, 327
Spinal cord compression, 362
Spinocerebellar ataxia, 340
Spironolactone, 183, 422, 440
Spleen
    blood supply to, 298
    injury to, 290
Splenic sequestration, 286
Sporozoites, 95
St. Louis encephalitis virus, 72,
        113
Stab wound, subclavian, 313
Stapes, 346
Staphylococcus aureus, 82, 93, 109,
        154, 155, 346, 423, 460
Staphylococcus saprophyticus, 419
Statins, 25
Status epilepticus, 120, 121, 359
Steatosis, 238
Stevens-Johnson syndrome, 359

Stomach cancer, 240
Streptococcus
    group A, 346
    group B, 68, 82
        in infant, 68, 82
Streptococcus epidermidis, 154
Streptococcus pneumoniae, 82, 154,
        346, 460, 469
    histologic findings of, 461
Streptococcus viridans, 154, 460
Stroke, 286, 360–361
    embolic, 368
    lacunar, 373
    recurrent, 373
Strongyloides stercoralis, 107
Strongyloidiasis, 107
Struma ovarii, 189, 271
Sturge-Weber syndrome, 363
Subacromial bursa, 314, 315
Subacute sclerosing
        panencephalitis, 57, 87
Subarachnoid hemorrhage,
        364–365
Subdural hematoma, 366
Subperiosteal abscess, 93
Substantia nigra, neuronal loss in,
        355
Succimer, 129
Succinylcholine, 132
Superantigens, 110
Superior mesenteric artery (SMA),
        obstruction of, 164–165
Swan-neck deformity, 310
Swimmer's itch, 103
Sydenham's chorea, 340
Syncope, 367
Syndrome of inappropriate
        secretion of antidiuretic
        hormone (SIADH), 275,
        411, 425, 475
Syndrome X, 192–193
Syphilis, 56, 159
    congenital, 56
Systemic lupus erythematosus
        (SLE), 154, 163, 316, 420,
        421, 474
    associated renal disease, 420, 421
Systemic sclerosis (scleroderma),
        317, 474

T

T-cell deficiency, 24
Taenia solium, 59

Tarasoff decision, 9
Tardive dyskinesia, 340, 395
Tay-Sachs disease, 40
Telangiectasia, 317
  gastrointestinal, 452
Temporal arteritis, 170
Teratoma, 271
Terrible triad, 303
Testicular atrophy, 226
Testicular cancer, 291
Testicular feminization syndrome, 432
Testicular torsion, 407, 451
Tetralogy of Fallot, 171
β-Thalassemia, 252–253, 286
Thecoma tumors, 282
Therapeutic index, 133
Thiamine (vitamin B_1) deficiency, 41, 226, 379
Thoracentesis, 468
Thoracic outlet obstruction, 477
Thoracic outlet syndrome, 477
Thoracotomy, 476
Thrombocytopenia, 261
Thrombotic thrombocytopenic purpura, 292
Thrush, oral, 51, 119
Thymoma, 329, 354
Thymectomy, 123, 354
Thyroglossal duct cyst, 201
Thyroid
  cancer, 202
  development, 201
  medullary carcinoma of, 194
  papillary carcinoma of, 345
Thyroid-stimulating hormone (TSH), 200, 358
Thyroid storm, 189
Thyroidectomy, 203, 204
Tinea capitis, 100
Tinea corporis, 100
Tinea cruris, 100
Tinea pedis, 100
Tinea unguium, 100
TORCH infections, 60, 111, 146
ToRCHeS infections, 56
Torticollis, 395
Tourette's disorder, 387, 396
Toxic megacolon, 52, 55, 236
Toxic multinodular goiter, 189, 204–205
Toxic shock syndrome, 109–110
Toxoplasma gondii, 111
Toxoplasmosis, 60, 111, 146, 263

Tracheobronchitis, *Haemophilus influenzae*, 466
Tracheoesophageal fistula, 221
Transient ischemic attack, 367, 368–369
Transplant immunology, 426
Transplant reaction, 112
Treponema pallidum, 101
Tricarboxylic acid (TCA) cycle, 39
  thiamine in, 41
Trichomonas vaginitis, 65, 433
Trichophyton, 100
Tricyclic antidepressants, 385, 389
Trisomy 21, 26–27, 221, 321
Trousseau's sign, 199
Truncus arteriosus (TA), 172–173
Trypanosoma cruzi, 52, 77
Trypanosoma gambiense, 77
Trypanosoma rhodesiense, 77
Tryptophan, 233
Tsetse fly, 77
Tuberculosis, 111, 114–115, 181, 476
Tuberous sclerosis, 370–371
Tubo-ovarian abscess, 67, 441
Tumor lysis syndrome, 258
Tumor suppressor gene, 378
Turcot's syndrome, 344
Turner's syndrome, 145, 201, 452
"Two-hit hypothesis," 285, 378
Typhus, endemic, 101
Tyrosine kinase, 196, 259
Tzanck smear, 70, 105

U

Ulcerative colitis (UC), 228
Ulnar nerve damage, 372, 477
Unhappy triad, 303
Uremia, 163, 241
Urinary reflux, 427
Urinary tract infection (UTI), 98, 419
Urticaria, 74
Urushiol, 96
Uterine fibroids, 444
Uveitis, 228, 474

V

Vaginitis, 51
  bacterial, 65
  Trichomonas, 65

Valproic acid, 359, 384
Valve replacement, 139
Vancomycin resistance, 155
Vardenafil, 440
Varicella-zoster virus (VZV), 70, 71, 105–106
Vascular dementia, 373
Vascular endothelial growth factor (VEGF), 76
Vasculitis, 170
Ventricular septal defect (VSD), 171
  uncorrected, 284
Ventricular system, anatomy of, 339
Verapamil, 157
Vertebral compression fractures, 312
Vestibular pathways, principal, 375
Vestibulo-ocular reflex, 374–375
Vibrio cholerae, 53
Virchow's node, 240
Virchow's triad, 151
Vitamin B_1 (thiamine) deficiency, 41, 226, 379
Vitamin B_3 (niacin)
  deficiency, 233
  overdose, 233
Vitamin B_6, 32, 115
Vitamin B_{12}
  deficiency, 6, 226, 242–243, 264, 276
  role of in nucleic acid and myelin metabolism, 243
Vitamin C deficiency, 309
Vitamin D, 6, 190, 199, 412, 423
  deficiency, 6, 412
  intoxication with, 190
  renal activation of, 423
Vitamin K deficiency, 261, 293
Vitreous humor, 325
Volume of distribution, 133
von Gierke's disease, 42
von Hippel–Lindau (VHL) disease, 378
von Reckinghausen's disease (neurofibromatosis type 1), 352–353
von Willebrand factor (vWF), defect in, 293
von Willebrand metalloproteinase (ADAMTS-13) deficiency, 292

von Willebrand's disease (vWD), 261, 270, 293

W

Waldenström's macroglobulinemia, 403
Wallenberg's syndrome, 336
Warfarin, 141, 293, 470
Warthin-Finkeldey cells, 87
Waterhouse-Friederichsen syndrome, 181
Watershed zone, 326
Weber test, 357
Wegener's granulomatosis, 176, 405, 474
Wermer's syndrome, 186, 244
Wernicke-Korsakoff syndrome, 41, 379

Wernicke's aphasia, 360, 368
Wernicke's encephalopathy, 41, 226, 379
   mammillary bodies in, 379
West Nile virus, 62, 113
Western blot, 86
Whiff test, 433
Whipple's procedure, 222
White matter disease, diffuse, 373
Wilms' tumor, 278
Wilson's disease, 223, 226, 307, 340
Wolff-Parkinson-White (WPW) syndrome, 174–175
Woolsorter's disease, 47
Wrist drop, 274
Wuchereria bancrofti, 64

X

X-linked hypophosphatemic rickets (XLH), 412
Xanthelasma, 234
Xanthomas, 25
Xeroderma pigmentosum, 297

Y

Yellow fever, 113
Yersinia enterocolitica, 252

Z

Ziehl-Neelsen stain, 114
Zollinger-Ellison syndrome, 222, 241, 244
Zygomycosis, 89

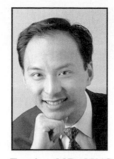

Tao Le, MD, MHS

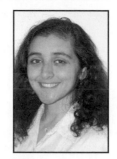

Vinita Takiar, MS, MPhil

Tao Le, MD, MHS   Dr. Le has been a well-recognized figure in medical education for the past 14 years. As senior editor, he has led the expansion of *First Aid* into a global educational series. In addition, he is the founder of the *USMLERx* online test bank series as well as a cofounder of the *Underground Clinical Vignettes* series. As a medical student, he was editor-in-chief of the University of California, San Francisco *Synapse,* a university newspaper with a weekly circulation of 9000. Dr. Le earned his medical degree from the University of California, San Francisco, in 1996 and completed his residency training in internal medicine at Yale University and fellowship training at Johns Hopkins University. At Yale, he was a regular guest lecturer on the USMLE review courses and an adviser to the Yale University School of Medicine curriculum committee. Dr. Le subsequently went on to cofound Medsn and served as its chief medical officer. He is currently conducting research in asthma education at the University of Louisville.

Vinita Takiar, MS, MPhil   Vinita is currently completing her sixth year in the MD/PhD Medical Scientist Training Program at the Yale University School of Medicine. Originally from Baltimore, Maryland, she graduated Phi Beta Kappa from Johns Hopkins University in 2003, where she studied Biophysics and English. She has extensive experience in tutoring and teaching, including leading the Yale Anatomy Training Program. She is currently working towards a PhD in Cellular and Molecular Physiology, focusing on a potential treatment for patients with Autosomal Dominant Polycystic Kidney Disease. This year is her fourth year as a member of the *First Aid* team. In her spare time, Vinita enjoys traveling, listening to all kinds of music, and trying to make some of her own.

ABOUT THE AUTHORS

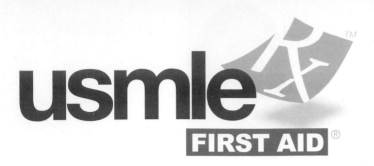
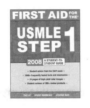